Musculoskeletal MRI

Tarek M. Hegazi • Jim S. Wu

Musculoskeletal MRI

A Case-Based Approach to Interpretation and Reporting

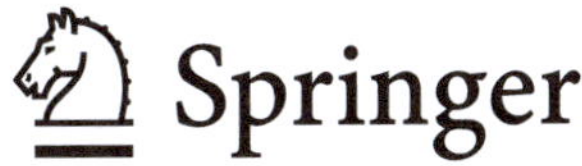

Tarek M. Hegazi
Assistant Professor of Radiology
Radiology Residency Program Director
Imam Abdulrahman Bin Faisal University
Dammam
Saudi Arabia

Jim S. Wu
Chief, Musculoskeletal Imaging and
Intervention
Associate Professor in Radiology,
Harvard Medical School
Beth Israel Deaconess Medical Center
Boston, MA
USA

ISBN 978-3-030-26776-6   ISBN 978-3-030-26777-3   (eBook)
https://doi.org/10.1007/978-3-030-26777-3

This Springer imprint is published by the registered company Springer Nature Switzerland AG
The registered company address is: Gewerbestrasse 11, 6330 Cham, Switzerland

To my parents, Mohammed and Dalal, for always being there for me; to my late brother, Mahmoud, i miss you so much, to my wife, Nuha for her continuous love and support, without which I would be lost; and to my kids, Mahmoud and Ascia, for making me a better person.

–T.M.H

To Ann, Alex, and Sonie, thanks for everything.

–J.S.W

Preface

The amount of knowledge needed to practice radiology can be daunting. Understanding the nuances of each disorder and knowing the crucial findings to describe for each case in order to guide clinical and surgical treatment effectively can be overwhelming. Moreover, with the ever-increasing demands on radiologists, concise, accurate, and efficient reports are critical. Interpreting musculoskeletal (MSK) MRI studies is particularly challenging since there is complex anatomy and concepts that can be difficult for radiologists, especially for those who are not MSK fellowship trained.

The goal of this book is to teach the reader how to interpret and dictate MSK MRI studies accurately and efficiently through a series of high-yield cases. We have included the most common disorders that you are likely to encounter in your everyday clinical practice. Each case begins with a short clinical history, similar to what could be present on the ordering/requisition form and several carefully selected MRI images. We then provide a concise dictation that highlights the correct terminology to use in order to fully describe the disorder, including the important pertinent negatives of the case. When relevant, we also provide clinical recommendations since many disorders require direct communication with the ordering physician, such as a newly discovered aggressive tumor or certain fractures. Next, we include a detailed discussion of the important characteristics of the case to provide the reader with in-depth knowledge of the disorder. When helpful, we have included relevant normal anatomy images and supplemental cases to help with understanding the details of the case. These discussions are organized similar to the teaching that occurs at workstations with our MSK fellows. Lastly, we provide a "report checklist" to ensure that important findings are included in the final report. The first sets of cases are organized by joint (shoulder, elbow, wrist/hand, pelvis/hip, knee, and foot/ankle). Three additional sets of cases focus on tumor, arthropathy, and miscellaneous conditions. We have also included a section containing normal report templates that can be used to create structured reports for many existing dictation systems.

This book is an ideal guide for anyone who interprets MSK MRI on a regular basis, including general radiologists, MSK radiologists, and MSK radiology fellows/residents. Orthopedic and sports medicine physicians and nurse practitioners will also find this book useful. We hope that this book can be used as a useful reference tool for all readers of MSK MRI.

Introduction

The written radiology report is perhaps the most critical service we provide as radiologists. It is the formal documentation of the findings of each imaging study and consolidates our interpretation of the findings in order to provide a diagnosis or supporting evidence to guide treatment. The importance of the radiology report cannot be understated. It serves as a medicolegal document and is invariably the most important item scrutinized during lawsuits against radiologists. However, we should produce quality reports not out of fear of litigation; but instead, we should create complete and accurate reports out of a desire to perform to the best of our abilities and in order to best treat our patients. Reports can differ in style, understandability, and effectiveness. It can be frustrating for radiologists, referring clinicians, and patients to see poorly worded radiology reports that have limited utility. Although we acknowledge that there is no singular "correct" way to write a radiology report, the ramblings provided below have aided us in our clinical practice over the years, and we hope that you will find some of these points useful in producing concise, complete, and effective MSK MRI reports that fit your style.

Most reports are divided in various subheadings. We like to use five distinct subheadings: Indication, Technique, Comparison, Findings, and Impression. Using subheadings ensures that we do not forget to include certain items in the final report. If a subheading is listed in the report template, you are less likely to forget to include important information. Also, many dictation systems can autopopulate a variety of information directly into the report, such as the study name, patient demographics, and clinical history. Depending on your referral base, it can be a good idea to discuss your report subheadings and style with your most common referring orthopedists and physicians in order to arrive at a mutually helpful reporting style.

The indication for the study should always be included in the report. Oftentimes, the provider may provide a useless history such as "pain" or "r/o pain." However, we should not take out our frustration on the patient and simply read the study with limited clinical information. We are more likely to miss an important finding if we do not know their complete history. It is important to review the clinical notes to determine the specific injury and symptoms leading to the reason for the MRI. Often, the assessment and plan of the last clinical note will state the reason for the MRI. Moreover, it is of utmost importance to determine if a patient has had prior surgery, which can prevent the radiologist from appearing careless and, at worse, incompetent. This is especially true for knee MRI exams. For instance, after meniscal repair, there can be abnormal signal contacting an articular surface that can be a normal postoperative finding for several years. However, in a native meniscus, the same appearance could constitute a new tear. In the shoulder, a common mistake is to report a biceps tendon rupture in someone with a biceps tenodesis or tenotomy. Knowledge of prior treatments and procedures is also important. We have seen bone marrow aspiration sites being mistakenly reported as tumors and gas in a joint from recent joint aspiration being overcalled as an acute septic joint. Knowing more information about the patient will only help you in interpreting the MRI exam. Moreover, we should always answer the clinical question given to us by the referring clinician. Read it! If the requisition asks to "evaluate for lymphadenopathy" on a routine shoulder MRI exam, then be sure to include the presence or absences of lymphadenopathy in the Findings and Impression sections of the report. If the provided clinical history specifically asks if there is osteonecrosis on a routine hip MRI, then be sure to comment on this in the final report. There have been numerous times when we have reread the indication and realized that the exact disorder is actually present. This often occurs when the findings are not part of our routine search pattern.

For the Technique section, we like to keep it short but informative as to what MR protocol was used. Most institutions have specific protocols for different indications: routine knee, tumor/infection, Morton's neuroma, or pectoralis tear protocols are some examples. Including the protocol and actual MR sequences can aid in future protocols for comparison studies and to document the use of intravenous or intra-articular contrast. Occasionally, special sequences such as in-and-out-of-phase images or diffusion-weighted images maybe performed to help elucidate certain findings.

The Comparison section should always be included, mostly as a reminder for us to look at old studies. For every case, we should either (1) compare to a prior study; (2) compare to the prior report, if the images are not available; or (3) state that there are no comparison exams. At times, patients are referred to our institution for MRI due to findings seen on outside hospital imaging studies. We make a point to state in this section that those outside hospital films are not available to us in the Comparison section. Furthermore, many PACS systems will bring up old comparison studies when the study is "launched." However, this can be misleading depending on how the studies are coded in the PACS system. Slight variations can make an appropriate old study not appear as a comparison, making the radiologist think that there are no comparison studies. We make a point to quickly look at the entire list of cases in the patient's folder to be sure the old comparison studies are reviewed. You should also look for studies that may not be identical but will include the anatomic area of interest. For instance, sagittal images from a CT scan of the abdomen and pelvis are excellent for evaluating the spine and sacrum. CT scans of the chest can include portions of the shoulders and are very helpful in diagnosing calcific tendinitis or loose bodies. Comparison studies can greatly aid in determining whether a finding is new and worrisome or old and of doubtful clinical significance. Seeing the identical finding unchanged over several years is often reassuring.

The Findings subheading is the meat of the report. In this section, one should comment on the important anatomic structures of each MRI exam, both abnormal findings and pertinent negatives. We find it helpful to divide this subheading into anatomic parts in order to ensure that each structure is reviewed carefully and completely. Structures are often listed in order of most importance or commonly abnormal areas. For instance, in the shoulder, we start with the rotator cuff; and in the knee, we start with the menisci. In this subheading, each finding should be described clearly. Personally, we prefer full sentences as opposed to sentence fragments; however, this is personal preference. If using full sentences, try to avoid exceedingly long run-on sentences. Remember that these reports will be read by many people including your colleagues, referring physicians, and patients. It is important to be definitive when possible without using ambiguous terms. When appropriate, give the actual dimensions of the findings, such as the size of an enlarged tendon, soft tissue mass, or ganglion. This can help the reader understand the severity of the process or lesion. When it is not possible for actual measurements, quantifying findings as mild, moderate, or severe can be helpful, such as "mild degenerative changes of the tibiotalar joint," "moderate tendinosis of the quadriceps tendon," or "severe tenosynovitis of the posterior tibialis." For each important finding that can impact patient care, it is important to comment on whether it was present on prior studies, as this will affect the final conclusion and whether treatment is needed.

The last subheading of the report is the Impression and is the culmination of your thoughts and your synthesis of the case. Past studies have shown that only the Impression of the radiology report is read by referring physicians in 40–50% of the time. This is clearly not ideal for patient care as important information can be found in the Findings subheading, but it does highlight the importance of the Impression section. Note that this subheading is not called Diagnosis. The Impression is exactly your impression of what is occurring in the patient based on your assessment of the imaging findings and clinical history. Oftentimes, an actual diagnosis cannot be made, so it would be inaccurate to have a Diagnosis section for each report. In these cases, a differential diagnosis may need to be given. For instance, if you see nonspecific marrow edema in the femoral head, this could represent infection, tumor, trauma, or a myriad of other disorders. It is of no use to the reader to simply list a whole slew of disorders without guidance as to which one is most likely to be the cause of the patient's symptoms. Give the most likely diagnosis first, and then discuss the other less likely disorders next. This is your impression, not something that is set in stone. Also, avoid listing new items in the impression. Any item in the Impression should have been discussed in the Findings subheading. Lastly, it is important to make any recommendations based on your impressions of the case, and this may require direct communication with the referring physician or medical provider. For instance, a new stress fracture on the tensile side of the femoral neck should be directly discussed with referring physician and recommendations for limited weight-bearing be made so that the patient does not complete the fracture. A newly discovered aggressive tumor should also be communicated and recommendations on whether the lesion is amenable to percutaneous biopsy be made. Oftentimes, these are common sense questions that the referring physician will need to know, and good radiologists will anticipate these questions and answer them in the report.

Hopefully, these tips will help you in interpreting MSK MRI studies and generate quality reports. Again, we realize that there are many ways to write a radiology report, and each radiologist will arrive at his or her own style, often changing it throughout their career. It could be argued that the basic aspects of the radiology report could be summarized in this quote by Leonard Berlin, Professor of Radiology at Rush University and the University of

Illinois, Chicago: "You should ask yourself four questions: what do I see on the images, what do I think the findings mean, what do I want the referring physician to conclude from my report, and what do I think the referring physician should do next." Now on to the cases!

Dammam, Saudi Arabia   Tarek M. Hegazi
Boston, MA, USA   Jim S. Wu

Acknowledgments

This book would not be possible without the assistance and guidance of my many mentors, colleagues, and friends. I would especially like to thank Andrew Haims, Lee Katz, Neil Rofsky, Wing Chan, Ferris Hall, Seward Rutkove, Mary Hochman, Corrie Yablon, Colm McMahon, Jennifer Ni Mhuircheartaigh, Justin Kung, Suzanne Long, Daniel Siegal, Yu-Ching Lin, Yulia Melenevsky, Ron Eisenberg, Clotell Forde, and of course my coauthor Tarek Hegazi. I would also like to thank all the residents and fellows that I have had the pleasure of teaching. Seeing their enthusiasm for our specialty and watching them mature as radiologists provides me with great joy.

Jim S. Wu

I would like to thank all the attending staff at the MSK division of Thomas Jefferson University, especially Diane Deely, Bill Morrison, Adam Zoga, Suzanne Long, Kristen McClure, Paul Read, and Johannes Roedl. It has been a privilege to work with such a talented and creative group. I would also like to thank Jim Wu for agreeing on taking this endeavor of writing this book together and for his continuous support and guidance throughout this journey. Lastly, to my residents and fellows from whom I learn everyday, Shukran!

Tarek M. Hegazi

Contents

Case 1.1

Indication A 37-year-old woman with nontraumatic right shoulder pain. Evaluate for rotator cuff tear.

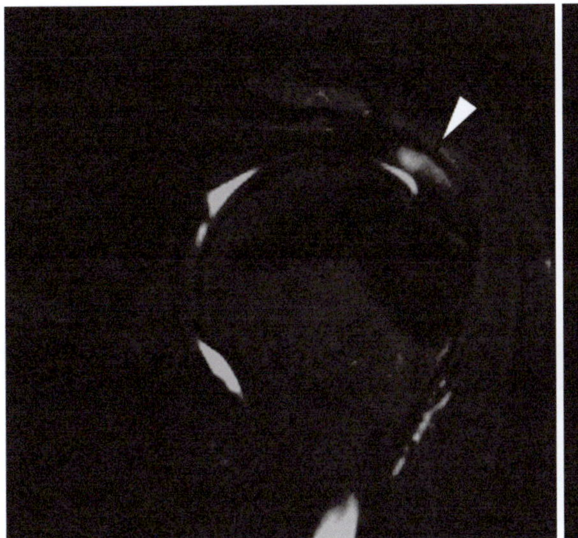

Coronal T2 fat saturated

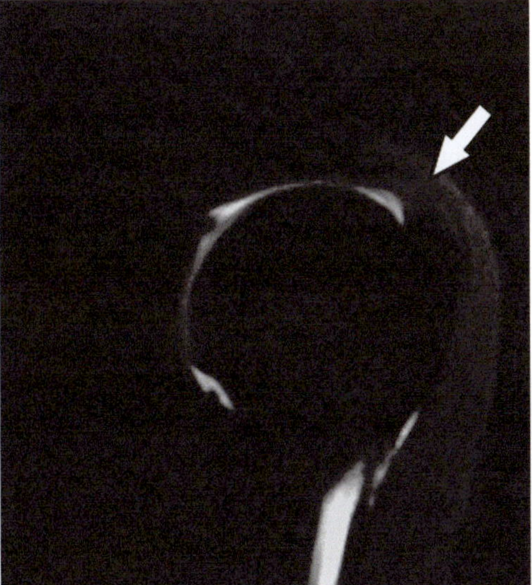

Coronal T1 fat saturated arthrogram

Findings

On the T2-weighted images, there is hyperintense signal in the supraspinatus tendon just proximal to its footprint (arrowhead) compatible with moderate tendinosis. The signal intensity is not as bright as fluid, thus excluding a focal tear. On the T1-weighted post-arthrogram images, there is no contrast extending into the tendon substance (arrow) to indicate an articular surface tear. There is no fluid in the subacromial/subdeltoid bursa. There is no subacromial spur or os acromiale.

Impression/Recommendation

Tendinosis of the supraspinatus tendon without focal tear.

© Springer Nature Switzerland AG 2020
T. M. Hegazi, J. S. Wu, *Musculoskeletal MRI*, https://doi.org/10.1007/978-3-030-26777-3_1

Discussion: Rotator Cuff Tendinosis

The rotator cuff (RTC) is made up of four separate muscles and tendons that act to stabilize the shoulder. They consist of the supraspinatus, infraspinatus, teres minor, and subscapularis tendons. They arise from the scapula and join on the tuberosities of the humeral head. The footprint of the supraspinatus tendon inserts onto the superior facet of the greater tuberosity, just posterior to the bicipital groove. The infraspinatus tendon footprint is much larger, and the anterior fibers of the infraspinatus tendon interdigitate with the posterior fibers of the supraspinatus tendon and insert on the posterior aspect of the superior facet. The remainder of the infraspinatus tendon inserts onto the middle facet of the greater tuberosity. The teres minor tendon inserts on the inferior facet. The subscapularis tendon is multipennate and inserts broadly on the lesser tuberosity. On MRI, the normal RTC tendons show uniform hypointense signal intensity on all pulse sequences since they are composed of dense collagen bundles. The supraspinatus and infraspinatus tendons are best evaluated on the coronal and sagittal oblique sequences, while the subscapularis and teres minor tendons are best assessed on the axial and sagittal sequences.

RTC tendinosis refers to chronic degeneration of the tendons. The exact etiology is controversial, with two common theories. In the extrinsic theory, there is external impingement of the subacromial bursa and the bursal surface of the rotator cuff by hypertrophic changes of the acromion (subacromial spur), osteophytes from the acromioclavicular joint, type 3 (hooked) acromion, or an os acromiale. In the internal theory, intratendinous degeneration of the tendons occurs due to advancing age and chronic overuse. RTC tendinosis is a common finding seen on routine MRI of the shoulder and may or may not be associated with shoulder pain. On MRI, RTC tendinosis appears as mild to moderate diffuse thickening of the tendon and diffuse intermediate signal intensity within the substance of the tendon on T1- and T2-weighted images. It is important to differentiate tendinosis from low-grade partial tears. The T2 signal intensity in RTC tendinosis should not reach the intensity of fluid signal, while tendon tears should demonstrate fluid signal intensity. This is best seen on a T2-weighted fat-suppressed sequence. One should compare the signal intensity in the tendon with fluid in the joint space or subacromial/subdeltoid space. Furthermore, the signal in RTC tendinosis is more globular and typically less linear in appearance than the signal abnormalities seen in RTC tears. Tendinosis is often associated with fluid in the subacromial/subdeltoid bursa indicating bursitis. Moreover, there has been confusion about the terms: tendinosis, tendinitis, tendinopathy, and tendonitis. Tendinosis is tendon degeneration due to chronic overuse, whereas tendinitis indicates inflammation of the tendon with an inflammatory response, often due to microtears or arthropathies. Tendinopathy is the broader term that includes both tendinosis and tendinitis. We have used the term tendinosis here as it is likely the more common process occurring in rotator cuff pathology, but the term tendinopathy would also be appropriate. Tendinosis and tendinitis cannot be distinguished based on imaging. Lastly, tendonitis is simply a misspelled word and should not be used; however, it is unclear why the "o" was replaced by the "i" in these terms (see Suggested Reading).

Most patients with RTC tendinosis respond well to physiotherapy, nonsteroidal anti-inflammatory medication, and heat/ice therapy. Infrequently, surgery may be required.

Report checklist
1. Which rotator cuff tendons are involved?
2. What is the degree of tendinosis (mild, moderate, or severe)?
3. Is there an associated rotator cuff tear (i.e., is there fluid signal in the tendon substance)?
4. Are there findings to suggest external impingement (subacromial spurs, os acromiale, hooked acromion, or inferior osteophytes with acromioclavicular joint osteoarthritis)?
5. Is there subacromial/subdeltoid bursitis?

Suggested Reading

Ahmad Z, Ilyas M, Wani GM, Choh NA, Gojwari TA, Ahmad Kazime MJ. Evaluation of rotator cuff tendinopathies and tears with high-resolution ultrasonography and magnetic resonance imaging correlation. Arch Trauma Res. 2018;7:15–2.

Kyff R. Who took tendon out of tendinitis? The Hartford Courant. 8 Mar 2000.

McMonagle JS, Vinson EN. MRI of the shoulder: rotator cuff. Appl Radiol. 2012;41:20–7.

Case 1.2

Indication A 46-year-old male with chronic shoulder pain and impingement. Evaluate for rotator cuff tear.

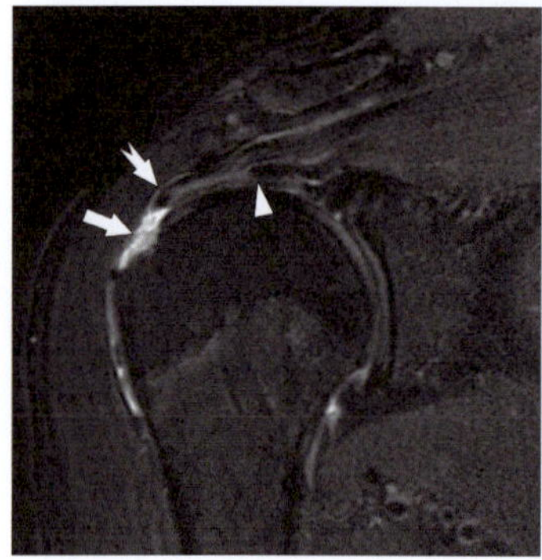

Coronal T2 fat saturated

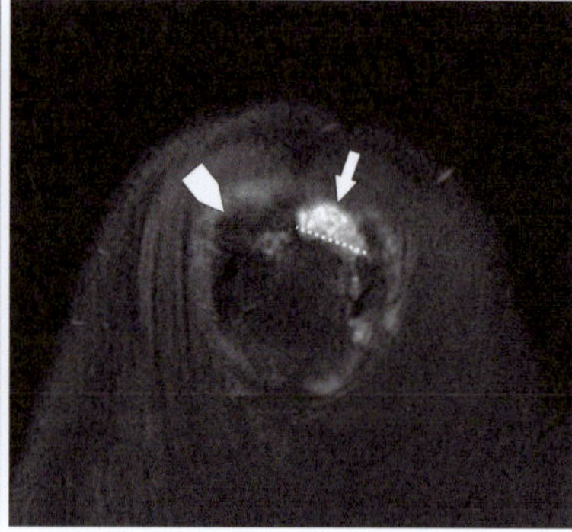

Sagittal T2 fat saturated

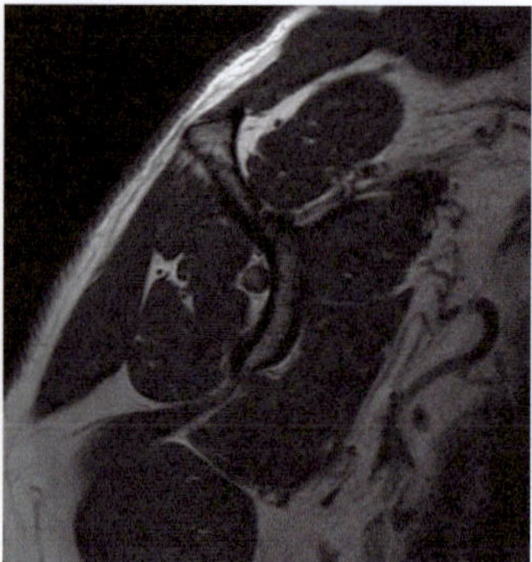

Sagittal T1

Findings

There is a full-thickness tear (arrows) of the anterior fibers of the supraspinatus tendon at its humeral insertion with fluid filling the tendon defect. The tear measures 1.5 cm (dashed line) in anterior to posterior dimension. There is retraction of the superior tendon fibers (notched arrow) by 1.5 cm and of the undersurface fibers (arrowhead) by 3.2 cm. There is no muscle atrophy on the sagittal T1-weighted images. There is no subacromial spur, os acromiale, or significant AC arthropathy to cause impingement on the rotator cuff tendons. The infraspinatus (block arrow) and the remainder of the rotator cuff tendons are normal.

Impression/Recommendation

Full-thickness tear of the anterior fibers of the supraspinatus tendon with 3 cm of tendon retraction.

Discussion: Rotator Cuff – Full-Thickness Tear

Tendons connect muscles to the bone and are extremely strong. In general, tendons do not tear unless abnormal. In the shoulder, rotator cuff tears are extremely common and are the result of degeneration, often beginning as tendinosis. A full-thickness rotator cuff tear is a tear that involves the entire craniocaudal depth (thickness) of the tendon from superior to inferior with communication between the glenohumeral joint and the subacromial-subdeltoid bursa. These tears are most commonly seen at the most anterior fibers of the supraspinatus tendon and can either extend posteriorly to involve the infraspinatus tendon or extend anteriorly to involve the superior fibers of the subscapularis tendon. A "complete" tear is defined as a full-thickness tear that involves the entire width of the tendon in the anterior to posterior dimension. These types of tears are usually associated with retraction of the torn tendon fibers medially.

On MRI, a full-thickness tear is seen as a region of hyperintense fluid signal on the T2-weighted images extending through the entire thickness of the tendon. Tears of the supraspinatus and infraspinatus tendons are best evaluated on the coronal and sagittal oblique sequences. The size of the tear should be reported in the anterior to posterior dimension, measured on the sagittal plane, and in the medial to lateral dimension measured on the coronal plane. At times, it can be hard to distinguish where the posterior fibers of the supraspinatus tendon terminate and where the anterior fibers of the infraspinatus tendon begin. If there is any tendon retraction, this should also be stated in the report and measured. If there is more than 3 cm of tendon retraction, then this indicates a poorer prognosis for surgical repair and should be clearly stated. The distal free edge of the tendon should also be described. If the free edge is frayed or has extensive tendinosis, this can have implications for surgery as the tendon free edge may have to be debrided to allow for adequate bony reattachment (*see supplementary images*). The presence of a tendon stump on the humerus should also be reported to aid in surgical planning. Assessment for RTC fatty muscle atrophy is important. This is seen as fatty areas of high signal intensity in the muscle on the T1-weighted images (best seen in the sagittal plane). The *Goutallier* classification (although initially created for CT) is commonly used to quantify the amount of fatty atrophy of the rotator cuff muscles: grade 0, normal muscle; grade 1, some fatty streaks; grade 2, less than 50% fatty muscle atrophy; grade 3, 50% fatty muscle atrophy; and grade 4, greater than 50% fatty muscle atrophy (*see supplementary images*). The degree of fatty atrophy is important to include in the report since grade 3 or 4 fatty atrophy has poor surgical outcome, and these patients often will not undergo surgical repair. A pitfall to avoid is that rotator cuff muscles can have decreased bulk when compared to the others; however, if there is no internal hyperintense fatty intensity on the T1-weighted images, then this should only be described as "loss of muscle bulk" and not fatty atrophy as decreased muscle bulk can be reversible. These patients can still benefit from surgical repair. Finally, it is important to discuss your reporting criteria with your orthopedists to use common language.

A massive rotator cuff tear is defined as a full-thickness tear that either involves more than two tendons or measures greater than 5 cm in the anterior to posterior dimension. These types of tears are usually associated with superior migration of the humeral head (high riding humeral head) that may be seen articulating with the undersurface of the acromion and usually results in accelerated glenohumeral joint osteoarthritis.

The majority of full-thickness tears are treated surgically. Relative contraindications for surgery are muscle atrophy or significant tendon retraction.

Supplementary Images

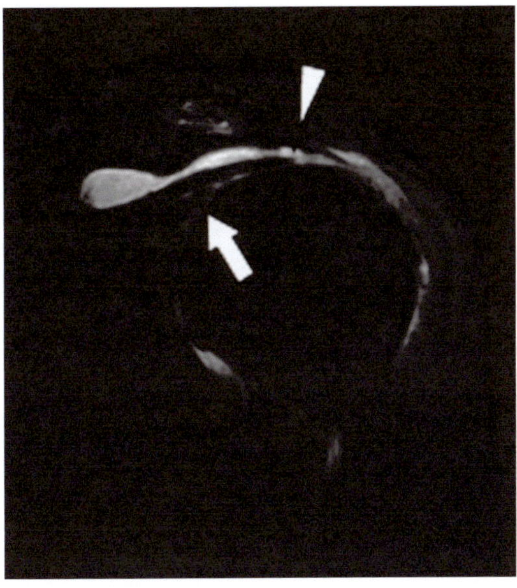

Coronal T2 fat saturated

Full-thickness supraspinatus delaminating tear with retraction of 4 cm of the undersurface (arrow) fibers but only 2.5 cm retraction of the bursal surface (arrowhead) fibers

Report checklist
1. Which tendon(s) are involved?
2. Is there a partial-thickness, full-thickness, or complete (full-thickness, full-width) tear?
3. What is the size of the tear in the anterior to posterior (AP) dimension? Does the tear involve the anterior, central, or posterior fibers?
4. Does the tear involve the adjacent tendon(s) (i.e., extension of a posterior supraspinatus tear to the anterior fibers of infraspinatus)?
5. What is the extent of the medial tendon retraction if present?
6. How is the tendon free edge (frayed, tendinosis, interstitial tearing)? Is there a tendon stump on the humerus?
7. Is there any associated muscle fatty atrophy? (Use Goutallier classification or check with your referring orthopedists.)
8. Are there findings to suggest external impingement (subacromial spurs, os acromiale, hooked acromion, or inferior osteophytes from acromioclavicular joint osteoarthritis)?

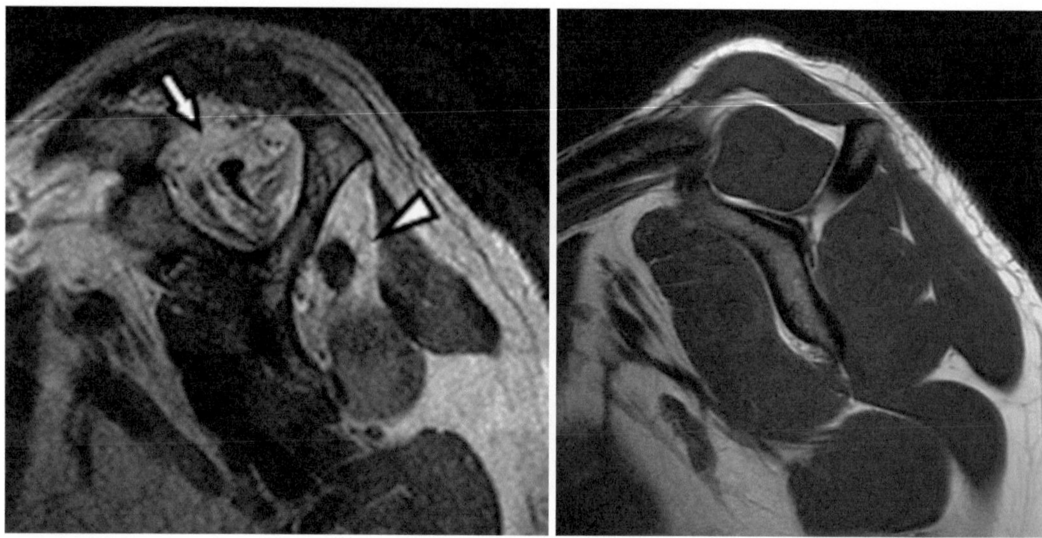

Sagittal T1

Sagittal T1

First image shows severe fatty atrophy (Goutallier grade 4) and loss of muscle bulk of the supraspinatus (arrow) and infraspinatus (arrowhead) muscles. Second image shows normal muscle bulk of the rotator cuff in a different patient

Suggested Reading

Ahmad Z, Ilyas M, Wani GM, Choh NA, Gojwari TA, Ahmad Kazime MJ. Evaluation of rotator cuff tendinopathies and tears with high-resolution ultrasonography and magnetic resonance imaging correlation. Arch Trauma Res. 2018;7:15–23.

Morag Y, Jacobson JA, Miller B, et-al. MR imaging of rotator cuff injury: what the clinician needs to know. Radiographics. 2006;26(4):1045–65.

Case 1.3

Indication   A 43-year-old woman with shoulder pain for 6 months, not improved with physical therapy.

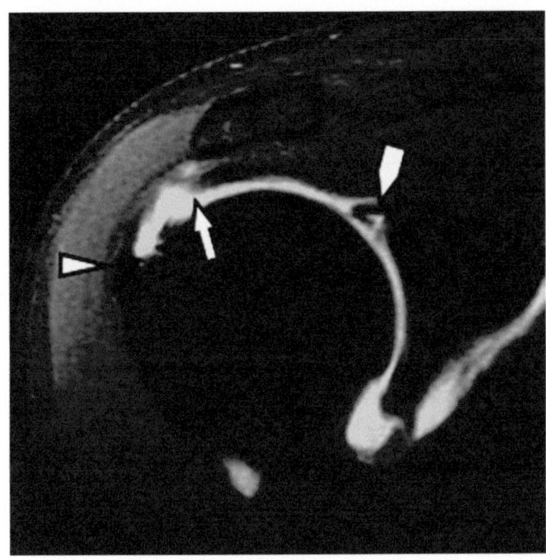

Coronal T1 fat saturated (MR arthrogram)

Findings

There is a high-grade undersurface (articular) tear of the supraspinatus. The free edge of the articular tendon fibers (arrow) is retracted by 2 cm, and there is contrast filling the tendon gap. There remain a few intact bursal surface fibers still attaching to the humeral head (arrowhead). There is no contrast in the subacromial/subdeltoid space to indicate a full-thickness tear. There is also a superior labrum anterior to posterior (SLAP) tear with contrast in the substance of the labrum (block arrow).

Impression/Recommendation

1. High-grade partial (undersurface) tear of the supraspinatus tendon
2. SLAP tear

Discussion: Rotator Cuff – Partial-Thickness Tear

Rotator cuff tears occur secondary to chronic tendinosis and weakening of the rotator cuff tendons which result in a focal defect in the normal contour of the rotator cuff that is filled with fluid signal. A rotator cuff tear is defined as either being partial thickness or full thickness based on the depth of the involved tendon from superior to inferior (*please refer to Case 1.2 for discussion on full-thickness rotator cuff tears*). Partial RTC tears can be articu-

lar, bursal, or interstitial. Articular tears involve the undersurface or deep fibers of the rotator cuff and connect to the joint space, bursal tears involve the superficial fibers and connect with the subacromial/subdeltoid space (*see supplementary images*), and interstitial tears involve the central fibers and do not extend to either the bursal or articular surfaces.

On MRI, a partial tear is differentiated from tendinosis by the degree of high signal on the T2-weighted images. Tendinosis has high signal but does not reach fluid signal intensity as seen in a tear (*please refer to Case 1.1 for discussion on rotator cuff tendinosis*). The majority of partial-thickness tears occur at the anterior insertional fibers of the supraspinatus tendon just posterior to the long head of biceps tendon, and special attention to this region should be made on every MRI so as not to miss these small tears. A partial-thickness tear of the rotator cuff is generally seen as focal fluid signal on the T2-weighted images extending partially through the thickness of the tendon touching either the bursal or articular fibers or remaining entirely intrasubstance (interstitial). This means that fluid or contrast will not extend from the joint surface to the subacromial/subdeltoid space. The extent of involvement of the tendon thickness should be reported as either being low grade (<25% of the tendon thickness), moderate (25–50% of the tendon thickness), or high grade (>50% of the tendon thickness). Also, the extent of the tear in the anterior to posterior dimension should be measured on the sagittal plane similar to full-thickness tears.

A particular type of partial-thickness tear called a "rim-rent tear" has been described in the literature which represents an articular-sided acute avulsion usually occurring at the insertion of the supraspinatus tendon at the bone-tendon interface (*see supplementary images*). They appear as a small focal linear discontinuity deep to the footprint of the tendon. This has also been termed a PASTA lesion in the orthopedic literature (partial articular side supraspinatus tendon avulsion).

Treatment of partial tears varies between surgeons; however most low-grade partial-thickness tears are treated conservatively with NSAIDs and physiotherapy. High-grade partial-thickness tears can be treated surgically.

Supplementary Images

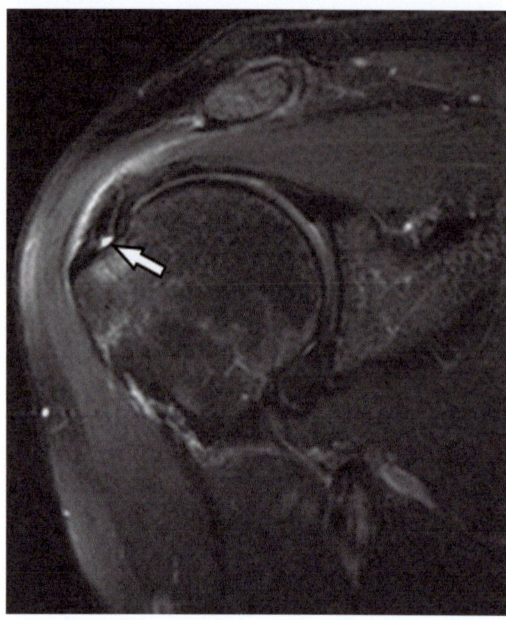

Coronal T2 fat saturated

"Rim-rent" tear of the anterior fibers of the supraspinatus tendon (arrow)

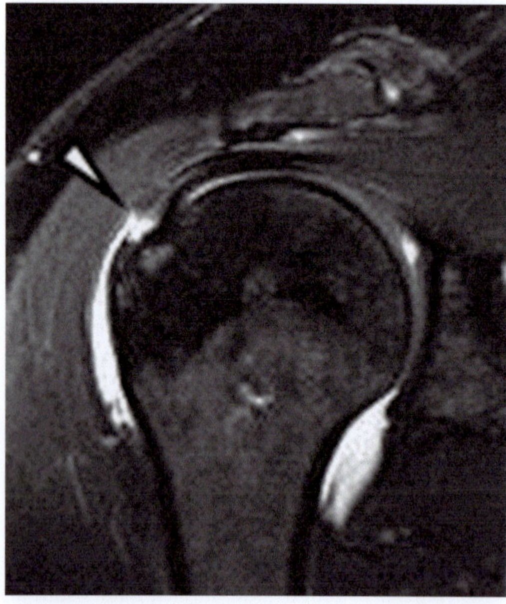

Coronal T2 fat saturated

Bursal-sided tear (arrowhead) of the supraspinatus tendon with tendon defect filled with fluid from the subacromial/subdeltoid space

Suggested Reading

Lee JH, Yoon YC, Jung JY, Yoo JC. Rotator cuff tears noncontrast MRI compared to MR arthrography. Skeletal Radiol. 2015;44(12): 1745–54.

Smith TO, Daniell H, Geere JA, et al. The diagnostic accuracy of MRI for the detection of partial- and full-thickness rotator cuff tears in adults. Magn Reson Imaging. 2012;30(3):336–46.

Case 1.4

Indication A 54-year-old male with prior rotator cuff repair 2 years ago. Returning with recurrent shoulder pain and weakness. Rule out rotator cuff tear.

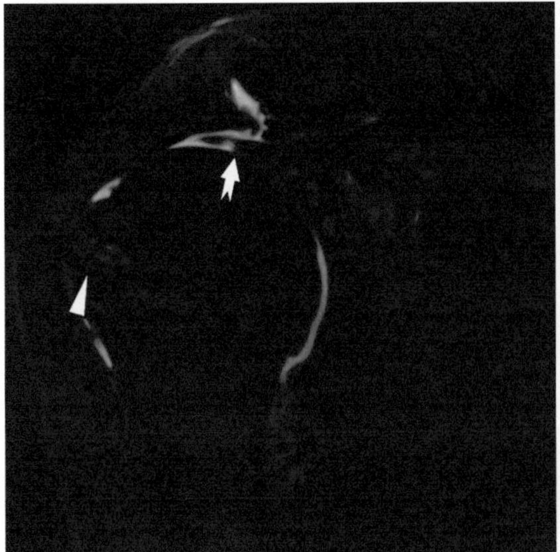

Coronal T2 fat saturated

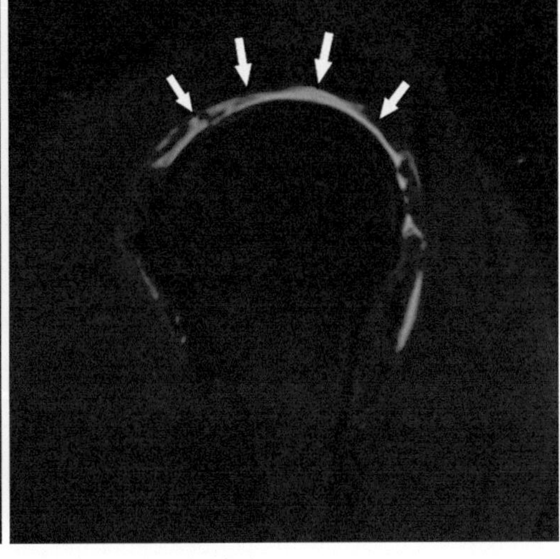

Sagittal T2 fat saturated

Findings
A suture anchor is seen at the greater tuberosity related to prior rotator cuff repair (arrowhead). There is however a new full-thickness re-tear involving the entire width of both the supraspinatus and infraspinatus tendons (arrows) with retraction of the torn tendon stump (notched arrow) by about 3 cm. There is no muscle atrophy.

Impression/Recommendation
Full-thickness re-tear at the insertion of the supraspinatus and infraspinatus tendons.

Discussion: Postoperative Shoulder
The number of rotator cuff-related surgery is increasing annually. Evaluation and interpretation of the postoperative MRI of the shoulder can be a daunting and challenging task for the radiologist; however, understanding the common surgical procedures performed and their appearance can make interpreting these studies easier. The most common surgeries performed are (1) subacromial decompression for impingement with subacromial bursectomy and acromioplasty, (2) rotator cuff debridement or repair, and (3) labral repair for glenohumeral instability.

The first challenge with postoperative MRI is susceptibility artifact from surgical material used during surgery. There are multiple ways of decreasing these artifacts to evaluate the underlying anatomy better. This includes using thinner slices, increasing matrix, increasing bandwidth, increasing NEX, using STIR sequences instead of fat-suppressed sequences, and avoiding using GRE sequences. Imaging on a 1.5 versus a 3.0 Tesla system can also reduce metal artifact.

Subacromial decompression has become the treatment of choice for extrinsic impingement with the goal being to increase the subacromial space to allow more room for the cuff tendons. The surgery includes resection of a portion of the anterolateral acromion, shaving the undersurface of the acromion, resection of the coracoacromial ligament, and resection of any inferior osteophytes arising from the acromioclavicular joint. If required, the distal aspect of the clavicle can also be resected (Mumford procedure). The normal postoperative appearance includes a flat undersurface of the acromion with a slight change in morphology, mainly anteriorly. There should be no osteophytes directed inferiorly, and there is usually lack of visualization of a normal coracoacromial ligament. If a Mumford procedure has been performed, there is widening of the acromioclavicular distance by approximately 1–2 cm and should not be mistaken for acromioclavicular joint separation. Evaluation of the coracoacromial arch is essential in patients with signs of impingement in the postoperative setting. Any residual osteophytes are best seen on the sagittal sequences. Fluid in the region of the resected subacromial bursa is a normal finding and should not be reported as bursitis.

The type of rotator cuff repair depends on many factors depending on the patient's age, activity level, and the location, type, and size of the tear. Low-grade partial-thickness rotator cuff tears involving less than 30% of the tendon thickness are usually treated with debridement only. Partial-thickness tears involving 30–70% of the tendon thickness are treated with debridement of the cuff and suture of the tendon (tendon-to-tendon). High-grade partial-thickness tears extending more than 70% of the tendon thickness are usually completed and repaired similar to a full-thickness rotator cuff repair. This includes reattachment of the tendon at the greater tuberosity using suture anchors. The typical MRI appearance of the postoperative cuff includes intermediate T1 and T2 signal abnormalities related to granulation tissue and fibrosis; however, it should not reach fluid signal intensity. It is normal to see fluid in the subacromial/subdeltoid bursa after shoulder surgery, and this is a nonspecific finding. Also, after surgery, the shoulder joint is no longer water-tight; thus contrast or joint fluid in the glenohumeral joint may enter into the subacromial/subdeltoid space and does not necessarily indicate a full-thickness tear. The majority of the suture anchors used are biodegradable, and you can normally see osteolysis and cystic changes around them which represents an inflammatory reaction. MRI findings of a full-thickness re-tear include abnormal fluid-filled signal tendon defect or nonvisualization of the tendon. Partial-thickness re-tears are very difficult to diagnose. Biceps tenodesis can be performed in the setting of a rotator cuff repair if there is severe tendinosis or tearing. This involves resection of the intra-articular portion of the tendon (tenotomy) with reattachment of the biceps tendon to the proximal humeral shaft.

There are many different procedures for repairing a labral tear; however, the most common is a Bankart labral repair which involves placing suture anchors at the anteroinferior glenoid at the 3, 4, and 5 o'clock positions and suture material to re-attach the torn labrum. A capsulorrhaphy is often performed in addition to the labral repair to tighten the joint capsule. An osseous Bankart is usually repaired by placing a screw through the osseous fragment. Following a labral repair, the labrum usually appears irregular and frayed related to labral debridement, and it is difficult to evaluate for a labral re-tear due to susceptibility artifact from the adjacent suture anchors. However, MR arthrogram is very helpful in these situations. There should be no fluid or contrast undermining the repaired labrum in an intact labral repair. If contrast extends beneath the labrum or there is detachment of the repaired labrum, then this suggests a recurrent labral tear. Other complications include loosening of the suture anchors which can be displaced into the glenohumeral joint (*see supplementary images*).

Supplementary Images

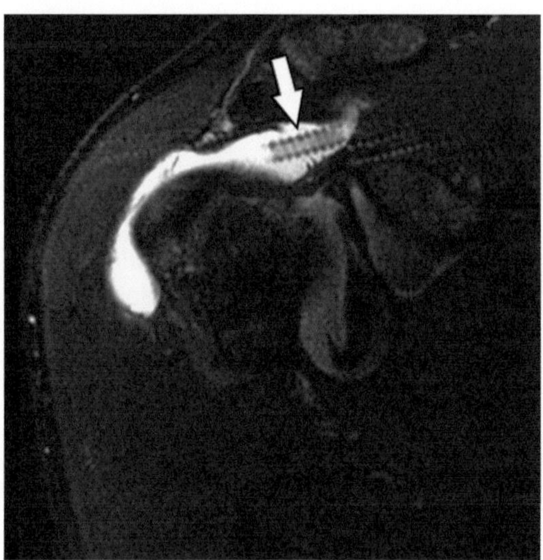

Coronal T2 fat saturated

A 28-year-old man with persistent pain after rotator cuff repair 1 year earlier. Displaced suture anchor (arrow) is seen in the subacromial space. Ghosting artifact of the screw is also seen

Report checklist

1. What type of surgery has been performed (subacromial decompression, rotator cuff repair, or labral repair, etc.)?
2. If subacromial decompression, are there residual subacromial spurs or inferior osteophytes impinging on the rotator cuff? Is there worsening rotator cuff tendinosis or new rotator cuff tear?
3. If there has been a rotator cuff repair, then what tendons have been repaired? Are there findings to suggest a partial- or full-thickness re-tear? Is there muscle atrophy? Is there a new rotator cuff tear in another location?
4. How is the long head of biceps tendon? Has there been tenodesis?
5. If labral repair, which portion of the labrum has been repaired? Is there thickening and irregularity of the anterior capsule to suggest prior capsulorrhaphy? Are there findings to suggest a labral re-tear? Is there loosening or malpositioning of the suture anchors?

Suggested Reading

Hayashida K, Tanaka M, Koizumi K, Kakiuchi M. Characteristic retear patterns assessed by magnetic resonance imaging after arthroscopic double-row rotator cuff repair. Arthroscopy. 2012;28:458–64.

Khazzam M, Kuhn JE, Mulligan E, et al. Magnetic resonance imaging identification of rotator cuff retears after repair: interobserver and intraobserver agreement. Am J Sports Med. 2012;40:1722–7.

Wu J, Covey A, Katz LD. MRI of the postoperative shoulder. Clin Sports Med. 2006;25(3):445–64.

Case 1.5

Indication A 44-year-old female with left shoulder pain and decreased range of motion. X-rays show calcification adjacent to the greater tuberosity.

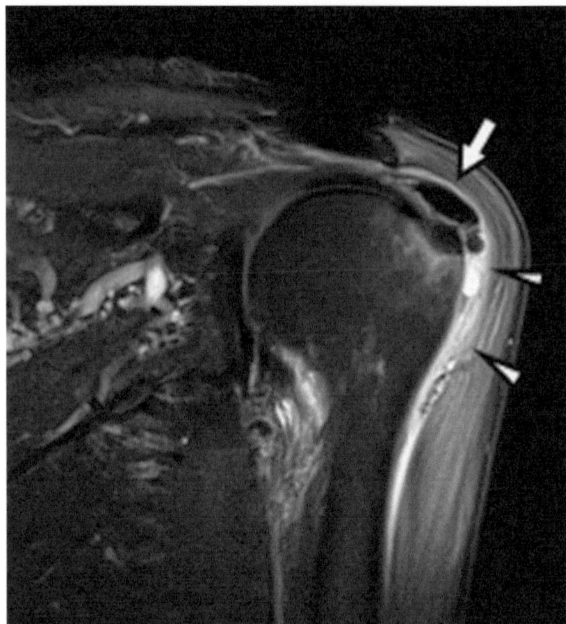

Coronal T2 fat saturated

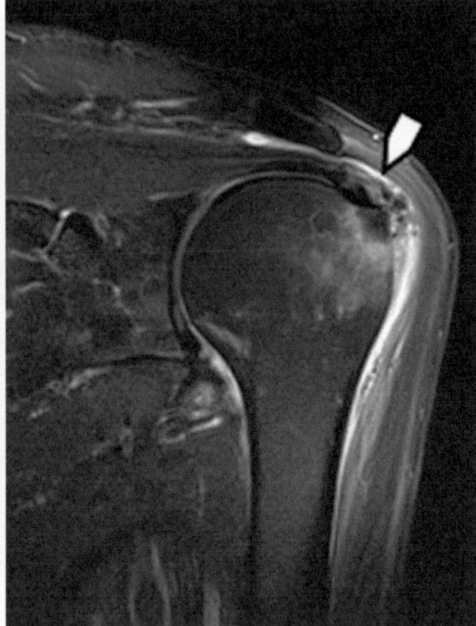

Coronal T2 fat saturated

Findings

There is well-defined low signal intensity focus in the supraspinatus tendon at its humeral insertion measuring about 1.5 cm (arrow) corresponding to calcifications seen on the prior radiographs (not shown). This is associated with surrounding soft tissue edema as well as a moderate subacromial/subdeltoid bursitis (arrowheads). There is also mild fraying and low-grade partial-thickness bursal-sided tear at the insertion of the supraspinatus tendon (block arrow) with adjacent reactive bone marrow edema at the greater tuberosity. There is no shoulder joint effusion.

Impression/Recommendation

Calcific tendinitis (resorptive/active phase) of the supraspinatus tendon and moderate subacromial/subdeltoid bursitis.

Discussion: Calcific Tendinitis

Deposition of calcium hydroxyapatite in the tendon can lead to calcific tendinitis. The etiology is unknown but thought to result from microtrauma and decreased oxygen tension, leading to secondary mineralization. Calcific tendinitis can affect any tendon in the body but is typically seen in the rotator cuff, especially the supraspinatus tendon (80%). It can also involve the periarticular soft tissues such as the glenohumeral ligaments, bursae, and joint capsule.

These calcifications are best seen on radiographs but can also be visualized on MRI. They typically appear as well-defined oval or lobular foci in the rotator cuff about 1 cm from their insertion on the humerus and are of low signal intensity on all pulse sequences. They can range from a few millimeters to several centimeters in size.

Sometimes the calcifications are tiny and difficult to detect on routine MRI. The use of gradient echo sequences is helpful as the small calcifications can be exaggerated by the blooming artifact and hence better detected. If no dedicated gradient sequence is performed, it is always helpful to go back to the localizer sequences as these are gradient echo sequences and the blooming artifact can sometimes be visualized. Obtaining new or scrutinizing old radiographs can be very helpful (*see supplementary images*). When in the resorptive or active phase, there can be surrounding inflammatory changes resulting in soft tissue edema and insertional marrow edema. When the process leads to distension of fluid within the subacromial/subdeltoid bursa, it can be called calcific bursitis. It is not uncommon for these calcific deposits to cause fraying and partial-thickness tears at the bursal surface of the rotator cuff tendons. Clinically, patient often presents with nontraumatic acute shoulder pain with mild elevation in inflammatory markers. This acute phase can mimic a septic joint where a joint effusion is often present but uncommon with calcific tendinitis.

It is important to consider incidental calcifications and loose bodies associated with chondral defects and secondary osteoarthritis; however, these are usually intra-articular in location, rather than within the rotator cuff tendon.

Potential treatments for calcific tendinitis of the rotator cuff include oral analgesic/anti-inflammatory medication; however, ultrasound-guided barbotage with or without steroid injection has become the treatment of choice.

Supplementary Images

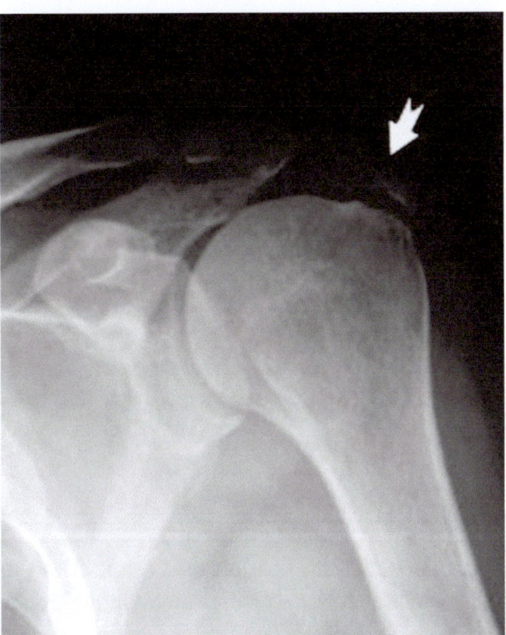

Multiple foci of calcifications (notched arrow) are seen adjacent to the greater tuberosity most compatible with calcium hydroxyapatite deposition (calcific tendinitis).

Report checklist
1. Which tendon is involved? What are the size and location of the calcification?
2. Is there surrounding soft tissue edema and subacromial/subdeltoid bursitis indicating the resorptive/active phase?
3. Is there any associated rotator cuff fraying or tear?
4. Did you compare to radiographs to confirm diagnosis?
5. Is there an associated joint effusion?

Suggested Reading

ElShewy MT. Calcific tendinitis of the rotator cuff. World J Orthop. 2016;7(1):55–60.

Nörenberg D, Ebersberger HU, Walter T, Ockert B, Knobloch G, Diederichs G, Hamm B, Makowski MR. Diagnosis of calcific tendonitis of the rotator cuff by using susceptibility-weighted MR imaging. Radiology. 2016;278(2):475–84.

Siegal DS, Wu JS, Newman JS, Del Cura JL, Hochman MG. Calcific tendinitis: a pictorial review. Can Assoc Radiol J. 2009;60(5):263–72.

Case 1.6a

Indication A 48-year-old female with chronic left anterior shoulder pain and impingement.

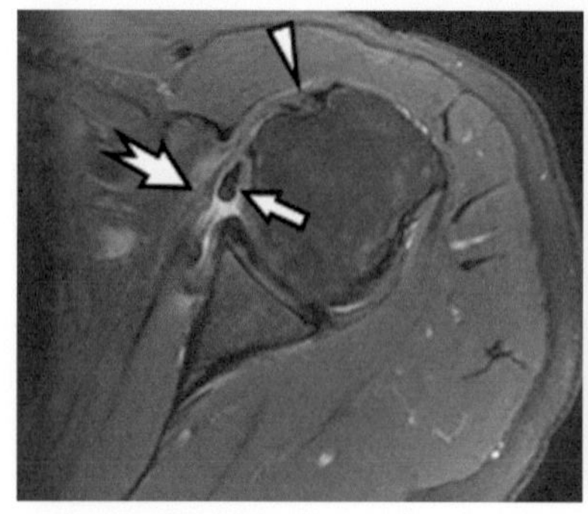 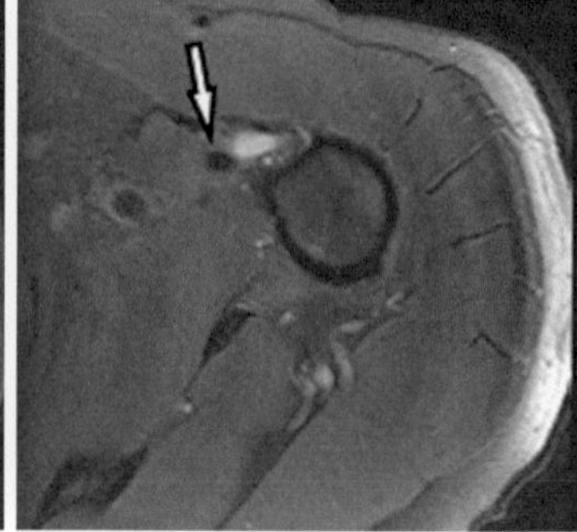 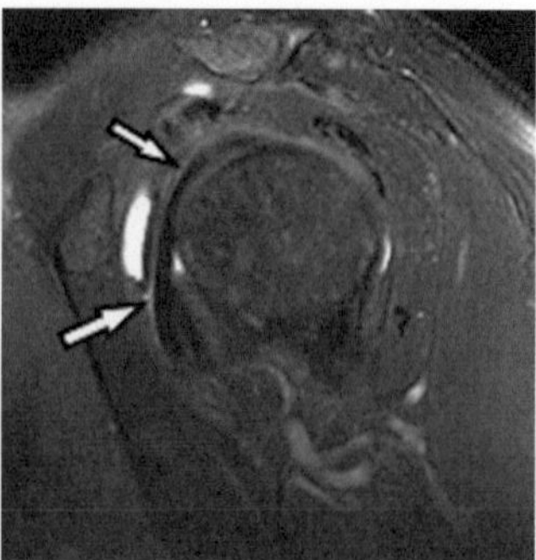

Axial T2 Fat saturated   Axial T2 Fat saturated   Sagittal T2 Fat saturated

Findings

There is medial dislocation of the long head of biceps tendon (arrows) from the bicipital groove (arrowhead) beneath the subscapularis tendon into an intra-articular location. There is no focal tear of the biceps tendon. There is rupture of the subscapularis tendon (notched arrow) at its insertion with tapering of the tendon free edge.

Case 1.6b

Indication A 42-year-old male with anterior shoulder pain over the biceps tendon.

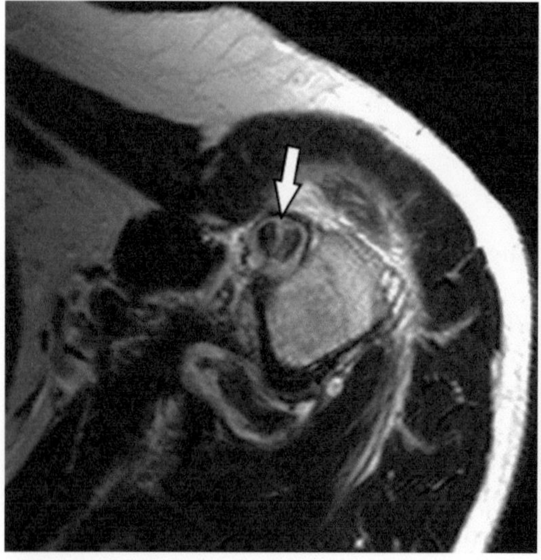 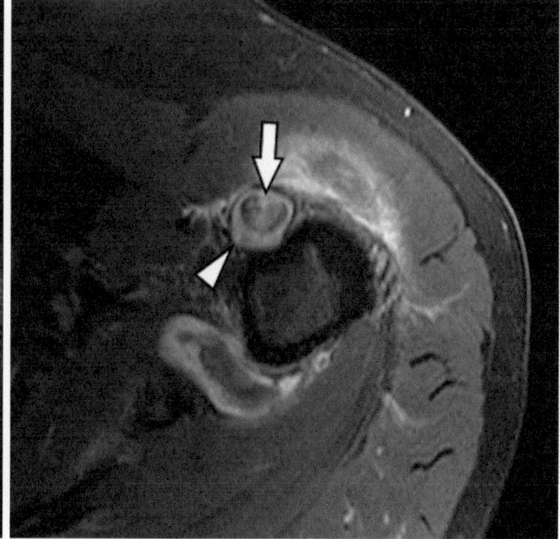

Axial T2   Axial T1 fat saturated post contrast

Findings

There is moderate tendinosis of the extra-articular portion of the long head of biceps tendon with a longitudinal T2 hyperintense cleft within the tendon substance compatible with a longitudinal split tear (arrows). There is also a moderate amount of fluid and synovial proliferation in the biceps tendon sheath out of proportion to the amount of glenohumeral joint fluid and peripheral enhancement compatible with moderate tenosynovitis (arrowhead).

Impression/Recommendation

- **Case 1.6a:** Intra-articular dislocation of the long head of biceps tendon related to complete rupture of the subscapularis tendon.
- **Case 1.6b:** Moderate tendinosis and tenosynovitis of the long head of the biceps tendon with longitudinal interstitial tearing.

Discussion: Pathology of the Long Head of Biceps Tendon

Proximally, the biceps tendon is composed of two heads: the long head of the biceps tendon (LHBT) and short head of the biceps tendon. The short head arises from the tip of the coracoid process. The LHBT originates from the supraglenoid tubercle and the superior glenoid labrum. From there, the long head traverses obliquely along the anterosuperior part of the humeral head and then turns caudally into the bicipital groove. The LHBT is initially intra-articular but becomes extra-articular as it enters the bicipital groove. At the transition between the intra-articular and extra-articular portions of the tendon at the lateral aspect of the rotator interval, the superior glenohumeral ligament (SGHL), the coracohumeral ligament (CHL), as well as some fibers of the supraspinatus and subscapularis tendons wrap around the biceps tendon to form the "biceps pulley" which help to strengthen this portion of the tendon and prevent it from medial subluxation.

The normal LHBT has dark signal on all MRI pulse sequences. Utilization of orthogonal imaging planes is needed to appropriately asses the biceps tendon in its entirety (*see supplementary images*). The biceps anchor is best visualized on coronal images, while the distal intra-articular portion of the LHBT within the rotator interval and the biceps pulley are best seen on sagittal images. Axial images are best for evaluating the LHBT at the level of the bicipital groove.

The long head of biceps tendon may undergo progressive degeneration due to repetitive use as well as associated rotator cuff tears which puts the biceps tendon under further stress. This will lead to tendinosis as well as tenosynovitis of the surrounding tendon sheath. Later, delaminating tears and complete tendon rupture can ensue. On MRI, tendinosis is visualized as diffuse thickening of the intra-articular portion of the tendon with intermediate signal intensity within the tendon substance. The extra-articular portion of the tendon may have a small amount of fluid in the tendon sheath given that the glenohumeral joint and the tendon sheath are in direct communication. However, when the amount of fluid in the tendon sheath is out of proportion to the amount of glenohumeral joint fluid, then this suggests tenosynovitis. Partial thickness tears are seen as either diffuse thinning or attenuation of the tendon or linear high T2 fluid signal clefts traversing the substance of the tendon suggesting longitudinal tears. These tears are usually seen at the distal aspect of the intra-articular portion of the tendon about 2–3 cm from its origin, given that this area is relatively hypovascular; however, tears can be seen in the extra-articular portion of the tendon as well. A pitfall is mistaking the normal mesotendon which encircles the biceps tendon and attaches to the tendon sheath as a focal tear or synovial proliferation or loose body in the tendon sheath (*see supplementary images*). A complete rupture is relatively straightforward; there is nonvisualization of the tendon in the bicipital groove, "empty groove" sign, with distal retraction of the extra-articular portion of the tendon. There has been description in the literature of severe tendinosis and hypertrophy of the intra-articular portion of the LHBT termed the "hourglass biceps" which prevents normal sliding of the tendon in the groove and can cause biceps tendon entrapment. This is usually only seen in conjunction with full-thickness rotator cuff tears.

Certain injuries can result in displacement of the tendon from its normal position in the bicipital groove. Displacement of the tendon but with continued contact with the bicipital groove is known as subluxation. These are usually harder to diagnose but often seen as medial migration of the LHBT on the medial ridge of the intertubercular groove. More severe displacement with complete loss of contact with the bicipital groove is considered a dislocation. Displacement of the LHBT is often associated with tears of the subscapularis tendon as well as injury to the biceps pulley. The biceps tendon can be displaced into one of three locations. First, if there is a tear of the biceps pulley as well as tear of the subscapularis tendon, then this usually results in intra-articular dislocation of the LHBT. If there is a tear of the biceps pulley but the subscapu-laris tendon remains intact, then the tendon tends to dislocate medially but lies superficial to the subscapularis tendon. Lastly, if there is a tear of the biceps pulley but both the subscapularis tendon and the transverse humeral ligament are intact, then the LHBT dislocates into the substance of the subscapularis tendon and can cause interstitial tearing.

Tendinosis and low-grade injuries to the LHBT are usually treated conservatively. Ultrasound-guided injections into the tendon sheath can be performed in the setting of tenosynovitis. Severe injuries and dislocations can be treated by either tendon debridement or tenodesis.

Supplementary Images

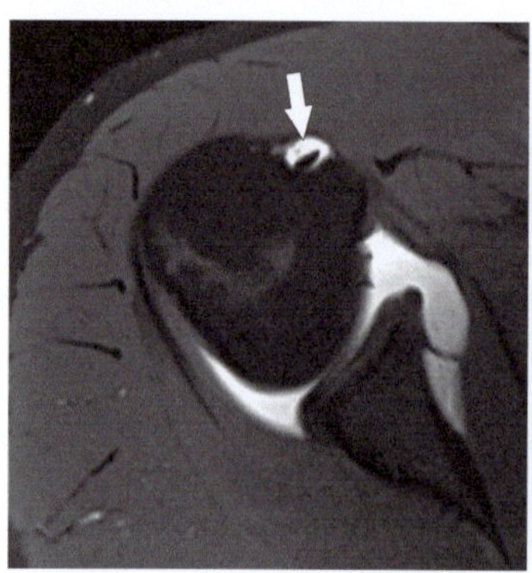 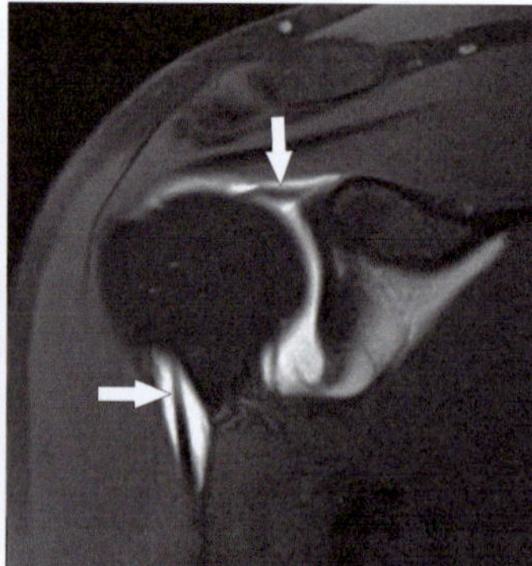 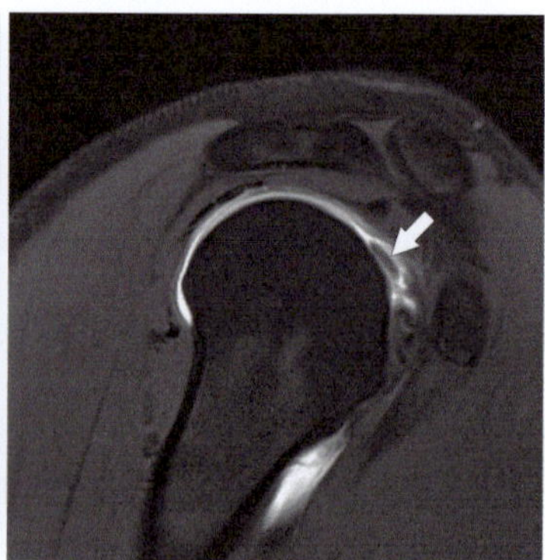

Axial T1 fat saturated arthrogram   Coronal T1 fat saturated arthrogram Sagittal T1 fat saturated arthrogram

Normal appearance of the long head of the biceps tendon (arrows) on MR arthrography. Contrast is seen distending the joint space as well as the biceps tendon sheath

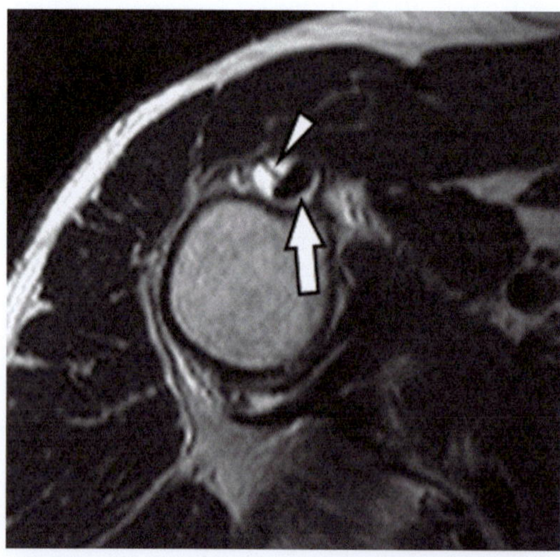

The normal mesotendon (arrowhead) encircles the biceps tendon (arrow) and runs longitudinally along tendon sheath. It should not be mistaken for a tendon tear or synovitis in the tendon sheath

Report checklist

1. Is there tendinosis of the long head of biceps tendon? Which portion (intra-articular or extra-articular)?
2. Is there tenosynovitis of the tendon sheath? Is there longitudinal interstitial tearing of the tendon substance?
3. Is the biceps tendon visualized in its normal position in the intertubercular groove? If it is not visualized at all, is there a complete rupture (or prior surgery)?
4. If the tendon is dislocated from the intertubercular groove, is it located beneath the subscapularis tendon (intra-articular location), superficial to the subscapularis tendon, or within the substance of the subscapularis tendon? Is the subscapularis torn?
5. Are there rotator cuff tears?
6. Can you visualize an injury to the biceps pulley (coracohumeral ligament or superior glenohumeral ligament)?

Suggested Reading

Morag Y, Jacobson JA, Shields G, et al. MR arthrography of rotator interval, long head of the biceps brachii, and biceps pulley of the shoulder. Radiology. 2005;235:21–30.

Nakata W, Katou S, Fujita A, Nakata M, Lefor AT, Sugimoto H. Biceps pulley: normal anatomy and associated lesions at MR arthrography. Radiographics: a review publication of the Radiological Society of North America, Inc. 2011;31(3):791–810.

Case 1.7

Indication   A 24-year-old male with right shoulder pain for 6 months after a fall. Evaluate for labral tear.

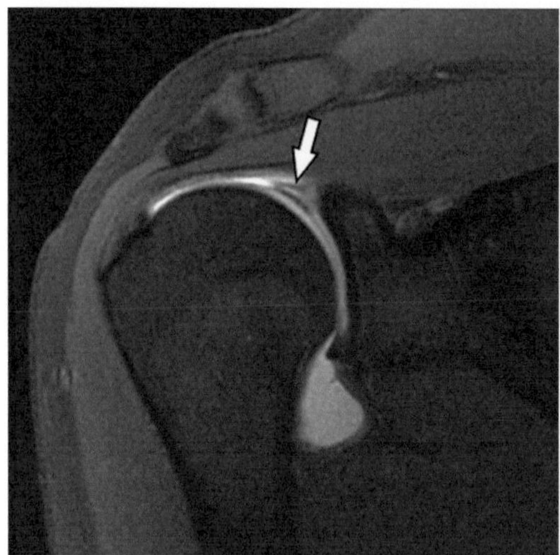

Coronal T1 fat saturated MR arthrogram

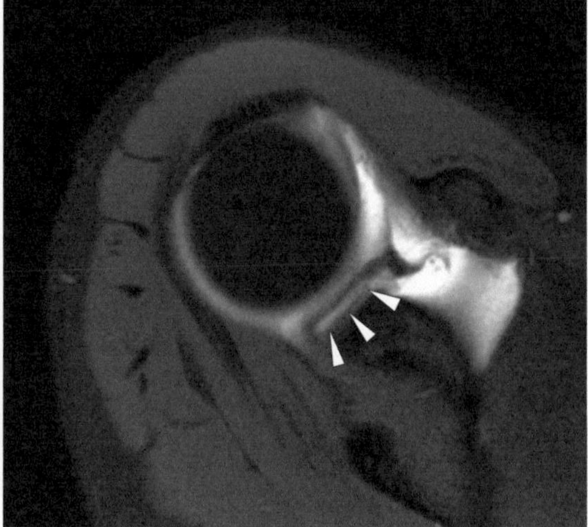

Axial T1 fat saturated MR arthrogram

Findings

There is intra-articular contrast in the substance of the superior labrum compatible with a SLAP tear (arrow). On the axial images, the tear extends anterior to posterior to involve the entire superior labrum (arrowheads). The tear extends from the 10 to 1 o'clock position. There is no displaced bucket handle fragment, and the tear does not extend into the proximal long head of the biceps tendon. There are no paralabral cysts and the articular cartilage surface is intact.

Impression/Recommendation

Superior labral anterior posterior (SLAP) tear, type II.

Discussion: Superior Labral Anterior Posterior (SLAP) Tear

The superior glenoid labrum is approximately 4 mm broad and triangular and demonstrates low signal intensity on all pulse sequences. A SLAP lesion describes a focal tear within the superior labrum centered at the origin of the long head of the biceps tendon that extends in an anterior to posterior dimension. The tear can also extend into the periarticular soft tissues, including the long head of biceps tendon (LHBT), glenohumeral ligaments, and rotator interval. There are a few normal variants of the superior labrum which need to be discussed in order to differentiate them from a true labral tear. These include the sublabral recess, sublabral foramen, and the Buford complex. Most of the labral variants are seen between 11 and 3 o'clock positions. (The clockface is commonly used to describe the location of various pathology in the shoulder with the 12 o'clock position being the most superior, the 3 o'clock position being the most anterior (regardless of right or left side), the 6 o'clock position being the most inferior, and the 9 o'clock position being the most posterior.) First, the sublabral recess is the most common labral variant and is defined as a potential recess beneath the free margin of the superior labrum and the underlying glenoid bone at the 11 to 1 o'clock position. On MRI, this is seen as a linear high signal intensity fluid cleft that has smooth margins and extends medially paralleling the glenoid margin, without extension into the substance of the labrum *(see supplementary images)*. Any extension of abnormal signal into the labrum not paralleling the glenoid is considered a labral tear and not a recess. The second variant is related to focal detachment of the labrum from the underlying glenoid, called a sublabral foramen (*see supplementary images*). This is only seen at the anterosuperior aspect of the glenoid from 1 to 3 o'clock position. Any extension inferior to the 3 o'clock position or posterior to the LHBT insertion at the 11 o'clock position is considered a labral tear rather than a variant. A rare variant, the Buford complex, is related to a congenital absence of the anterosuperior labrum from the 1 to 3 o'clock position with a thickened cord-like middle glenohumeral ligament (MGHL) which can be easily mistaken for a labral tear (*see supplementary images*). This can be avoided by following the thick MGHL on the axial plane which will blend with the underlying subscapularis tendon, rather than just floating within the anterior joint recess.

SLAP tears are frequently seen in throwing sports or related to a fall onto an outstretched arm. Snyder and colleagues initially described four patterns of injury from arthroscopic findings:

- Type I: wearing and fraying of the superior labrum which is often asymptomatic and seen in elderly individuals
- Type II: separation of the biceps anchor and the superior labrum from the underlying glenoid, the most frequent type
- Type III: displaced bucket handle tear of the superior labrum without extension into the long head of biceps tendon
- Type IV: an extension of a bucket handle tear into the long head of biceps tendon

The classification of SLAP tears has been expanded to include ten different subtypes and counting. They all describe tears of the superior labrum at the origin of the LHBT which extend to involve the adjacent soft tissue structures. It is not crucial to delineate the exact SLAP subtype when reporting; rather it is more important to accurately describe the extent of the labral tear and involvement of adjacent structures.

On MRI, the main anatomic plane for evaluating the superior labrum is the coronal plane; however, the axial plane helps to delineate the extent of the tear as well as evaluate the extension of the tear to the adjacent structures. A tear is diagnosed when there is abnormal high signal intensity within the substance of the labrum or when there is a displaced labral fragment. MR arthrography offers higher accuracy of detecting SLAP tears (75–90%) when compared to conventional MRI, and hence MR arthrograms are the examination of choice in these clinical situations. This would be seen as irregular areas of intra-articular contrast extending into the labral substance with or without a bucket handle component (vertical as well as horizontal tears at the base of the superior labrum) or extension of contrast into the proximal aspect of the LHBT.

When describing SLAP tears in your report, it is first important to differentiate between a labral variant and a true labral tear. If it does represent a tear, then describe the extent of the tear in the anterior to posterior direction with respect to the clockface position and whether the tear extends into the adjacent soft tissue structures. Then describe if the tear results in an inferiorly displaced bucket handle fragment. The status of the biceps anchor and the proximal aspect of the LHBT should be commented on. Lastly, report if there are any associated injuries, including fractures, chondral injuries, rotator cuff tears, and paralabral cysts.

Treatment of SLAP tears varies depending on the type and extension of the labral tear and includes labral debridement, labral repair, or LHBT tenodesis.

Supplementary Images

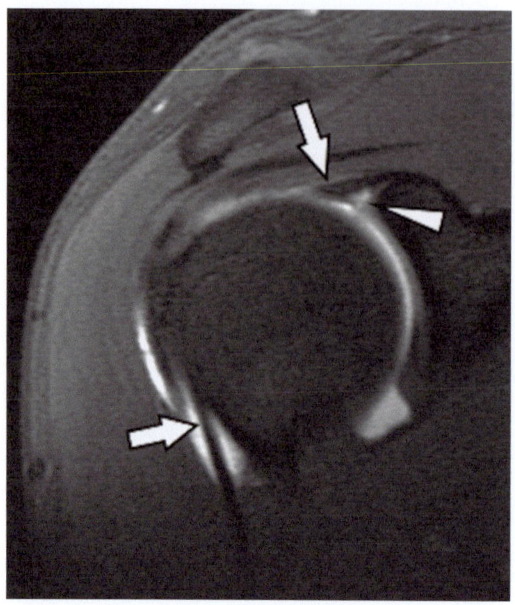

Coronal T1 fat saturated (MR arthrogram)

Normal appearance of the sublabral recess. Small amount of contrast (arrowhead) is seen at the junction of the biceps tendon (arrow) and anterior labrum in the 1 o'clock position paralleling the glenoid margin

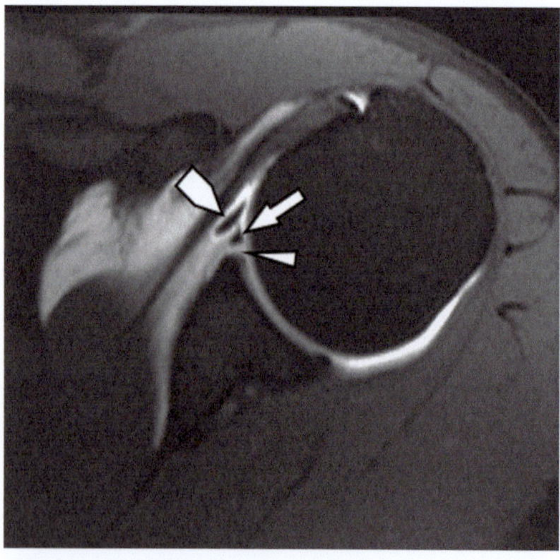

Axial T1 fat saturated (MR arthrogram)

There is a separation of the anterosuperior labrum (arrow) from the underlying glenoid with fluid between them, compatible with a sublabral foramen (arrowhead). This should not be confused with a labral tear since it is localized to the anterosuperior quadrant (1–3 o'clock position).The normal middle glenohumeral ligament (block arrow) is seen anterior to the labrum

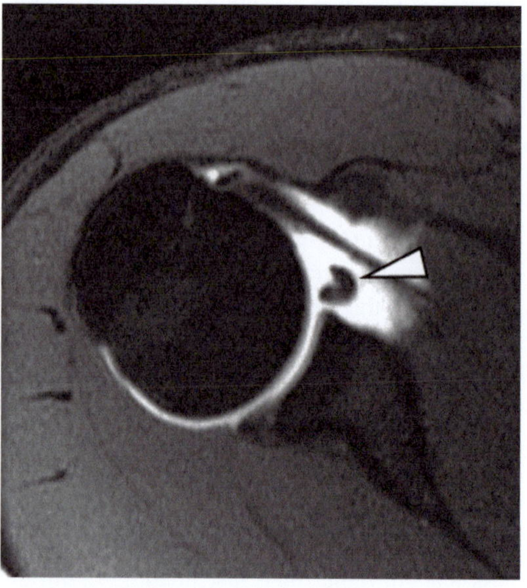

Axial T1 fat saturated (MR arthrogram)

There is absence of the anterosuperior labrum with a thickened cord-like MGHL (arrowhead) compatible with a Buford complex. This should not be confused for a labral tear. When scrolling through the axial plane, the MGHL will attach to the undersurface of the subscapularis tendon and anterior joint capsule

Report checklist

1. Does the abnormal signal intensity within the superior labrum represent a normal variant (sublabral recess, sublabral foramen, Buford complex) or a SLAP tear?
2. What is the extent of the labral tear in the anterior to posterior direction (use clockface position)?
3. Is there a displaced bucket handle tear or flap fragment?
4. Does the tear extend into the LHBT?
5. Does the tear extend into other adjacent soft tissue structures (inferior labrum, glenohumeral ligaments, rotator interval)?
6. Are there any associated injuries (bone marrow edema, chondral injury, paralabral cysts, or rotator cuff tears)?

Suggested Reading

Mohana-Borges AV, Chung CB, Resnick D. Superior labral anteroposterior tear: classification and diagnosis on MRI and MR arthrography. AJR Am J Roentgenol. 2003;181(6):1449–62.

Popp D, Schöffl V. Superior labral anterior posterior lesions of the shoulder: current diagnostic and therapeutic standards. World J Orthop. 2015;6(9):660–71.

Case 1.8

Indication A 35-year-old male with recent history of anterior shoulder dislocation to assess for labral tear.

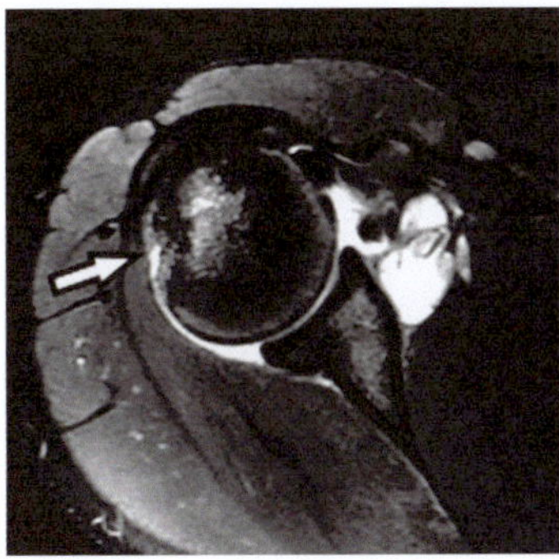

Axial T2 fat saturated

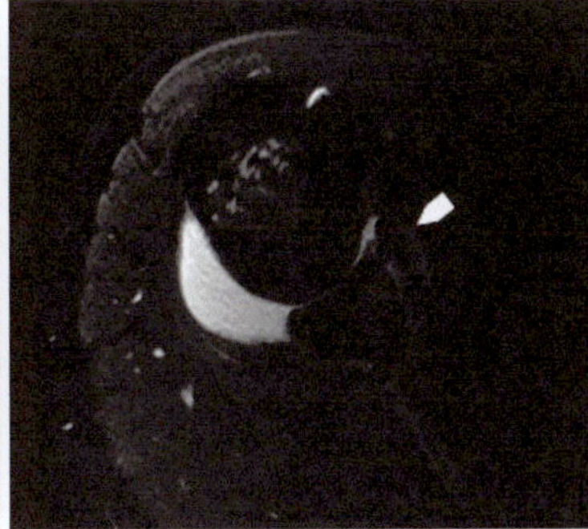

Axial T2 fat saturated

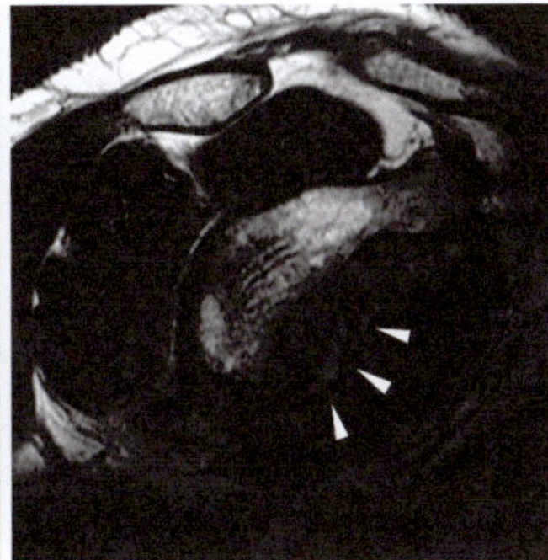

Sagittal T1

Findings

There is an impaction fracture at the posterolateral aspect of the humeral head (Hill-Sachs deformity) with underlying bone marrow edema (arrow) compatible with a recent anterior glenohumeral joint dislocation. There is detachment of the anteroinferior labrum from the underlying glenoid (block arrow) as well as tear of the adjacent periosteum extending from the 3 to 6 o'clock position. There is also a fracture of the adjacent glenoid rim (arrowheads) compatible with a bony Bankart lesion. The amount of bone loss measures 3 mm and involves about 20% of the glenoid articular surface.

Impression/Recommendation

Bony Bankart lesion and Hill-Sachs deformity compatible with prior anterior glenohumeral joint dislocation.

Discussion: Bankart Lesion

Glenohumeral joint dislocation can lead to instability due to injury of the static and dynamic stabilizers of the joint. An anterior dislocation can result in disruption of the labroligamentous complex in the anteroinferior quadrant of the glenoid located in the 3–6 o'clock position. The most common lesion that results from an anterior dislocation is the classic Bankart lesion (*please refer to Case 1.9 for further discussion of Bankart*

variants). It is a consequence of the humeral head being compressed against the anterior labrum and associated ligaments.

A Bankart lesion is an avulsion of the anteroinferior glenolabral complex along with disruption of the associated scapular periosteum. Typically, the anteroinferior labrum appears triangular in shape on MRI with a sharp free margin; this is best evaluated on the axial imaging plane. Although the majority of large labral tears can be seen on conventional MRI, MR arthrography offers better sensitivity and specificity in detecting subtle labral tears and should be the modality of choice in these clinical situations.

Following an injury, the anteroinferior labrum can lose its normal triangular shape and appear slightly amorphous or abnormally small in size. There can be stripping of the medial scapular periosteum with abnormal linear high T2 signal or intra-articular contrast extending into the labral substance creating a labral tear. Alternatively, there can be focal detachment of the labrum at the glenolabral junction with fluid or contrast beneath the avulsed labrum and a bare glenoid rim. When only the labrum is torn, this injury is termed a soft tissue Bankart lesion. However, when there is an anteroinferior labral tear associated with a fracture of the adjacent glenoid rim, then this is termed a bony Bankart lesion. Although most surgeons prefer CT for evaluating the amount of glenoid bone loss, this can also be evaluated on MRI, and it is essential to state the amount of bone loss of the anteroinferior glenoid (*see supplementary images*). This is usually best calculated off the sagittal plane. A best-fit circle is drawn that approximately represents the normal glenoid articular surface. A line measuring the diameter of the circle is made. Then, a horizontal line is measured between the anterior margin of the circle and the anterior margin of the glenoid. This measurement represents the amount of glenoid bone loss. This glenoid bone loss distance is then divided by the diameter of the circle to give a percentage of glenoid bone loss. If the glenoid bone loss is >7 mm or > 20–30% of the total glenoid surface area, then this may result in recurrent dislocations, and surgery is likely needed.

When the humeral head impacts upon the anteroinferior aspect of the glenoid, this can result in an impaction fracture of the posterolateral aspect termed a Hill-Sachs deformity. On MRI, it can range from minimal chondral injury to a large osteochondral defect in the posterolateral humeral head. It is best identified on the axial images at or just above the level of the coracoid process. A Hill-Sachs deformity should not be confused with the normal humeral groove on the posterior aspect of the humerus that is usually seen >2 cm from the top of the humeral head (*see supplementary images*). The coracoid process is a reliable anatomic landmark to differentiate between the two, and if there is a defect on the humeral head while the coracoid process still visualized, then this will most likely represent a Hill-Sachs deformity.

Bankart lesions predispose patients to further dislocations, and because the labrum is displaced away from the glenoid rim, they are unlikely to heal on their own, and hence surgical repair of the labrum is required. If there is significant bone loss at the glenoid, bone grafting may be necessary.

Supplementary Images

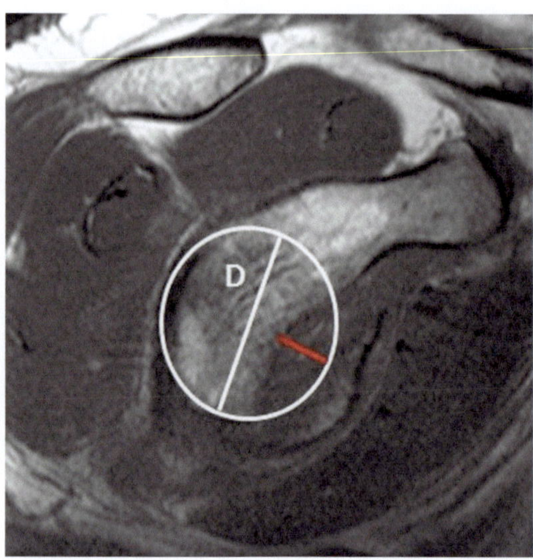

Sagittal T1

To calculate the percentage of glenoid bone loss, a best-fit circle is drawn. The width of the bone loss is divided by the diameter of the circle. There is 34% glenoid bone loss in this case

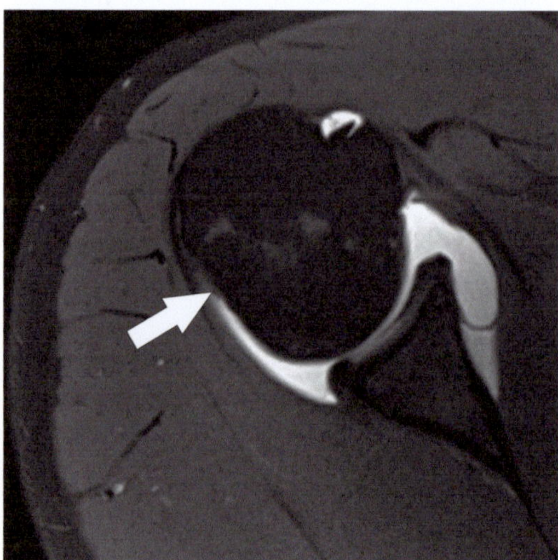

Axial T1 fat saturated (MR arthrogram)

There is normal flattening on the posterior aspect of the humeral head (arrow) that occurs below the coracoid process. This should not be mistaken for a Hill-Sachs impaction fracture

Report checklist

1. Is there a tear of the anteroinferior labrum and tear of the adjacent periosteum (Bankart lesion)?
2. What is the extent of the labral tear using the clockface position?
3. Is there a fracture of the adjacent glenoid rim (bony Bankart lesion)?
4. What are the size of glenoid bone loss and percentage of involvement of the glenoid articular surface?
5. Is there adjacent chondral injury?
6. Presence and size of osteochondral impaction at the humeral head (Hill-Sachs deformity). And if present, is there underlying bone marrow edema to suggest a more recent injury?

Suggested Reading

De Coninck T, Ngai SS, Tafur M, Chung CB. Imaging the glenoid labrum and labral tears. Radiographics. 2016;36(6):1628–47.

Robinson G, Ho Y, Finlay K, et-al. Normal anatomy and common labral lesions at MR arthrography of the shoulder. Clin Radiol. 2006;61(10):805–21.

Case 1.9a

Indication A 25-year-old female with history of anterior shoulder dislocation. Rule out labral tear.

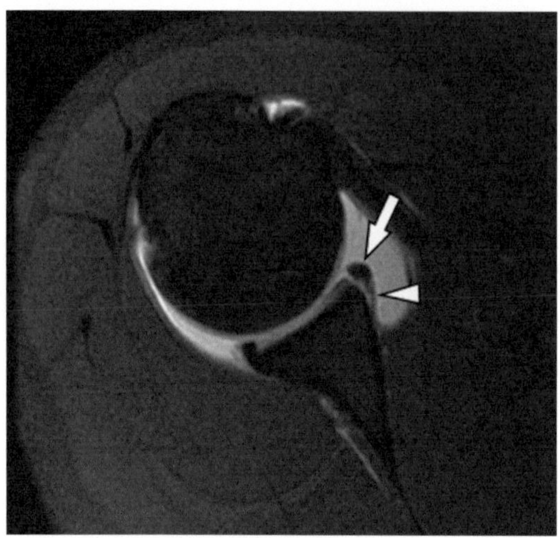

Axial T1 fat saturated (MR arthrogram)

Findings

There is an avulsed anteroinferior labral tear extending from the 3–5 o'clock position (arrow). Intra-articular contrast undermines a medially stripped but intact scapular periosteum (arrowhead). The labrum is not significantly displaced. The adjacent articular cartilage is intact. There is no glenoid fracture.

Case 1.9b

Indication A 27-year-old male with recurrent shoulder dislocation and instability. Assess labrum.

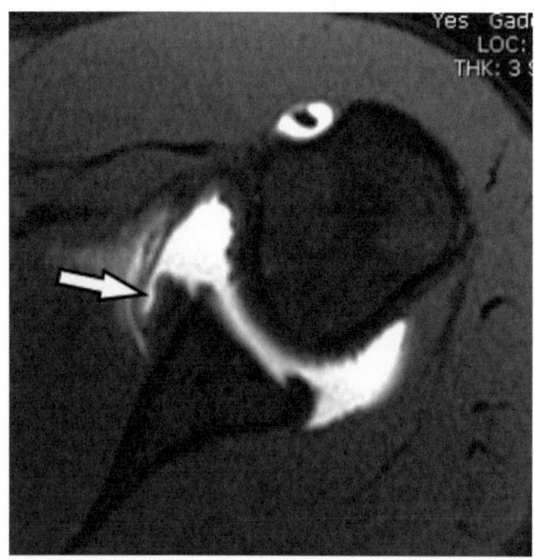

Axial T1 fat saturated (MR arthrogram)

Findings

There is tearing and detachment of the anteroinferior labrum from the 3–5 o'clock position with medial displacement of the labrum (arrow) along the anterior aspect of the glenoid. The scapular periosteum remains intact. The adjacent articular cartilage is intact. There is no glenoid fracture.

Impression/Recommendation
- **Case 1.9a:** Perthes lesion
- **Case 1.9b:** Anterior labroligamentous periosteal sleeve avulsion (ALPSA) lesion.

Discussion: Bankart Variants

Following anterior glenohumeral joint dislocation, there can be injury to the anterior stabilizers of the glenohumeral joint. The most common lesion is the classic Bankart lesion (*please refer to Case 1.8 for further discussion on Bankart lesions*). Other, less common but clinically significant lesions to the anterior soft tissues have been described which includes Perthes, anterior labroligamentous periosteal sleeve avulsion (ALPSA), and glenoid labral articular defect (GLAD) lesions. These lesions have been collectively called the Bankart variants. Although all these lesions share a common finding of a labral tear at the anteroinferior quadrant of the glenoid from the 3–6 o'clock positions. They differ from the classic Bankart lesion in that the adjacent scapular periosteum remains intact and not torn.

The Perthes lesion has also been referred to as the nondisplaced Bankart lesion. It represents a small focal tear of the anteroinferior labrum with stripping of the medial scapular periosteum but remains continuous. It is challenging to detect these lesions given that the labrum is usually normal in morphology and remains in its normal anatomic position. It may go undetected on conventional MRI sequences; however, a small cleft of high signal intensity at the antero-inferior labrum might be seen without significant displacement of the labrum. If faced with a clinical situation where the referring surgeon questions glenohumeral instability but MRI is normal, performing MR arthrography with the patient in abduction and external rotation (ABER) position on the MRI table can be helpful. This creates tension on the anterior band of the inferior glenohumeral ligament and highlights potential tears. This would be seen as linear contrast extension between the labrum and the underlying glenoid.

The anterior labroligamentous periosteal sleeve avulsion (ALPSA) lesion has been referred to as the medialized Bankart lesion. Similar to the Bankart and other variant lesions, it arises between the 3 and 6 o' clock position of the glenoid labrum. It is described as a detachment of the anteroinferior labrum from the glenoid, with an unruptured but stripped scapular periosteum. Instead of staying in its normal anatomic position as in a Perthes lesion, the labral fragment undergoes medial rotation adopting a position along the anterior surface of the osseous glenoid. The ALPSA lesion usually arises as a result of chronic injury due to multiple anterior dislocations of the humeral head. Due to its chronic nature, the ALPSA lesion may be missed on conventional MRI, especially in the absence of joint effusion. Therefore, MR arthrography is also useful in identifying these lesions. On MR arthrography, the classic finding is abnormal morphology of the anteroinferior labrum that is inferiorly and medially displaced along the anterior aspect of the osseous glenoid.

Glenolabral articular disruption (GLAD) lesion is a rare injury occurring secondary to the humeral head impacts on the glenoid which causes a tear of the anteroinferior labrum and an injury to the adjacent articular cartilage. Again, MR arthrography is the optimal study for evaluating these injuries, but they can also be seen on conventional MRI when larger and more apparent. This would be demonstrated as focal area of contrast or high T2 signal intensity at the anteroinferior labrum that extends into the adjacent articular cartilage as a small flap tear (*see supplementary images*).

It is essential to notify the referring surgeon on these Bankart variant lesions as they may not be easily seen during arthroscopy. The majority of these injuries are treated similarly to the classic Bankart lesion by repairing the torn labrum and debridement of the adjacent articular cartilage.

Supplementary Images

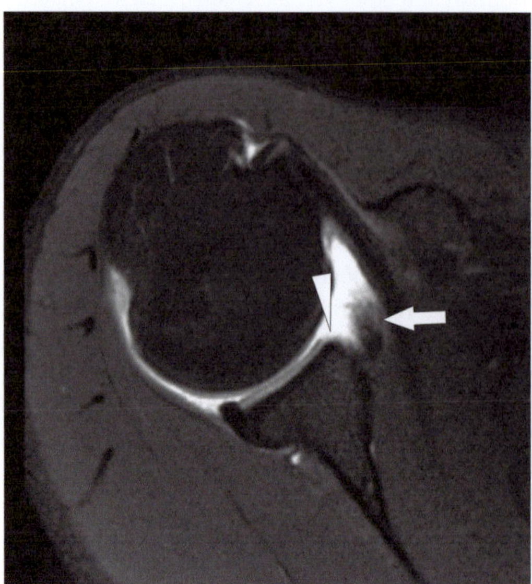

Axial T1 fat saturated (MR arthrogram)

There is a tear of the anteroinferior labrum (arrow) and injury to the adjacent articular cartilage (arrowhead) compatible with a GLAD lesion

Report checklist
1. Is there a tear of the anteroinferior labrum but the scapular periosteum remains intact (Perthes)?
2. Is the torn labrum nondisplaced or displaced medially along the anterior surface of the osseous glenoid (ALPSA)?
3. What is the location of the labral tear using the clockface position?
4. Is there adjacent chondral injury (to suggest a GLAD lesion)?
5. Presence and size of osteochondral impaction at the humeral head (Hillsachs deformity). And if present, is there underlying bone marrow edema to suggest a more recent injury?

Suggested Reading

De Coninck T, Ngai SS, Tafur M, Chung CB. Imaging the glenoid labrum and labral tears. Radiographics. 2016;36(6):1628–47.

Wischer TK, Bredella MA, Genant HK, Stoller DW, Bost FW, Tirman PF. Perthes lesion (a variant of the Bankart lesion): MR imaging and MR arthrographic findings with surgical correlation. AJR Am J Roentgenol. 2002;178:233–7.

Case 1.10

Indication A 38-year-old male with chronic shoulder pain and weakness. History of fall down on shoulder 4 years ago.

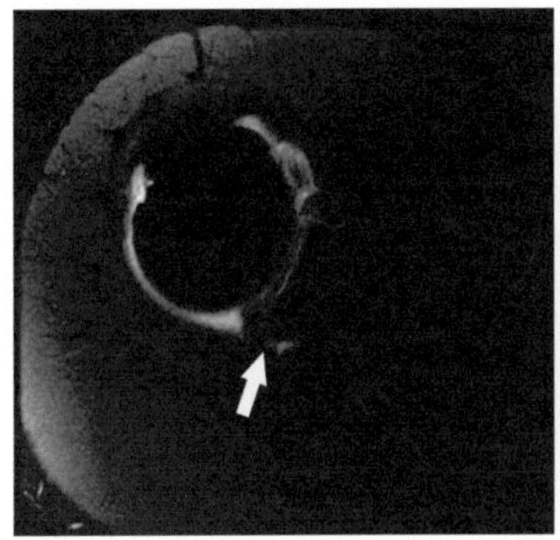
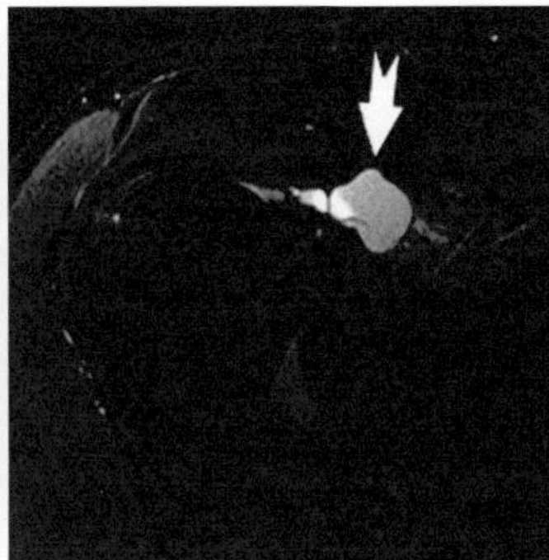
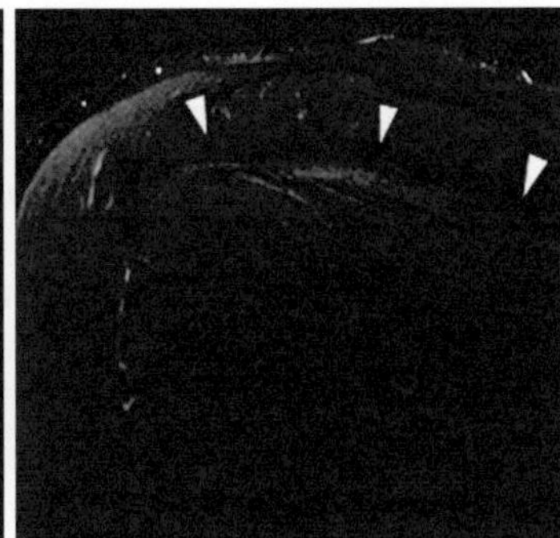

Axial T1 fat saturated(MR arthrogram)   Coronal T2 fat saturated   Coronal T2 fat saturated

Findings

There is intermediate signal and a full-thickness tear of the posterosuperior labrum (arrow). There is a large 3 × 2 cm multi-lobulated T2 hyperintense cystic structure in the suprascapular notch compatible with a paralabral cyst (notched arrow) arising from the labral tear. There is diffuse intramuscular edema of the infraspinatus muscle (arrowheads) without fatty atrophy, consistent with subacute muscle denervation most likely related to impingement of a branch of the suprascapular nerve.

Impression/Recommendation

Posterosuperior labral tear and paralabral cyst impinging on the suprascapular nerve causing denervation edema of the infraspinatus muscle.

Discussion: Paralabral Cysts

Paralabral cysts are ganglions that occur from the extension of synovial fluid through a glenoid labral tear into the adjacent soft tissues. They can occur in a variety of locations along the glenoid, most commonly at the posterosuperior aspect. Generally, they are small and asymptomatic in most individuals but should be appropriately identified and described, as larger cysts can impinge on the adjacent axillary or suprascapular nerves causing neuropathies.

On MRI, these cysts are well defined, unilocular or multilocular cystic lesions that are hypointense on T1-weighted images and hyperintense on T2-weighted images. Frequently, a small tail-like extension is seen extending to the adjacent labrum which points to the site of a labral tear. Even if no labral tear is seen, suspicion for a labral tear should be raised as the likelihood of an underlying tear is exceptionally high. On MR arthrography, these cysts may or may not fill with intra-articular contrast and are easily missed on T1-weighted fat-suppressed images, and therefore a T2-weighted sequence should always be performed.

When cysts are large enough (usually above 3 cm), they can extend into the suprascapular notch and/or spinoglenoid notch which can compress on the suprascapular nerve. This can cause denervation changes in the muscle which in the subacute phase demonstrate high signal intensity on the T2-weighted images due to muscle edema. As the process continues into the chronic phase, there can be fatty infiltration and atrophy of the affected muscle. The classic teaching describes that when the suprascapular nerve is impinged in the suprascapular notch, this will cause denervation of both the supraspinatus and infraspinatus muscles. However, if the nerve is impinged in the spinoglenoid notch, only the infraspinatus muscle is affected since the nerve branch innervating the supraspinatus has already exited. This, however, is not a strict rule and variations do occur.

It is essential to distinguish a paralabral cyst from other cystic soft tissue masses such as myxomas or nerve sheath tumors which would demonstrate internal enhancement on the post-contrast images, while paralabral cysts will only show thin peripheral enhancement. These tumors also should not be subjacent to the labral tear and are often in atypical locations. If there is doubt, it is good practice to have the patient return for additional pre- and post-contrast images to exclude an underlying solid tumor.

Most asymptomatic paralabral cysts are left alone without any intervention; however, when symptomatic, percutaneous aspiration under ultrasound guidance or arthroscopic decompression can be performed.

Report checklist

1. What are the size and location of the paralabral cyst?
2. Can an underlying labral tear be identified, and what is its location along the glenoid? If no labral tear can be seen, this still should still be suspected and mentioned in the report.
3. Is there edema or fatty atrophy of the rotator cuff muscles to suggest nerve impingement?
4. Is the presumed "cyst" in an unusual location for a paralabral cyst, and could it represent a T2 bright neoplasm such as a myxoma or nerve sheath tumor? Consider having the patient return for contrast enhanced images.

Suggested Reading

De Coninck T, Ngai SS, Tafur M, Chung CB. Imaging the glenoid labrum and labral tears. Radiographics. 2016;36(6):1628–47.

Tung GA, Entzian D, Stern JB, et al. MR imaging and MR arthrography of paraglenoid labral cysts. AJR Am J Roentgenol. 2000; 174(6):1707–15.

Case 1.11

Indication A 44-year-old male with recent fall while skiing. Severe shoulder pain and ecchymosis. Radiographs are normal. Assess for rotator cuff tear or occult fracture.

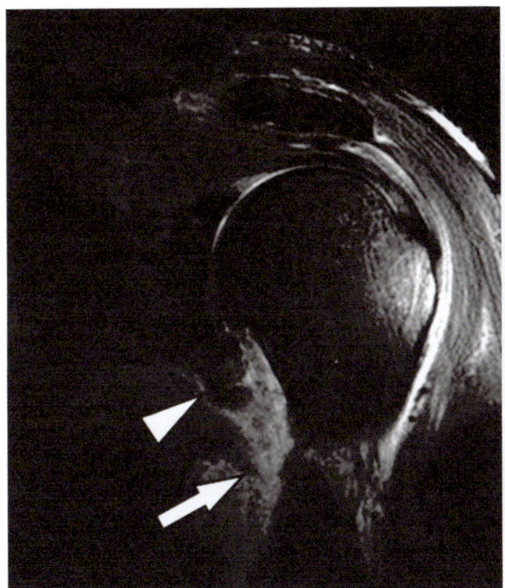

Coronal T2 fat saturated

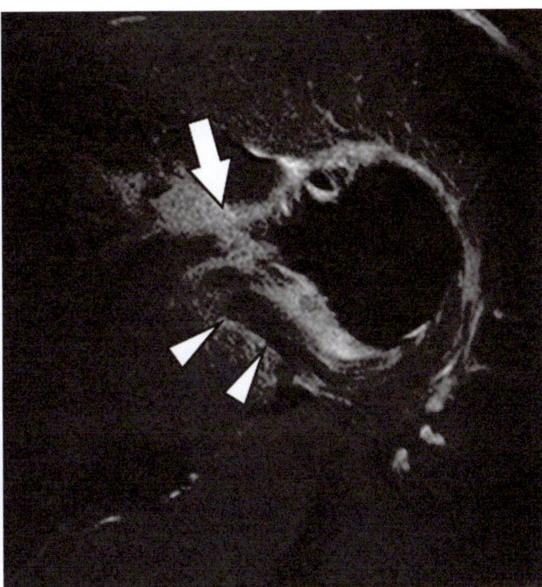

Axial T2 fat saturated

Findings

There is avulsion of the inferior glenohumeral ligament from its humeral insertion with a thickened and medially retracted ligament stump (arrowheads). The tear extends through the anterior, mid, and posterior portions of the inferior glenohumeral ligament. This is associated with extracapsular fluid within the soft tissues of the quadrilateral space related to leakage of joint fluid (arrows). There is no associated osseous avulsion fracture.

Impression/Recommendation

Acute humeral avulsion of glenohumeral ligament (HAGL).

Discussion: Humeral Avulsion of Glenohumeral Ligament (HAGL)

The capsuloligamentous complex at the glenohumeral joint includes the inferior glenohumeral ligament (IGHL), middle glenohumeral ligament, coracohumeral ligament, and the superior glenohumeral ligament. The IGHL is comprised of the anterior band, posterior band, and the axillary pouch of the capsule in between the two bands. The anterior and posterior bands arise from the anteroinferior and posterior inferior aspect of the glenoid respectively and attach at the surgical neck of the humerus. The IGHL in association with the anteroinferior labrum are essential structures for anterior shoulder stability, and a missed IGHL tear causes incompetence of the IGHL complex, which results in the instability of the glenohumeral joint.

Humeral avulsion of the IGHL (termed a HAGL lesion) usually occurs after a traumatic injury, most commonly from a shoulder dislocation. Avulsion of this ligamentous complex may occur in three locations: mid-substance, glenoid attachment, or more commonly from the humeral insertion. On MRI, an acute injury to the IGHL will be seen as a thickened and irregular ligament with increased signal intensity. Alternatively, if there is a frank tear, then there will be a focal discontinuity of the ligament with fluid tracking into the soft tissues along the humeral neck below the joint capsule. Normally, fluid should marginate a smooth inferior border of the axillary pouch (*see supplementary images*). MR arthrography can better detect subtle injuries since there will be extravasation of intra-articular contrast through the capsular defect into the surrounding soft tissues. A J-shaped configuration of the injured IGHL has been described related to inferior laxity of the normal U-shaped appearing capsule seen on the coronal images. In a small subset of patients, there can be associated small avulsion fracture from the humerus (referred to as bony HAGL). Chronic HAGL lesions commonly have torn edges on the humeral side which scar down to the capsule and therefore are difficult to visualize on MR imaging. Tears of the IGHL may have associated subscapularis tendon tears or labral injury, and these should be assessed for as well.

It is important to inform the surgeon of suspected IGHL tear since these injuries are easily overlooked on standard arthroscopic portals. Tears are usually surgically repaired since it has been found that it will reduce the chance of recurrent shoulder dislocations.

Report checklist

1. Is the IGHL sprained or completely torn?
2. Where is the tear (glenoid attachment, mid-substance, or humeral attachment)?
3. Is the tear localized to the anterior band, or does it extend posteriorly to involve the axillary pouch and posterior band?
4. Presence or absence of extracapsular fluid
5. On MR arthrography, is there a focal capsular defect with extravasation of intra-articular contrast?
6. Is there a bony avulsion fracture?
7. Is there an associated labral or subscapularis tendon tear?

Suggested Reading

Liavaag S, Stiris MG, Svenningsen S, et al. Capsular lesions with glenohumeral ligament injuries in patients with primary shoulder dislocation: magnetic resonance imaging and magnetic resonance arthrography evaluation. Scand J Med Sci Sports. 2011;21(6):e291–7.

Roy EA, Cheyne I, Andrews GT, Forster BB. Beyond the cuff: MR imaging of labroligamentous injuries in the athletic shoulder. Radiology. 2016;278(2):316–32.

Supplementary Images

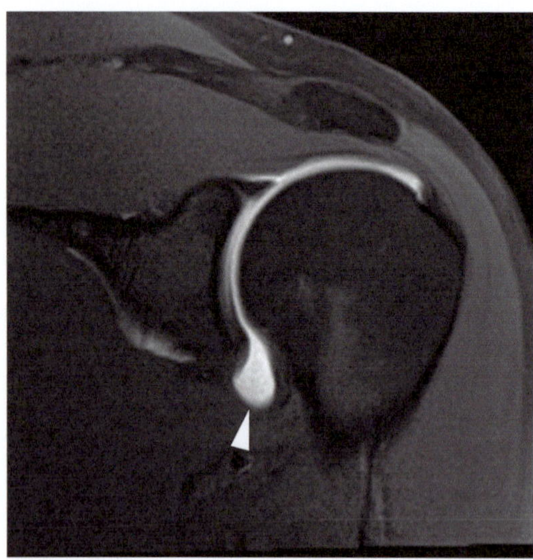

Coronal T1 fat saturated (MR arthrogram)

Normal appearing smooth, U-shaped, inferior margin of the IGHL (arrowhead)

Case 1.12a

Indication A 23-year-old male with pain and ecchymosis at the right chest wall after bench pressing injury. Assess pectoralis muscle.

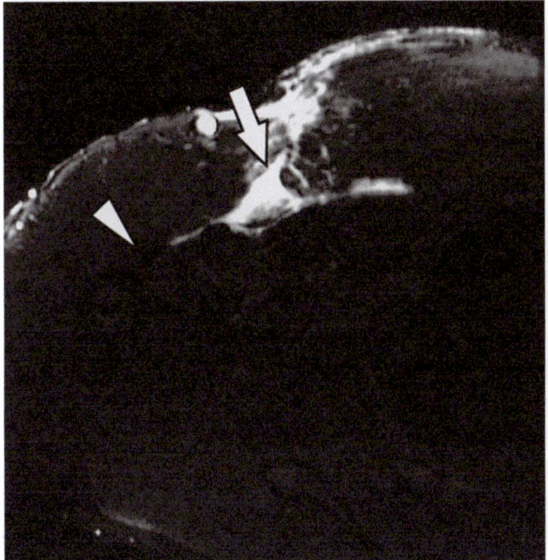

Axial T2 fat saturated

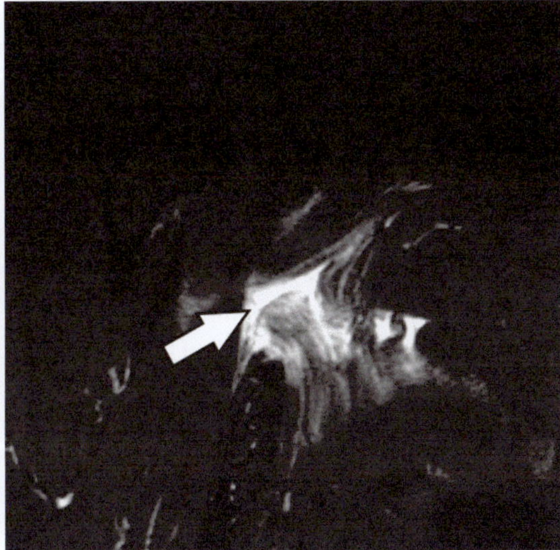

Coronal oblique T2 fat saturated

Findings
There is complete rupture (tear) at the myotendinous junction of the pectoralis major muscle (arrow) with retraction of the muscle with intramuscular/soft tissue edema and hemorrhage at the tendon gap. There is a 2 cm tendon stump on the humerus (arrowhead). There is no muscle fatty atrophy.

Case 1.12b

Indication A 24-year-old male with chest wall pain and pop sensation while bench pressing. Rule out pectoralis muscle tear.

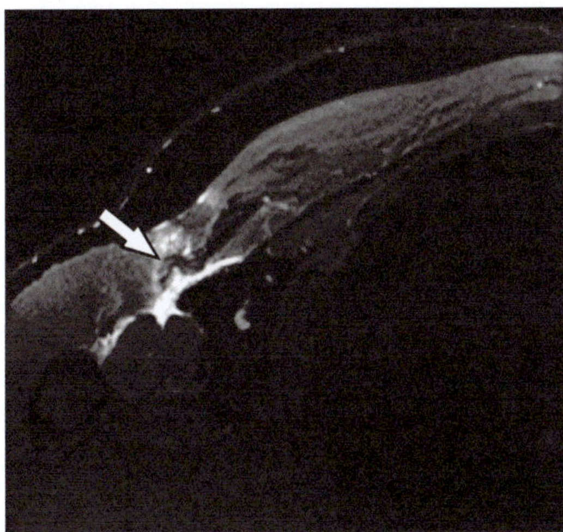

Axial T2 fat saturated

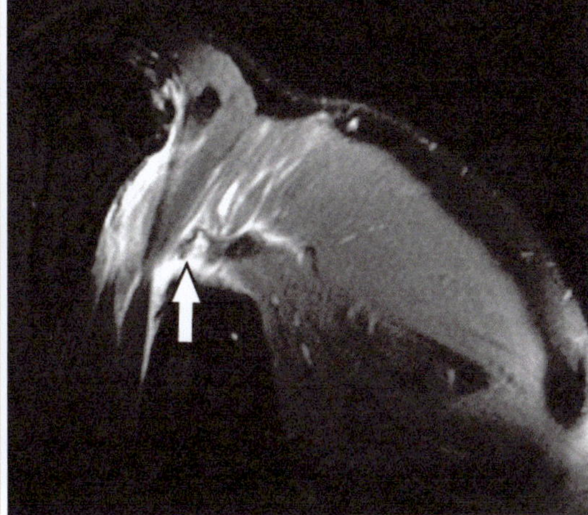

Coronal oblique T2 fat saturated

Findings

There is a complete tear of the pectoralis major at its tendinous insertion on the humerus with retraction of the torn tendon fibers (arrows) by 4 cm. No tendon stump on the humeral shaft is seen. This is associated with moderate intramuscular edema and surrounding soft tissue edema. No fatty atrophy is seen.

Impression/Recommendation

- **Case 1.12a:** Complete tear at the myotendinous junction of the pectoralis major muscle with 2 cm intact tendon stump.
- **Case 1.12b:** Complete rupture of the pectoralis major tendon from the humeral attachment.

Discussion: Tear of the Pectoralis Major Muscle

A proper understanding of the anatomy of the pectoralis major muscle is crucial to appropriately evaluate and describe these injuries. The pectoralis major is a thick, fan-shaped muscle at the anterior chest wall composed of three heads originating from clavicular, sternal, and abdominal origins. The largest of these heads is the sternal head which arises from the sternum and costal cartilages of the first six ribs. The smaller clavicular head originates from the anterior aspect of the medial clavicle. Few fibers form the inferior abdominal head which arises from the external oblique muscle. They all converge laterally to form a common tendon which inserts onto the humerus just lateral to the bicipital groove. This common tendon is about 1.5 cm in medial to lateral length and about 5 cm in craniocaudal dimension.

When planning MRI on patients suspected of pectoralis major muscle injuries, it is essential to obtain a large field of view axial sequence to assess the entire muscle; however, additional small field of view axial T1- and T2-weighted images centered at the tendon insertion site for more detailed evaluation of the tendon and myotendinous junction should be performed. Fluid-sensitive sequences are used to detect increased fluid signal intensity edema and hemorrhage, therefore helping localize the tear site. A coronal oblique view parallel to the muscle can be obtained for determining which part of the muscle is involved. Imaging the patient in the prone position may be preferred to help minimize respiratory motion.

Pectoralis major muscle tears are uncommon injuries typically occurring in weightlifters especially while bench pressing. Patients often mention hearing a "pop" and present with burning pain in the shoulder region and weakness with arm adduction. Pectoralis major tears are classified based on the extent of the injury (sprain, partial-thickness tear, or complete tears) and location of the tear (muscle belly, myotendinous junction, or tendon attachment). Majority of the tears are partial-thickness tears that occur at the myotendinous junction which would show edema and hemorrhage at that region. There may be slight retraction of the muscle belly; however, a normal-appearing tendon should still be seen at the humeral insertion. Complete tears usually occur at the tendon insertion which shows an edematous and retracted tendon as well as soft tissue edema anterior to the humerus. If there is any hematoma associated with the tear, this should be mentioned with its location and size. A common injury pattern is a complete tear of the sternal head with retraction of the myotendinous junction, while the clavicular head remains intact and unaffected. This is sometimes misinterpreted as a partial-thickness tear; however, it should be correctly diagnosed as full-thickness tear isolated to the sternal head since this would be an indication for surgical repair. Chronic tears may be seen on MRI as fibrosis and scarring with fatty atrophy of the muscle belly.

Most partial tears are treated conservatively; however complete tears at the tendon insertion are an indication for surgery.

Report checklist

1. Where is the location of the pectoralis major tear (muscle, myotendinous junction, tendon)?
2. Degree of injury (strain, partial-thickness tear, complete tear)
3. Measurement of tendon or muscle retraction
4. Is there a tendon stump and how long is it?
5. Is there an associated hematoma?
6. Is there fatty atrophy of the pectoralis major muscle?

Suggested Reading

Lee J, Brookenthal KR, Ramsey ML, Kneeland JB, Herzog R. MR imaging assessment of the pectoralis major myotendinous unit: an MR imaging-anatomic correlative study with surgical correlation. AJR Am J Roentgenol. 2000;174(5):1371–5.

Lee YK, Skalski MR, White EA, Tomasian A, Phan DD, Patel DB, Matcuk GR Jr., Schein AJ. US and MR imaging of pectoralis major injuries. Radiographics. 2017;37:176–89.

Case 2.1

Indication A 39-year-old male with chronic pain and tenderness at the lateral elbow. Assess for tendon tear.

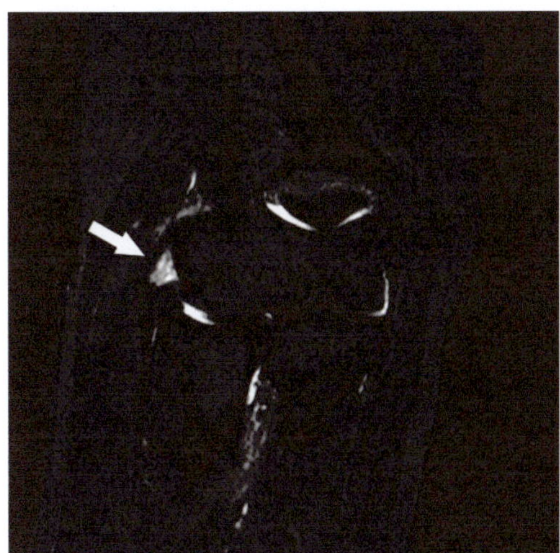

Coronal T2 fat saturated

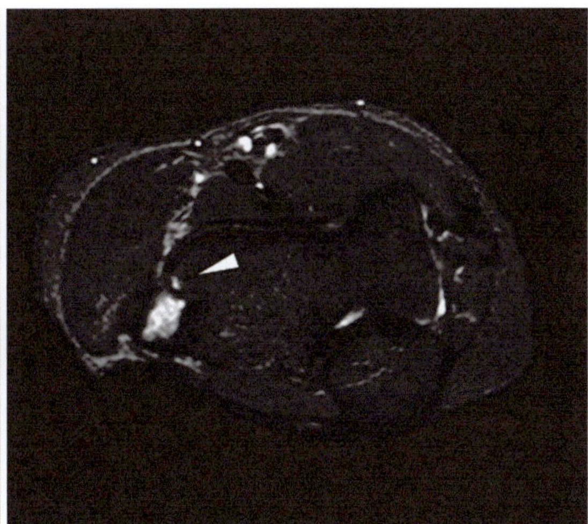

Axial T2 fat saturated

Findings

There is moderate tendinosis at the common extensor tendon origin at the lateral humeral epicondyle with a near full-thickness tear involving approximately 80% of the tendon thickness (arrow), best seen on the coronal images. A few lateral tendon fibers remain. There is a small amount of reactive marrow edema (arrowhead) in the lateral epicondyle. The lateral collateral ligament is intact.

© Springer Nature Switzerland AG 2020
T. M. Hegazi, J. S. Wu, *Musculoskeletal MRI*, https://doi.org/10.1007/978-3-030-26777-3_2

Impression/Recommendation

Near full-thickness tear of the common extensor tendon origin (lateral epicondylitis).

Discussion: Lateral Epicondylitis

At the lateral elbow, the extensor muscles of the forearm originate from the lateral humeral epicondyle via a common extensor tendon which is formed by the origins of the extensor carpi radialis brevis (ECRB), extensor digitorum communis, and the extensor carpi ulnaris. Lateral epicondylitis, also known as tennis elbow, is the most common overuse syndrome in the elbow and is related to a degenerative process of the common extensor tendon origin from repetitive varus stress resulting in tendinosis which can progress to tendon tear. The ECRB tendon is the most common tendon involved. Partial tearing may progress to a full-thickness tendon tear.

The diagnosis of lateral epicondylitis is usually evident clinically in patients presenting with lateral elbow pain and point tenderness at the lateral epicondyle. Usually, patients with lateral epicondylitis respond to conservative treatment. MRI is reserved for patients who do not respond to rest and pain medications, and can help establish the extent of tendon injury and evaluate for other causes of lateral elbow pain.

On MRI, the common extensor tendon is typically dark on all pulse sequences. Evaluation of the tendon is best done on coronal and axial T2-weighted fat-suppressed images. MRI findings of lateral epicondylitis are variable depending on the degree of tendon injury. Tendinosis is seen as abnormal diffuse thickening at the tendon origin with increased signal intensity on both the T1- and T2-weighted images; however, it does not reach fluid signal intensity. In cases of a partial- or full-thickness tear of the tendon, a fluid-filled gap with or without loss of fiber continuity will be seen with surrounding soft tissue edema. Other associated findings include reactive bone marrow edema at the lateral epicondyle, and in patients with chronic injury, there could be a concomitant injury to the lateral collateral ligament complex.

As mentioned earlier, most cases of tendinosis and partial tears respond to conservative treatment which can also include ultrasound-guided steroid injections. Surgery is usually reserved for patients who have failed conservative measures or if there is a full-thickness tear.

Report checklist

1. What is the degree of tendinosis (mild, moderate, severe)?
2. Is there a partial-thickness or full-thickness tear? And what is the size of the tendon defect?
3. Is there associated reactive bone marrow edema at the lateral epicondyle?
4. What is the integrity of the lateral collateral ligament complex?
5. Are there any cartilage defects or joint effusion?

Suggested Reading

Walton MJ, Mackie K, Fallon M, et al. The reliability and validity of magnetic resonance imaging in the assessment of chronic lateral epicondylitis. J Hand Surg Am. 2011;36:475–9.

Walz DM, Newman JS, Konin GP et-al. Epicondylitis: pathogenesis, imaging, and treatment. Radiographics. 2010;30(1):167–84.

Case 2.2

Indication A 44-year-old male with chronic medial elbow pain, started after a fall. Not responding to conservative treatment. Assess medial tendons.

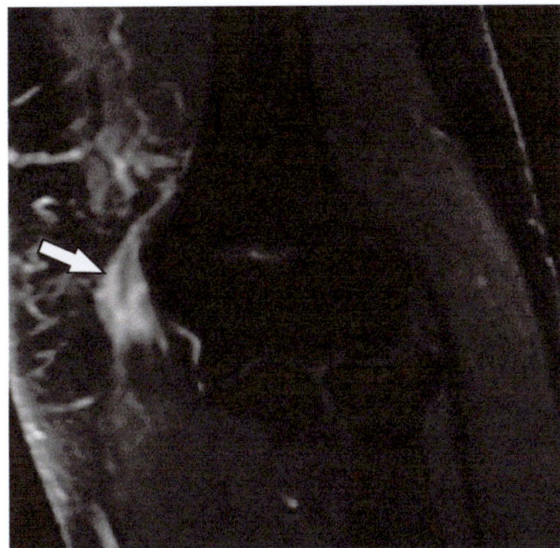

Coronal T2 fat saturated

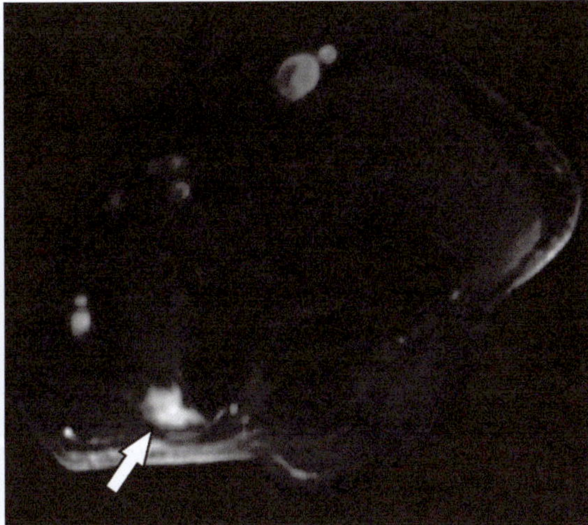

Axial T2 fat saturated

Findings

There is abnormal thickening and edema at the common flexor tendon origin with surrounding soft tissue edema compatible with severe tendinosis (arrows). There is no abnormal fluid signal intensity within the tendon substance to suggest a tear. The ulnar collateral ligament is normal. The ulnar nerve is normal in morphology and signal intensity. There is no joint effusion.

Impression/Recommendation

Severe tendinosis at the common flexor tendon origin (medial epicondylitis).

Discussion: Medial Epicondylitis

Medial epicondylitis, also known as golfer's elbow, is characterized by chronic medial elbow pain and point tenderness over the common flexor tendon origin that originates from the medial epicondyle. Medial epicondylitis results from common flexor tendinosis due to repetitive valgus stress which eventually progresses to partial-thickness and later full-thickness tears. It is commonly seen in activities that require frequent wrist flexion and forearm pronation generally occurring in the fourth to fifth decades of life. It is less common than lateral epicondylitis.

The diagnosis of medial epicondylitis is usually evident clinically and is treated conservatively. MRI is usually reserved for patients who do not respond to conservative treatment, which can help establish the extent of tendon injury and evaluate for other causes of medial elbow pain as ulnar collateral ligament injury or ulnar neuritis.

On MRI, the common flexor tendons are dark on all pulse sequences. Evaluation of the tendon is best done on coronal and axial T2-weighted fat-suppressed images. MRI findings of medial epicondylitis are variable depending on the degree of tendon injury. Tendinosis is seen as abnormal diffuse thickening at the tendon origin with increased signal intensity on both the T1- and T2-weighted images; however, it should not reach fluid signal intensity. This is usually associated with surrounding peritendinous soft tissue edema. The flexor carpi radialis and pronator teres tendons are usually the most affected components. In cases of a partial-thickness tear, there is a fluid-filled gap within the tendon substance or thinning and attenuation of the tendon. These are most commonly partial-thickness interstitial tears which appear as linear areas of high signal fluid within the tendon. In full-thickness tears, there is complete disruption of the tendon with a fluid-filled gap and retraction of the torn tendon stump. Other associated findings include reactive bone marrow edema at the medial epicondyle, and in patients with more severe injury, there could be a concomitant injury to the ulnar collateral ligament.

Attention should also be made to the ulnar nerve which can become affected in patients with medial elbow injuries. The ulnar nerve passes in the cubital tunnel which is located directly posterior to the medial epicondyle. Ulnar neuritis is manifested as thickening of the nerve with increased signal intensity on the T2-weighted images (*please refer to Case 2.9 for further discussion on ulnar neuritis*). There can also be inflammation and edema within the surrounding perineural fat.

Lastly, in young skeletally immature patients, medial epicondylitis should not be mistaken for medial epicondylar apophysitis which is known as "little leaguer's elbow." In these patients, the medial epicondylar apophysis is weaker than the medial elbow stabilizers and is more prone to injury with repetitive valgus stress. This is seen as high signal intensity within the physis with widening and slight irregularity as well as associated surrounding reactive bone marrow edema. In more advanced stages, there may be sclerosis and fragmentation of the apophysis.

Most cases of medial epicondylitis respond to conservative treatment which includes NSAIDs, ice, and physical therapy and, if needed, can also include ultrasound-guided steroid injections. Surgery is usually reserved for patients who have failed conservative measures.

Report checklist

1. What is the degree of tendinosis (mild, moderate, severe)?
2. Is there a partial-thickness or full-thickness tear? And what is the size of the tendon defect?
3. Is there associated reactive bone marrow edema at the medial epicondyle?
4. What is the integrity of the ulnar (medial) collateral ligament complex?
5. Are there signs of ulnar neuritis?
6. Are there any cartilage defects or a joint effusion?

Suggested Reading

Thornton R, Riley GM, Steinbach LS. Magnetic resonance imaging of sports injuries of the elbow. Top Magn Reson Imaging. 2003; 14:69–86.

Walz DM, Newman JS, Konin GP et-al. Epicondylitis: pathogenesis, imaging, and treatment. Radiographics. 2010;30(1):167–84.

Case 2.3

Indication A 28-year-old weight lifter presenting with sudden "popping sensation" in the elbow while exercising. Assess distal biceps tendon.

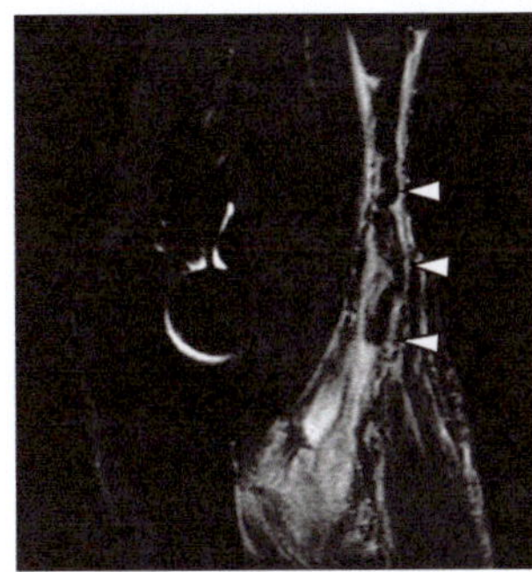 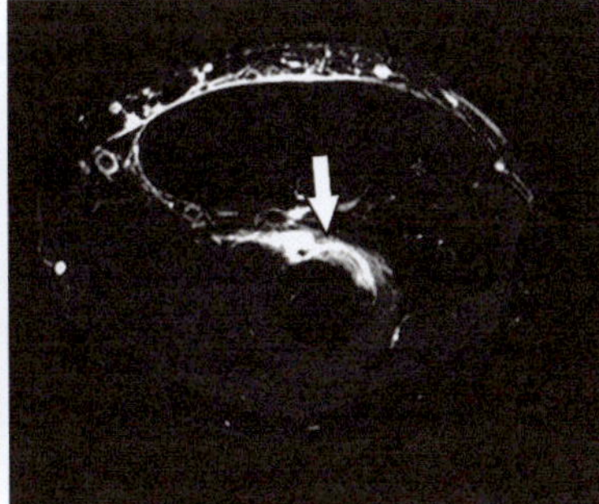 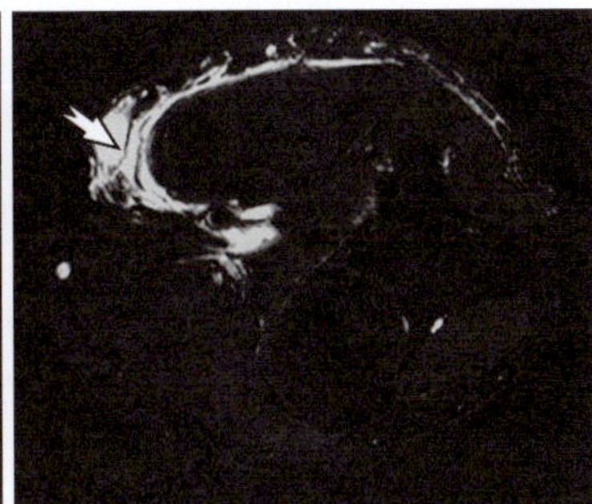

Sagittal T2 fat saturated   Axial T2 fat saturated   Axial T2 fat saturated

Findings

There is a complete rupture of the distal biceps tendon from its distal insertion on the radial tuberosity. The torn tendon stump is retracted 5 cm (arrowheads) with surrounding soft tissue edema and hemorrhage. The distal tendon stump is not frayed. Fluid is seen at the expected distal radial attachment of the biceps tendon (arrow). There is soft tissue edema superficial to the flexor pronator muscle group with irregularity of the lacertus fibrosus (notched arrow) suggesting that it is torn. There is no fatty atrophy of the muscle. The brachialis muscle is normal.

Impression/Recommendation

Complete rupture of the distal biceps tendon.

Discussion: Distal Biceps Tendon Rupture

The two heads (short and long heads) of the biceps muscle give rise to the common distal biceps tendon approximately 6–7 cm above the elbow joint, coursing obliquely in the cubital fossa until its attachment on the radial tuberosity. A small bicipitoradial bursa separates the distal biceps tendon from the adjacent radial tuberosity which is usually collapsed and not visualized on MRI of normal individuals. The bicipital aponeurosis (also termed the lacertus fibrosus) arises from the distal biceps tendon and blends with the fascia covering the common flexor muscle group.

Rupture of the distal biceps tendon is becoming an increasingly common injury; however, it is still much less common than injuries to the proximal biceps tendon. Injuries to the distal biceps tendon include tendinosis and partial-thickness and complete tendon ruptures (the most common type of injury). The majority of tendon tears occur at an area 1–2 cm above the radial tuberosity, which is a relatively hypovascular zone. This region is prone to degeneration secondary to hypoxic tendinopathy, which can lead to weakening and susceptibility to complete rupture. Patients usually experience a "pop" at the elbow when the tendon ruptures, followed by severe pain. On examination, visible swelling and ecchymosis at the elbow can be seen.

Complete rupture of the biceps tendon is often evident clinically; however, if the lacertus fibrosus remains intact following a complete rupture, then it may prevent retraction of the torn tendon stump and may make differentiation of a complete rupture from a partial tear difficult. The role of MRI hence is to confirm the clinical diagnosis and to help differentiate a complete from a partial tear and determine the location of the tear as well as the extent of tendon retraction for pre-surgical planning. If a patient is referred for MRI evaluation with a clinical suspicion of distal biceps pathology, it is important to obtain images in the axial plane that covers about 5 cm distal to the elbow joint line to accurately assess its insertion on the radial tuberosity. It is also important to comment on whether there is a bony avulsion of the distal tendon and the integrity of the tendon stump. Frayed tendon stumps may require more extensive debridement at surgery. Evaluation of the biceps tendon is best performed on both sagittal and axial T2-weighted images with fat suppression. The axial plane is best used for evaluating the tendon insertion, while the sagittal plane is used to assess the extent of tendon retraction. The oblique course of the tendon may make it difficult to obtain longitudinal images parallel to the tendon. Giuffrè and colleagues devised the FABS position, a novel way of positioning the patient, which helps overcome this difficulty. FABS is an acronym for flexed elbow, abducted shoulder, supinated forearm, with the thumb pointing superiorly. This way of positioning minimizes the partial volume-average effects due to the oblique course of the tendon and allows a longitudinal view of the tendon, often in one section. Ideally, both conventional and FABS views should be obtained.

If the lacertus fibrosus is intact, there is little or no significant tendon retraction (*see supplementary images*), which can be a pitfall for undercalling the injury. The normal lacertus fibrosus is best seen on the axial plane as a thin linear hypointense structure extending over the flexor pronator muscle group and extending obliquely to the distal biceps tendon. If soft tissue edema is seen superficial to the flexor pronator muscles with irregularity of the lacertus fibrosus, then this suggests it is torn. It is also common to see bicipitoradial bursitis which appears lobulated T2 hyperintense fluid collection within the bursa adjacent to the distal biceps tendon attachment site.

Biceps tendinosis is related to chronic intrasubstance degeneration and appears as thickening and intermediate signal intensity within the tendon substance but without a focal tear. In partial-thickness tears, there is attenuation of the tendon with abnormal contour and high fluid-like signal but has not completely torn. The FABS position helps in differentiating a partial from a complete tear.

Early surgical repair is the treatment of choice for biceps tendon rupture. Partial tears are often treated conservatively for symptomatic relief.

Supplementary Images

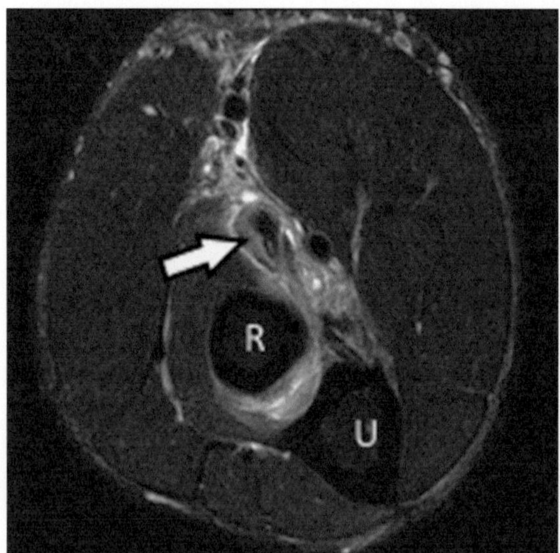

Axial T2 fat saturated

There is complete tear of the distal biceps tendon (arrow) from its insertion on the radial tuberosity with minimal retraction (<1 cm). Axial image more proximally shows normal appear-

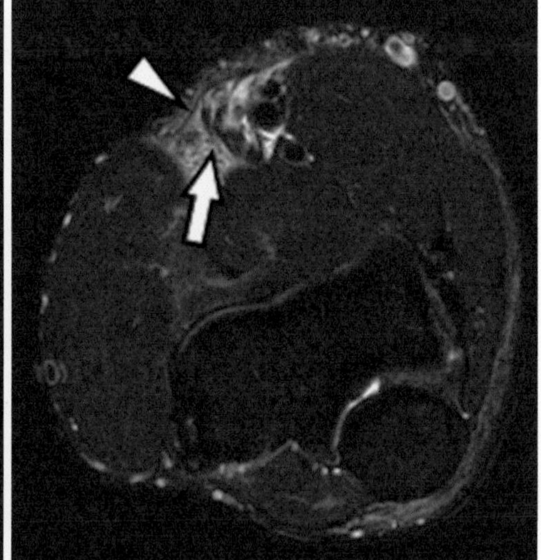

Axial T2 fat saturated

ance of the lacertus fibrosus (arrowhead) next to an irregular (interstitial tearing), but not fully retracted, biceps tendon. (R, radius; U, ulna)

Report checklist

1. Is there tendinosis or partial-thickness or complete tear of the distal biceps tendon?
2. Where is the tear located (at the radial tuberosity insertion, tendon substance, or the myotendinous junction)?
3. What is the amount of retraction of the torn tendon stump? Is the stump intact or frayed?
4. Is there a bony avulsion?
5. What is the integrity of the lacertus fibrosus, and is it preventing full tendon retraction?
6. Is there fatty atrophy of the biceps muscle?
7. Is there an associated injury to the brachialis muscle?

Suggested Reading

Chew ML, Giuffrè BM. Disorders of the distal biceps brachii tendon. Radiographics. 2005;25:1227–37.

Williams BD, Schweitzer ME, Weishaupt D, et al. Partial tears of the distal biceps tendon: MR appearance and associated clinical findings. Skeletal Radiol 2001;30:560–564.

Case 2.4

Indication A 49-year-old male with lateral elbow pain after a fall 6 months ago. Not responding to conservative treatment. Assess lateral collateral ligament injury or tendon tear.

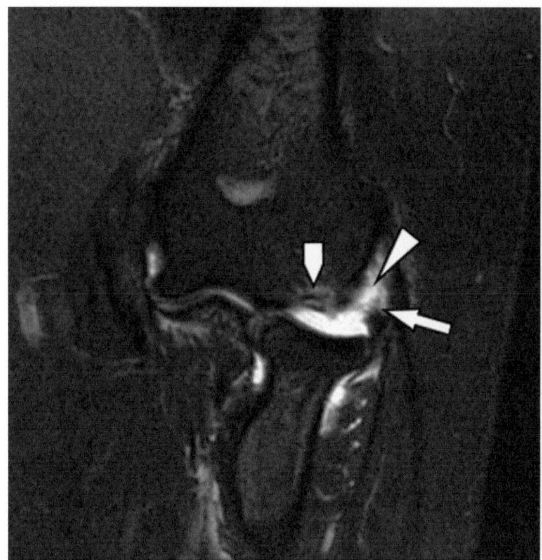

Coronal T2 fat saturated

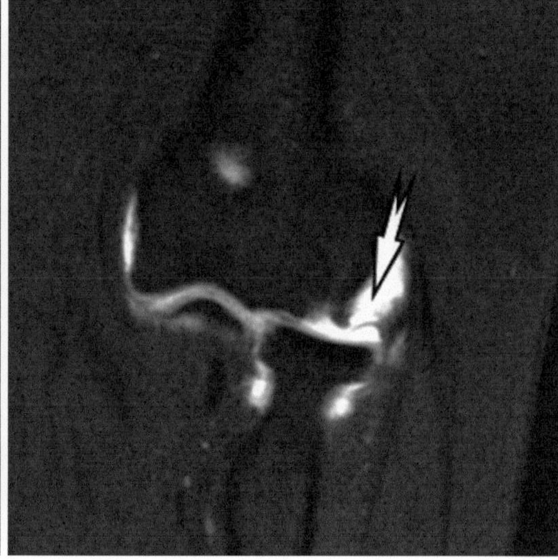

Coronal T1 fat saturated (MR arthrogram)

Findings

On the coronal T2 images, there is abnormal fluid signal (arrowhead) at the proximal attachment of the radial collateral ligament (arrow). On the T1 fat saturated post-arthrogram images, there is contrast medium extending into the ligamentous defect (notched arrow) compatible with full-thickness (complete) tear of the radial collateral ligament. There is also a small 5 mm osteochondral defect at the capitellum with underlying bone marrow edema (broad arrow). No intra-articular contrast extends beneath the osteochondral fragment, indicating a stable lesion. The common extensor and flexor tendons and the medial collateral ligament are intact.

Impression/Recommendation

1. Full-thickness (complete) tear of the radial collateral ligament
2. Stable 5 mm osteochondral lesion in the capitellum.

Discussion: Lateral Collateral Ligament Tear

The lateral collateral ligament complex has three primary components: the radial collateral ligament proper (RCL), the lateral ulnar collateral ligament (LUCL), and the annular ligament. The annular ligament encircles the head of the radius and keeps it in contact with the radial notch of the ulna, stabilizing the proximal radioulnar joint. The annular ligament is best visualized on the axial images. The RCL and LUCL have a common origin at the lateral epicondyle which lies deep to the common extensor tendon origin (*see supplementary images*). The anterior fibers represent the RCL which descends distally and merges with the annular ligament, while the posterior fibers represent the LUCL which extends from the lateral epicondyle and courses in an oblique fashion and passes posterolateral to the radial head forming a sling to insert medially and distally on the proximal ulna at the supinator crest. The LUCL is the primary stabilizer for preventing posterior subluxation or dislocation of the radial head. The RCL and LUCL are optimally assessed on the coronal plane.

Injuries to the LCL are often due to traumatic events such as a fall on an outstretched hand or dislocation of the elbow. Injuries to the RCL and LUCL are most commonly full thickness and occur at the proximal attachment. These are visualized as focal discontinuity of the normal hypointense ligament with fluid signal intensity gap as well as laxity of the ligament with periligamentous edema. It is important to know that the RCL and LUCL are not seen in their entirety on one slice, and scrolling through sequential MR images is necessary for complete assessment.

If the LCL complex fails to heal following injury (especially the LUCL), chronic instability may occur which is known as posterolateral rotatory instability (PLRI). Patients with PLRI complain of lateral-sided pain and tenderness, "clicking" with movement, and lateral instability. PLRI is usually diagnosed clinically; however, MRI may be used to guide the diagnosis and is commonly used to assist in surgical planning. On MRI, there is usually an injury to the proximal attachment of the LUCL on the coronal images. There may be posterior subluxation of the radius relative to the capitellum optimally assessed on the sagittal images.

In most cases, a partial-thickness tear is treated conservatively with rest, NSAIDs, and physical therapy, whereas a complete tear or patients with PRLI may require surgical reconstruction of the lateral collateral ligaments.

Supplementary Images

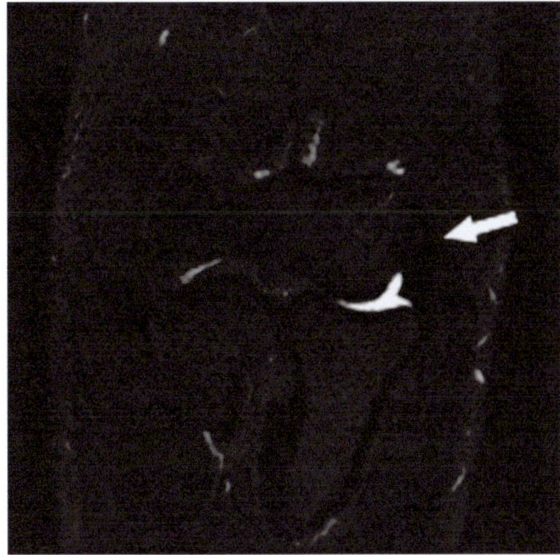

Coronal T2 fat saturated

Normal appearance of the lateral collateral ligament (arrow)

Report checklist
1. Which ligament is injured (RCL or LUCL)?
2. Location of the ligament injury (proximal, mid-substance, or distal)
3. Is the injury a low-grade sprain, partial-thickness tear, or complete tear?
4. Are there associated injuries to the overlying common extensor tendon origin?
5. What is the integrity of the ulnar collateral ligament?
6. Is there a joint effusion?

Suggested Reading

Conti Mica M, Caekebeke P, van Riet R. Lateral collateral ligament injuries of the elbow – chronic posterolateral rotatory instability (PLRI). EFORT Open Rev. 2016;1(12):461–8.

Reichel LM, Milam GS, Sitton SE, Curry MC, Mehlhoff TL. Elbow lateral collateral ligament injuries. J Hand Surg Am. 2013;38(1):184–201.

Case 2.5

Indication A 24-year-old baseball player with medial elbow pain and instability. Rule out ulnar collateral ligament tear.

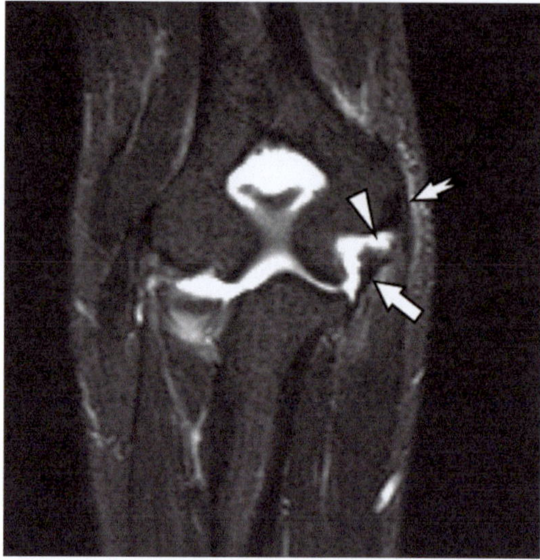

Coronal T2 fat saturated

Findings

There is linear fluid signal intensity (arrowhead) at the proximal attachment of the ulnar collateral ligament (arrow) compatible with a high-grade, near-complete tear. There is a moderate joint effusion. There is no edema or injury of the common flexor tendon (notched arrow).

Impression/Recommendation

High-grade partial-thickness ulnar collateral ligament (UCL) tear.

Discussion: Ulnar Collateral Ligament Tear

The ulnar collateral ligament (UCL) complex lies deep to the common flexor tendon origin and consists of three separate components: anterior bundle, posterior bundle, and the transverse bundle. The anterior bundle is the strongest component of the UCL and is the primary stabilizer against valgus stress at the elbow. The anterior bundle is also the only portion of the UCL complex that is easily identified on MRI. The anterior bundle arises from a broad-based origin at the inferior aspect of the medial epicondyle and inserts onto the sublime

tubercle at the medial coronoid margin. The posterior bundle is a fan-shaped area of capsular thickening and acts as a secondary stabilizer, while the transverse bundle does not significantly contribute to joint stability. The posterior and transverse bundles are not easily identified on MRI.

Injuries to the UCL most commonly occur in throwing athletes from chronic repetitive valgus stress. Early literature states that the most common injuries occur at either the mid-substance, however, this is untrue in daily clinical cases which is most commonly seen at either the proximal origin or distal attachment, with seldom cases seen involving the mid-substance. Patients usually present with medial joint instability and medial elbow pain. The clinical exam of these patients is often difficult, and hence MRI is critical for diagnosing these injuries for preoperative evaluation.

The normal anterior bundle of the UCL is most easily seen in the coronal plane as low signal intensity band on both T1- and T2-weighted images extending from the medial epicondyle to the sublime tubercle on the coronoid immediately adjacent to the articular cartilage. It is common to have high signal intensity striations at the proximal origin of the ligament due to the presence of interspersed fat, and this should not be mistaken for a tear. Injuries to the UCL range from minimal fraying to partial-thickness tear and lastly a complete tear.

Injuries to the UCL are best identified on coronal T2-weighted image with fat saturation; however, axial images are also helpful. A full-thickness tear is seen as a focal disruption of the ligament with a fluid signal gap and surrounding soft tissue edema. A partial-thickness tear manifests as abnormal morphology of the ligament (thickening or attenuation) with laxity and periligamentous edema. A partial tear is most commonly seen at the distal attachment site where there is a small avulsion of the deep fibers of the ligament from the sublime tubercle. Normally, no fluid is seen extending deep to the distal attachment of the UCL. However, when joint fluid (joint effusion or intra-articular contrast medium) is seen extending between the deep fibers of the UCL and its attachment on the bone, this is suggestive of a partial-thickness tear and has been described as the T sign (*see supplementary images*). Associated injuries to the elbow include bony contusions at the lateral (radiocapitellar) compartment as well as strains at the common flexor tendon origin.

In most cases, a partial thickness tear is treated conservatively with rest, NSAIDs, and physical therapy, whereas a complete tear requires surgical reconstruction of the ligament, especially in high-performing athletes.

Supplementary Images

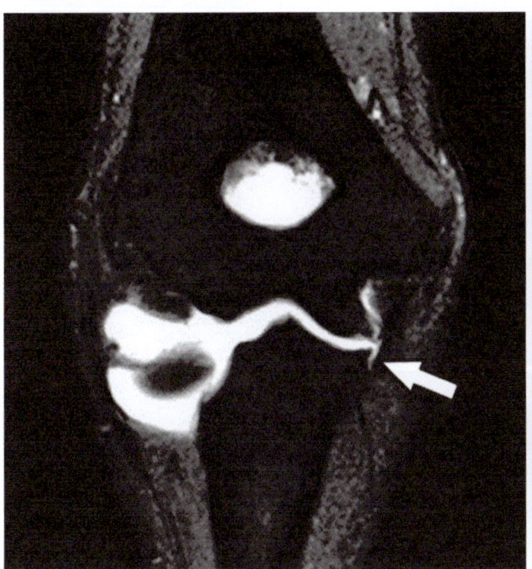

Coronal T2 fat saturated

First image shows extension of intra-articular contrast between the deep fibers of the UCL at its distal attachment onto the sublime tubercle of the ulna giving the sideways

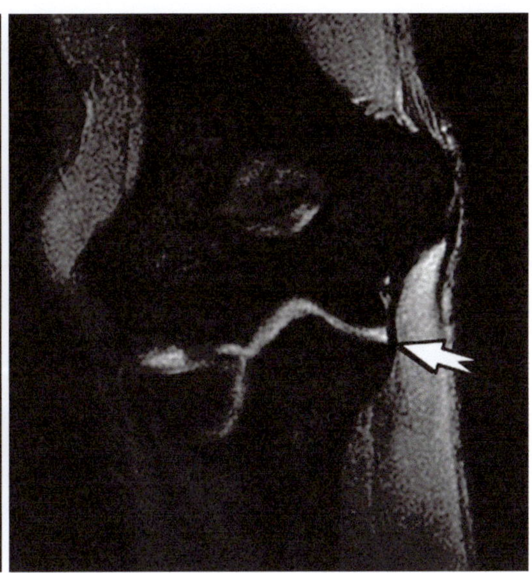

Coronal T2 GRE

"T sign" (arrow). Findings are consistent with a partial-thickness tear. Second image shows a normal UCL (notched arrow) for comparison in a different patient

Report checklist
1. What is the location of the ligament injury (proximal, mid-substance, or distal)?
2. Is the injury a low-grade sprain, partial-thickness tear, or complete tear?
3. Are there associated injuries to the overlying common flexor tendon origin?
4. What is the integrity of the other collateral ligaments?
5. Are there any bony contusions at the lateral (radiocapitellar) compartment?
6. Is there a joint effusion?

Suggested Reading

Delport AG, Zoga AC. MR and CT arthrography of the elbow. Semin Musculoskelet Radiol. 2012;16(1):15–26.

Munshli M, Pretterklleber ML, Chung CB, et al. Anterior bundle of the ulnar collateral ligament: Evaluation of anatomic relationships by using MR imaging, MR arthrography, and gross anatomic and histologic analysis. Radiology. 2004:231:797–803.

Case 2.6

Indication A 33-year-old female athlete with chronic elbow pain and locking. Plain radiographs show lucency and irregularity at the capitellum.

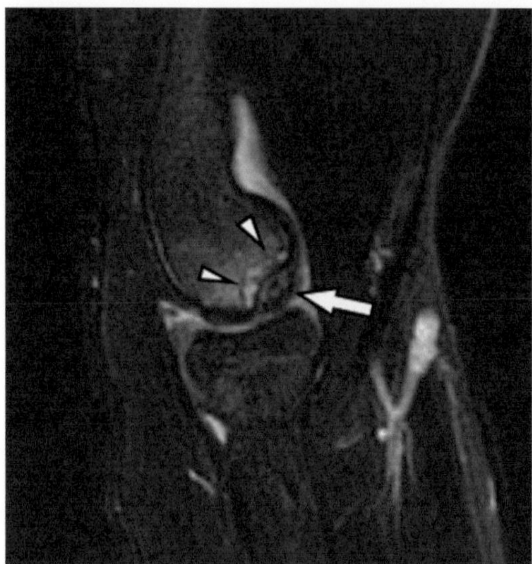

Sagittal T2 fat saturated

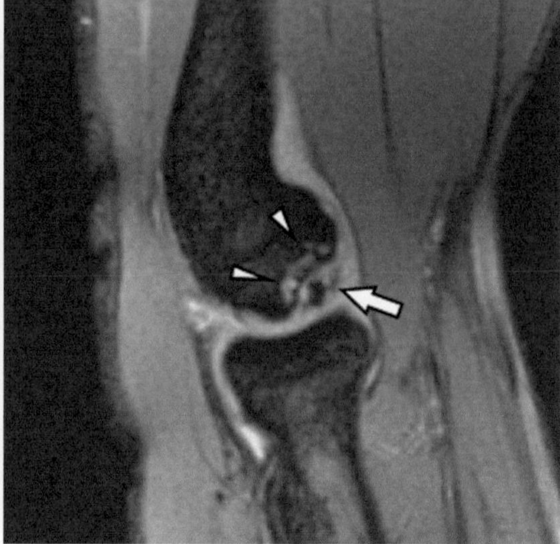

Sagittal T2 GRE

Findings

There is a 7 × 6 mm osteochondral lesion (arrows) at the anterior aspect of the capitellum that is seen separated from the underlying bone. There is high fluid signal beneath the osteochondral fragment with small underlying subchondral cysts (arrowheads) suggestive of an unstable lesion. There is no intra-articular displacement of the bony fragment. There is a small elbow joint effusion with mild synovitis posteriorly.

Impression/Recommendation

Osteochondritis dissecans of the capitellum.

Discussion: Osteochondritis Dissecans of the Capitellum

Osteochondritis dissecans (OCD) of the capitellum is an uncommon condition where a portion of the subchondral bone with overlying articular cartilage separates from the underlying capitellum with resultant fragmentation and osteonecrosis. It is typically seen in adolescent athletes from repetitive valgus stress at the elbow. OCD can occur at various locations in the elbow including the radial head and trochlea; however, it is most commonly seen in the capitellum. Patients typically present with elbow pain, swelling, and tenderness. The primary concern of referring surgeons is whether the osteochondral fragment is stable or unstable as the treatment can differ. MRI has high sensitivity for detecting these lesions; however, MR arthrography has been proven to provide better accuracy for staging OCD lesions.

The diagnosis is usually made on MRI when there are abnormal morphologic changes or abnormal signal intensity at the capitellum. In the early stages of the disease, there can be only nonspecific bone marrow edema at the anterior aspect of the capitellum, but as the disease progresses, there is usually a linear hypointense zone on the T1-weighted images and hyperintense signal on the T2-weighted images seen encircling the osteochondral fragment. The fragment itself may have normal bone marrow signal or may show diffuse low signal intensity indicating osteonecrosis. Stable lesions are usually characterized as signal changes within the subchondral bone, but there is a lack of high signal intensity at the lesion interface on the fluid-sensitive sequences. If high fluid signal intensity or intra-articular contrast is seen surrounding the osteochondral fragment, this indicates an unstable fragment. It has also been suggested that the presence of subchondral cysts beneath the osteochondral fragment is a sign of instability. Lastly, the osteochondral fragment can be displaced and become an intra-articular loose body. Essential features to describe in the report include the size and location of the osteochondral fragment, whether the fragment is stable or not and if there is a displaced osteochondral fragment into the joint. CT can also be helpful to further characterize the size of the OCD and degree of cystic changes.

Differentiating OCD from pseudodefect of the capitellum is important. Pseudodefects are normal anatomic findings that represent the normal interface between the articular cartilage and the non-articular surface at the posterior capitellum. The key finding differentiating the two entities is OCD which is usually located at the anterior capitellum, while pseudodefects are located posteriorly while viewing the sagittal sequences (*see supplementary images*).

OCD lesions that are small and stable are usually treated conservatively, while unstable lesions or stable lesions that have not responded to conservative treatment may need surgery.

Report checklist

1. What is the size and location of the osteochondral defect (OCD)?
2. Is there high signal fluid or intra-articular contrast (on MR arthrogram) encircling the osteochondral fragment?
3. Are there small subchondral cysts at the osteochondral interface?
4. Does the osteochondral fragment demonstrate normal marrow signal, or is it diffusely low signal on the T1-weighted images indicating osteonecrosis?
5. Is there displacement of the osteochondral fragment?
6. Is there an associated joint effusion?

Suggested Reading

Kijowski R, De Smet AA. MRI findings of osteochondritis dissecans of the capitellum with surgical correlation. AJR Am J Roentgenol. 2005;185:1453–9.

Wulf CA, Stone RM, Giveans MR, Lervick GN. Magnetic resonance imaging after arthroscopic microfracture of capitellar osteochondritis dissecans. Am J Sports Med. 2012;40:2549–56.

Supplementary Images

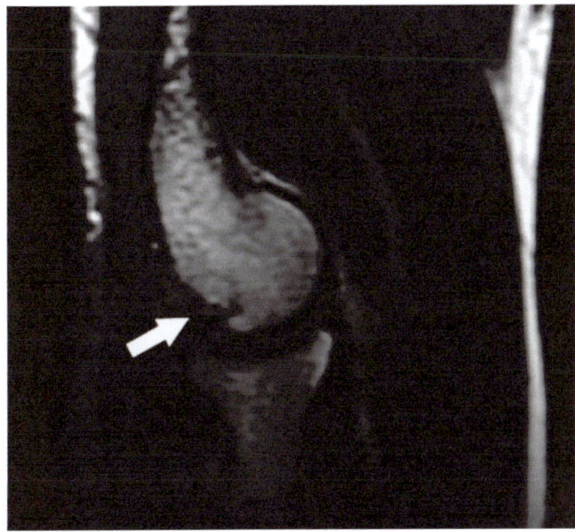

Sagittal T1

There is slight irregularity at the posterior aspect of the capitellum (arrow) which is a normal anatomic finding, compatible with pseudodefect of the capitellum

Case 2.7

Indication A 37-year-old male with posterior elbow pain and swelling. Evaluate for a fluid collection.

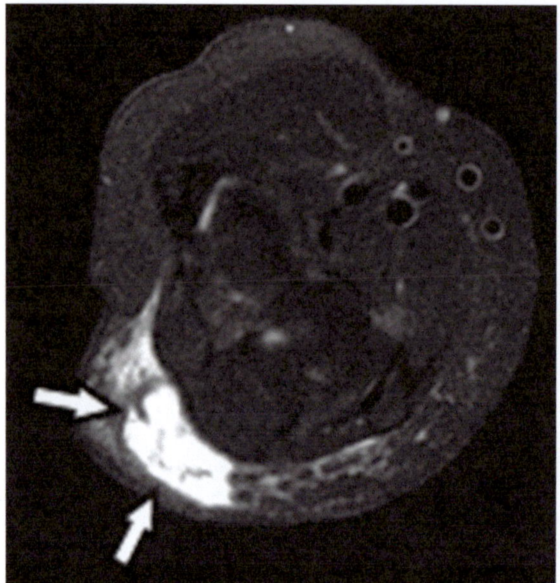

Axial T2 fat saturated

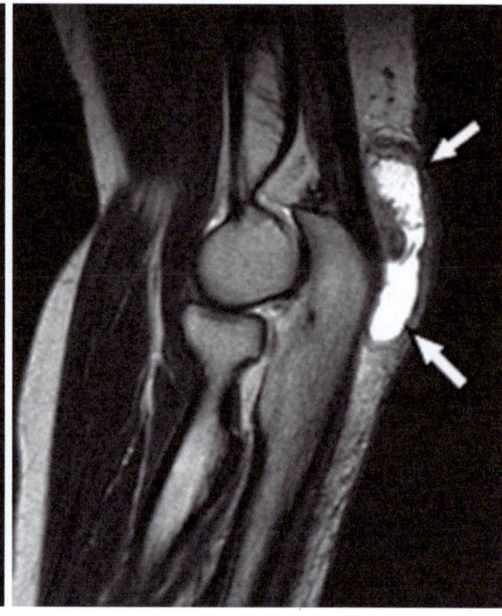

Sagittal T2

Findings
There is a well-defined cystic mass within the subcutaneous soft tissues overlying the olecranon process at the distal triceps insertion that measures 6 × 4 × 2 cm with thick peripheral wall (arrows), internal debris, and minimal surrounding soft tissue edema. There is rim enhancement on the post-contrast images (not shown). There is no significant bone marrow edema at the olecranon process, and there are no signs of osteomyelitis. The triceps tendon is normal. There is no elbow joint effusion.

Impression/Recommendation
Olecranon bursitis.

Discussion: Olecranon Bursitis
Olecranon bursitis is inflammation of the olecranon bursa located in the subcutaneous soft tissues between the skin and the olecranon process. Given its superficial location, it is a common location for injury, either acute or chronic. Olecranon bursitis can be classified as either due to septic or aseptic causes. The majority of cases are aseptic and are usually related to repetitive trauma or from an inflammatory arthropathy such as rheumatoid arthritis or gout. Septic bursitis is usually secondary to direct seeding from an open wound or in immunocompromised patients. The diagnosis is usually made clinically where there are focal swelling and tenderness at the posterior elbow. MRI is usually reserved for advanced cases or if there is a clinical concern of underlying osteomyelitis. It is, however, difficult to differentiate between septic and aseptic bursitis both clinically and on imaging, and aspiration of the bursa remains the gold standard.

Normally, the olecranon bursa is not visualized unless there is inflammation. Typical MRI findings of bursitis consist of a well-defined cystic mass within the subcutaneous soft tissues adjacent to the olecranon process and the triceps muscle insertion that is hyperintense on the

T2-weighted images and hypointense on the T1-weighted images; however, they can be complex-appearing in more advanced cases with surrounding soft tissue edema. On the post-contrast images, there is thick rim enhancement of the bursal margins. Other associated features include thickening and edema of the distal triceps muscle. Marrow edema within the olecranon process is usually reactive to the surrounding inflammation; however, scrutinizing the T1 non-fat-suppressed images for marrow replacement is essential to rule out osteomyelitis. There may also be an associated reactive joint effusion. Note should be made that no single feature is useful for discriminating septic from aseptic bursitis. However, with septic bursa, the wall of the collection is typically thicker, and there can be more soft tissue edema than with aseptic bursitis.

T2 hypointense fibrosis with granulation tissue nodularity along the periphery of the bursa suggests chronic bursitis. In rare cases, with chronic synovitis and repeated hemorrhage, the bursal inflammation can look very complex and may be difficult to distinguish from solid masses, and hence surgical consultation for possible excision is recommended in these cases.

Patients are treated according to the severity of the symptoms. Most cases can be treated conservatively; however advanced cases may need bursal excision surgically.

Report checklist

1. What is the size of the cystic collection within the subcutaneous soft tissues?
2. Are there rim enhancement and thickening of the bursal wall? Any surrounding soft tissue edema or enhancement? (These findings would favor septic over aseptic bursitis.)
3. Is there associated reactive bone marrow edema at the olecranon process? Any marrow replacement on the T1-weighted non-fat-suppressed images to suggest osteomyelitis? Any bony erosions?
4. Is there any internal enhancing nodularity within the cystic mass?
5. What is the integrity of the triceps insertion?
6. Any associated elbow joint effusion?
7. Does the patient have known rheumatoid arthritis or gout?

Suggested Reading

Floemer F, Morrison WB, Bongartz G, et-al. MRI characteristics of olecranon bursitis. AJR Am J Roentgenol. 2004;183(1): 29–34.

Stein JM, Cook TS, Simonson S, et-al. Normal and variant anatomy of the elbow on magnetic resonance imaging. Magn Reson Imaging Clin N Am. 2011;19(3):609–19.

Case 2.8

Indication A 58-year-old man with fall on outstretched hand. Now with acute pain, weakness, and swelling along the posterior elbow.

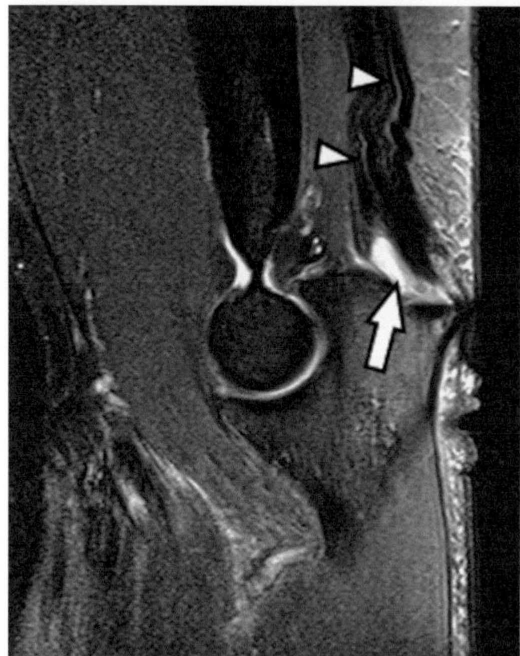

Sagittal T2 fat saturated

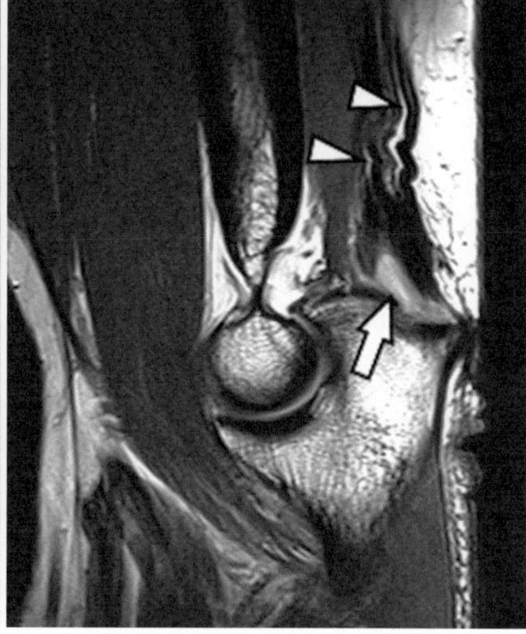

Sagittal T2

Findings

There is a high-grade (near-complete) tear of the distal triceps tendon from its distal attachment onto the olecranon with fluid (arrows) in between the tendon and olecranon. There are a few intact posterior fibers. There is mild thickening of the distal triceps with preservation of the normal striated appearance to the tendon (arrowheads). There is no marrow edema in the olecranon to indicate a bone contusion or fracture. There is no elbow joint effusion.

Impression/Recommendation

High-grade (near-complete) tear of the distal triceps tendon.

Discussion: Triceps Tendon Injuries

The triceps is a large muscle along the posterior aspect of the arm which extends the elbow joint. It is comprised of three heads (long, medial, lateral), and their distal fibers converge to form the triceps tendon insertion which is divided into the central tendon insertion onto the olecranon process and the lateral triceps expansion. The central tendon is comprised mostly of the medial and long head tendons. The lateral triceps expansion is thinner than the central tendon and covers the anconeus muscle and blends with the extensor carpi ulnaris and dorsal antebrachial fascia and has insertions onto the ulna. Tears of the triceps tendon are uncommon (1% of all tendon tears) and are more likely to occur in patients with prior tendinopathy and in anabolic steroid users. Systemic conditions including chronic renal disease, rheumatoid arthritis, Marfan syndrome, and diabetes can also increase risk for triceps injury. Patients complain of posterior elbow pain and weakness with elbow extension. If a full-thickness tear is present, a palpable gap near the triceps tendon attachment may be felt on physical exam.

On MRI imaging, the normal triceps tendon is low signal on all pulse sequences but can have a striated, laminated, appearance due to convergence of fibers from the three muscle heads. This should not be mistaken for a longitudinal tear. This striated appearance is similar to the quadriceps tendon of the knee. When evaluating for triceps tendon injury, edema-sensitive sequences (T2 fat saturated or STIR) are preferred and best assessed in the sagittal plane. The tendon can be enlarged and has high signal on T2 images and intermediate signal on T1 and proton density (PD) images. Focal tears will be replaced by fluid signal intensity. If no intact fibers are present, then a full-thickness (complete rupture) should be raised. One should describe whether the deep and/or superficial tendon fibers are injured. Isolated partial tears commonly involve the medial aspect of the tendon. Identifying the location of the tendon (bone-tendon, tendon substance, myotendinous junction) has implications on surgical treatment and should be mentioned in the report. The degree of tendon retraction, the presence of an avulsed olecranon fragment, and integrity of the tendon free edge should also be commented on in the report to aid with surgical repair. Although

MRI provides excellent assessment of triceps tendon injury, recent reports suggest that tendon injury can be overcalled as full-thickness tears when only partial tears are present.

Small partial tears or tendinopathy are treated conservatively with rest, analgesics, and physical therapy. Immobilization with the elbow in 30 degrees flexion can help with tendon healing and prevent further injury. Higher-grade tendon tears and those that do not improve with conservative therapy are managed with surgical repair. Typically, a bone tunnel is created in the olecranon, and the central triceps tendon is attached with high-tensile, braided sutures in a running, locked fashion. Rerupture occurs in 20% of repairs.

Report checklist
1. Where is the triceps tear located (avulsion, tendon substance, myotendinous junction)?
2. What is the integrity of the tendon free edge? Is there tendon retraction?
3. Is there associated olecranon fracture or bursitis?
4. Is the tear partial or complete? Does it involve the deep and/or superficial fibers?
5. Does the patient have predisposing conditions for tendinopathy?

Suggested Reading

Keener JD, Sethi PM. Distal Triceps Tendon Injuries. Hand Clin. 2015;31(4):641–50.

Kholinne E, Al-Ramadhan H, Bahkley AM, Alalwan MQ, Jeon IH. MRI overestimates the full-thickness tear of distal triceps tendon rupture. J Orthop Surg. 2018;26(2):1–5.

Case 2.9

Indication   A 67-year-old female with tingling and mild weakness of the ring and small fingers.

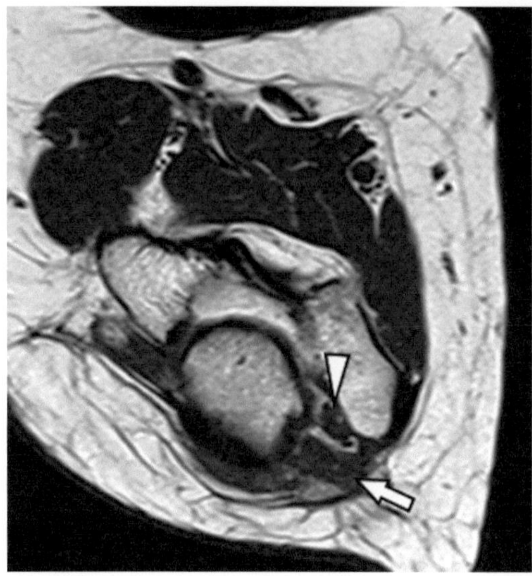

Axial T1

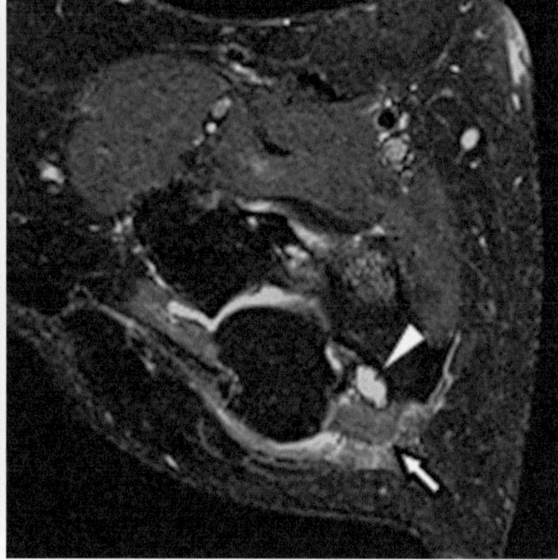

Axial T2 fat saturated

Findings

There is a soft tissue mass (arrows) in the cubital tunnel. The mass is low signal on the T1- and T2-weighted images similar to skeletal muscle. The structure is next to the ulnar nerve in the cubital tunnel and is most compatible with an accessory muscle. The ulnar nerve is enlarged and has high signal on the T2 fat saturated images (arrowheads). There is mild edema in the adjacent soft tissues. There is no marrow edema in the medical epicondyle, and the ulnar nerve is not subluxed or displaced from the cubital tunnel.

Impression/Recommendation

1. Ulnar neuritis due to compression from an accessory anconeus epitrochlearis muscle.
2. Please correlate with electromyographic (EMG) studies of ulnar nerve if clinically appropriate.

Discussion: Anconeus Epitrochlearis and Ulnar Nerve Impingement

The anconeus epitrochlearis (AE) is an accessory muscle that forms an arch covering the cubital tunnel with attachments to the medical epicondyle and olecranon. It is present in approximately 10–30% of the population. The AE has been implicated in impingement of the ulnar nerve leading to cubital tunnel syndrome. The floor of the cubital tunnel is formed by the posterior band of the ulnar collateral ligament, and the roof is formed by a retinaculum, Osborne's band (or ligament). The AE when present replaces the retinaculum, and its bulky size is believed to impinge upon the ulnar nerve leading to symptoms of ulnar neuritis or cubital tunnel syndrome. However, recent studies have suggested that having an AE may be protective for cubital tunnel syndrome. In a study by Wilson et al. (see reference below), 9.8% of patients with cubital tunnel syndrome requiring surgery had an accessory AE muscle, while 15.5% in the control group had an AE. The authors postulate that the AE muscle decreases the rigidity to the entrance to the cubital tunnel preventing cubital tunnel syndrome. Affected patients have tingling in the ring finger and small finger with elbow flexion. They can also have decreased hand grip strength and pain in the medial elbow.

On MRI, the AE is seen as a soft tissue structure overlying the roof of the cubital tunnel with signal intensity identical to skeletal muscle. The affected ulnar nerve can be enlarged and have increased T2 signal. It is also important to assess for other causes of ulnar nerve abnormalities leading to cubital tunnel syndrome (second most common compressive neuropathy). The ulnar nerve can sublux/dislocate from the cubital tunnel anteromedially (*see supplementary images*) and typically occurs with elbow flexion and thus may not be present if the elbow is scanned in extension. Bone spurs, synovitis, nerve sheath tumors, ganglia, and anomalous and hypertrophied triceps muscles can also irritate the ulnar nerve in the cubital tunnel.

Initial treatment is conservative with rest, splints, analgesics, and physical therapy. Steroid injections can help reduce pain and swelling. Lastly, surgery can be performed to release the structures, including the AE, that compress the ulnar nerve.

Report checklist
1. Is there a soft tissue mass forming the roof of the cubital tunnel with signal intensity the same as skeletal muscle?
2. Is the ulnar nerve located in the cubital tunnel, and does it have normal signal intensity?
3. Are there other reasons for ulnar nerve impingement (bone spurs, ganglia, synovitis, anomalous/hypertrophied triceps muscle)?

Suggested Reading

Park IJ, Kim HM, Lee JY, et al. Cubital Tunnel Syndrome Caused by Anconeus Epitrochlearis Muscle. J Korean Neurosurg Soc. 2018;61(5): 618–24.

Wilson TJ, Tubbs RS, Yang LJ. The anconeus epitrochlearis muscle may protect against the development of cubital tunnel syndrome: a preliminary study. J Neurosurg. 2016;125(6):1533–8.

Supplementary Images

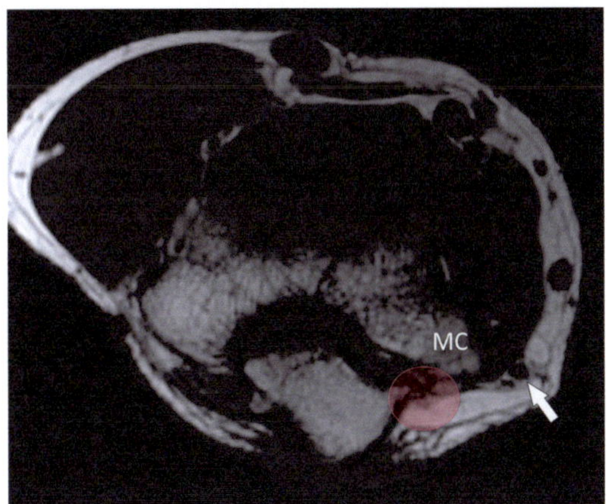

Axial T1

A 43-year-old man with dislocation of the ulnar nerve (arrow) anteromedially from the cubital tunnel (red circle), now lying medial to the medial epicondyle of the distal humerus (MC, medial epicondyle)

Wrist/Hand

Case 3.1

Indication A 28-year-old male with known scaphoid fracture and poor healing.

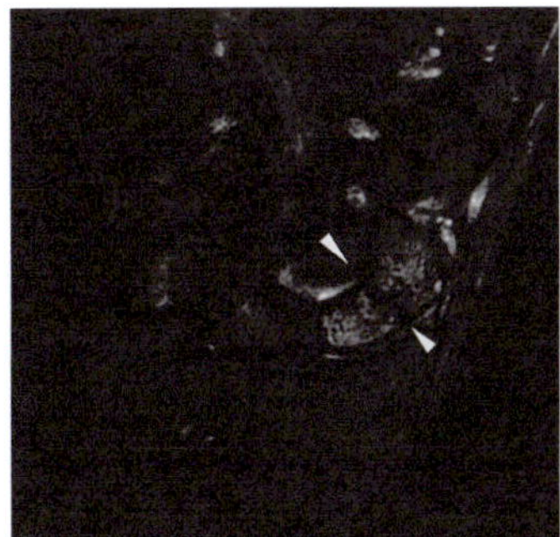
Coronal T2 fat saturated

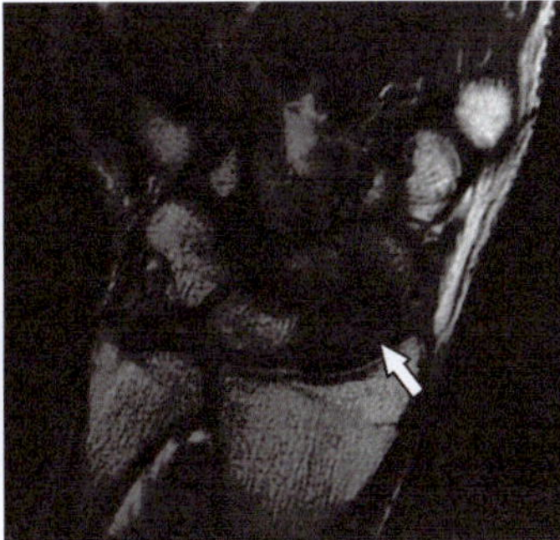
Coronal T1

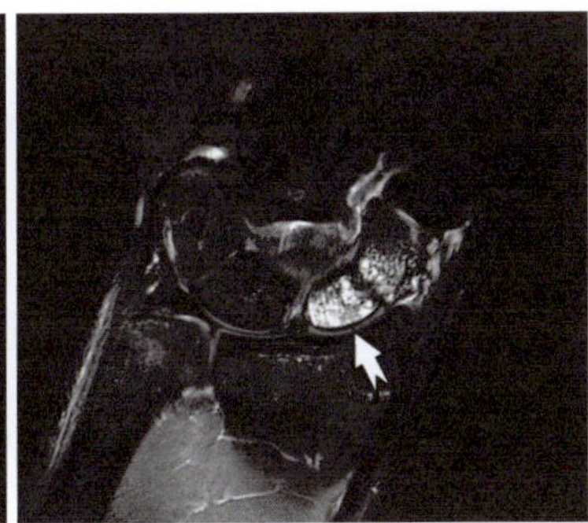
Coronal T1 fat saturated post contrast

Findings

There is a hypointense fracture line (arrowheads) running through the scaphoid waist with surrounding bone marrow edema as well as small subchondral cystic changes adjacent to the fracture site. There is diffuse low signal intensity of the proximal pole on the T1- weighted images (arrow); however, enhancement on the post-contrast images (notched arrow) indicates viable bone and no avascular necrosis. There is no collapse of the proximal articular surface or secondary osteoarthritis. The scapholunate ligament is intact.

Impression/Recommendation

Scaphoid fracture without AVN of the proximal pole.

Discussion: Scaphoid Fractures

The scaphoid is the most commonly fractured carpal bone accounting for 80% of all carpal fractures. It is typically the result of a fall on an outstretched hand (FOOSH) with most fractures occurring at the waist (70%). Tenderness in the anatomical snuffbox is characteristic of such a fracture. It is essential to promptly diagnose these cases as a delay in the diagnosis can result in avascular necrosis (AVN) of the proximal pole with resultant secondary osteoarthritis. The proximal 70% of the scaphoid bone receives its blood supply from a dorsal branch of the radial artery that enters the scaphoid distally with retrograde intraosseous extension. The distal 30% is supplied by a volar branch that enters at the distal pole.

© Springer Nature Switzerland AG 2020
T. M. Hegazi, J. S. Wu, *Musculoskeletal MRI*, https://doi.org/10.1007/978-3-030-26777-3_3

MRI is the modality of choice for evaluating radiographically occult fractures. Ideally, T1-weighted and fluid-sensitive sequences should be obtained in three planes (axial, sagittal, and coronal). On MRI, acute fractures show a low signal intensity band running through part or all of the scaphoid with significant surrounding bone marrow edema. If there is bone marrow edema but no clear hypointense fracture line visualized, this suggests a bone contusion. Fractures of the scaphoid waist could disrupt the blood supply to the proximal region of the bone, which may result in complications of delayed union or nonunion (approximately 15% of patients). Nonunion would be seen as a fluid-filled signal within the fracture line without significant marrow edema of the bone as well as low signal sclerosis at the fracture margins. This can later cause AVN of the proximal pole. AVN appears as diffuse low signal intensity of the necrotic region on both T1- and T2-weighted images; however, areas of ischemia without osteonecrosis can have a similar appearance, and caution should be taken in calling AVN in all cases. Gadolinium administration has been proven to help differentiate these cases. Homogeneous enhancement on the post-contrast images suggests intact blood supply and viability of the fragment. However, if there is only minimal heterogeneous enhancement, then this suggests AVN. When AVN becomes chronic, this can lead to collapse and fragmentation of the proximal pole and then secondary osteoarthritis.

Non-displaced scaphoid fractures can usually be managed with a closed cast. In cases of displaced fractures, or disrupted vascularity, surgical intervention is needed.

Report checklist
1. Is there marrow edema and/or a discrete low signal fracture line? Where is it located (waist, distal pole, proximal pole)?
2. Is there displacement of the fracture fragments?
3. Are there signs of delayed union or nonunion (fluid signal at the fracture site and/or low signal sclerotic fracture margins)?
4. Is there diffuse low signal intensity on T1- and T2-weighted images of the proximal pole? If yes, is there homogeneous enhancement on the post-contrast images?
5. Is there secondary osteoarthritis or fragmentation of the scaphoid articular surface?
6. What is the integrity of the scapholunate ligament?

Suggested Reading

Fox MG, Gaskin CM, Chhabra AB, Anderson MW. Assessment of scaphoid viability with MRI: a reassessment of findings on unenhanced MR images. AJR Am J Roentgenol. 2010;195:W281–6.

Fox MG, Wang DT, Chhabra AB. Accuracy of enhanced and unenhanced MRI in diagnosing scaphoid proximal pole avascular necrosis and predicting surgical outcome. Skeletal Radiol. 2015;44:1671–8.

Case 3.2

Indication A 34-year-old female status post fall 2 weeks ago with scapholunate widening on radiographs. Assess for scapholunate ligament tear.

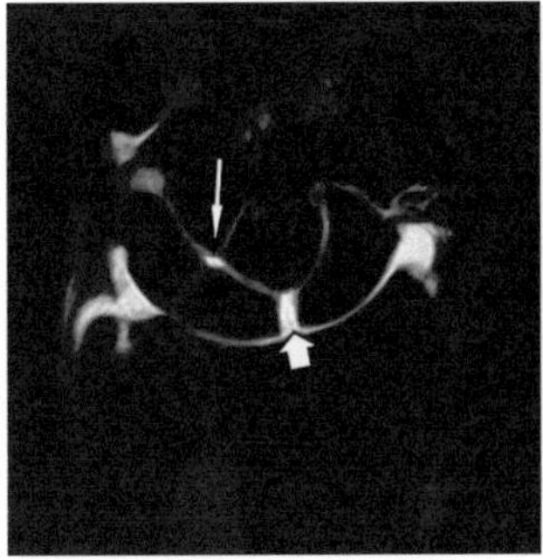
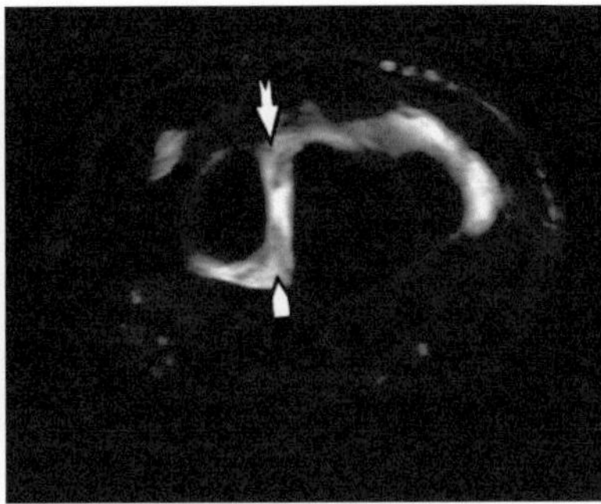
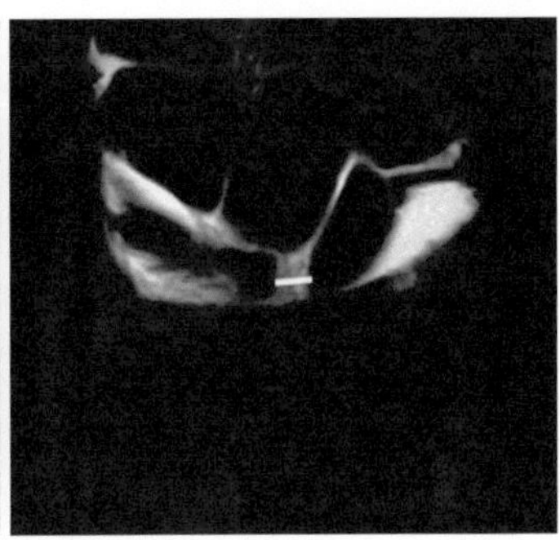

Coronal T1 fat saturated (MR arthrogram)

Axial T1 fat saturated (MR arthrogram)

Coronal T1 fat saturated (MR arthrogram)

Findings

On this MR arthrogram study, there is abnormal extension of intra-articular contrast through the scapholunate interval (short arrow) extending into the midcarpal compartment (long arrow) from a full-thickness tear of the scapholunate ligament. There is disruption and irregularity of all three components, dorsal (notched arrow), central, and volar (block arrow), compatible with a complete tear, best seen on the axial images. There is secondary widening of the scapholunate distance (white line) measuring 5 mm. The lunotriquetral ligament is intact. There is no proximal migration of the capitate to indicate a SLAC wrist and no radioscaphoid osteoarthritis.

Impression/Recommendation

Full-thickness tear of the scapholunate ligament involving all three components (complete tear).

Discussion: Scapholunate Ligament Tear

The scaphoid and lunate are bound together by a U-shaped scapholunate (SL) ligament complex, which acts to stabilize the proximal carpal row along with the lunotriquetral ligament. The SL ligament is divided into three components; dorsal, central (membranous), and volar, of which the dorsal segment is the thickest and most functionally important *(see supplementary images)*.

The thinner central component attaches on the articular cartilage of the scaphoid and lunate and can hence have high signal intensity at its insertion and should not be mistaken for a tear. The dorsal and volar components attach directly on the bone and have homogenous low signal intensity along their entire length. Although the dorsal and volar components can be visualized on coronal images, they are better evaluated on the axial images where band-like structures are seen. The coronal images better visualizes the central component which appears more triangular in shape.

It is important to realize that degeneration and perforations of the central (membranous) portion of the SL ligament can be seen in asymptomatic older patients. In younger individuals, tears are usually traumatic, commonly from a fall on an outstretched hand. Injury to the SL ligament can range from a low-grade sprain to partial-thickness tears and finally a full-thickness tear. A sprain appears as abnormal thickening of the ligament with increased intrinsic signal on the T2-weighted images, but if you can trace the entire length of the ligament, then this suggests that it is still intact. A tear is diagnosed when there is non-visualization of the ligament with abnormal fluid signal intensity seen traversing the ligament either partially (partial tear) or along the entire thickness of the ligament (full thickness). When a tear is seen, it should also be described as being complete (involving all three components) or partial (sparing at least one component).

MR arthrography increases the sensitivity and specificity of detecting subtle tears and should be the study of choice when there is a high index of suspicion for SL ligament tears. A tear is present when high signal intra-articular contrast is seen traversing the ligament. If there is a full-thickness tear, there will be extension of intra-articular contrast into the midcarpal compartment from a proxi-mal radiocarpal injection. If there is disruption of any two components of the SL ligament, there may be widening of the scapholunate distance which will then result in instability causing dorsal intercalated segmental instability (DISI). If a DISI deformity is left untreated, this may result in degenerative osteoarthritis at the radioscaphoid articulation and scapholunate advanced collapse (SLAC) *(see supplementary images)*.

SL ligament tears are usually treated initially with immobilization and surgery if symptoms persist.

Supplementary Images

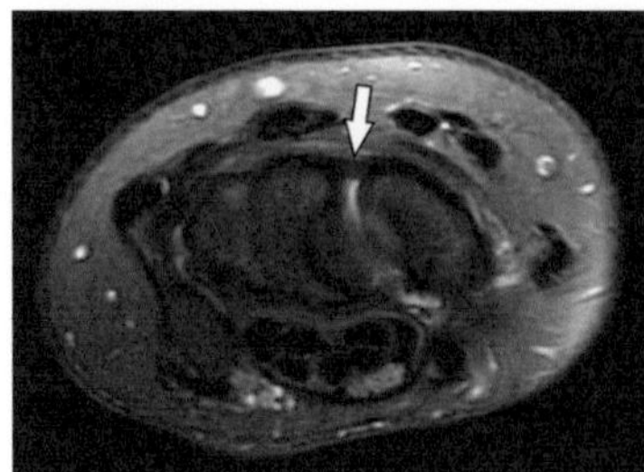 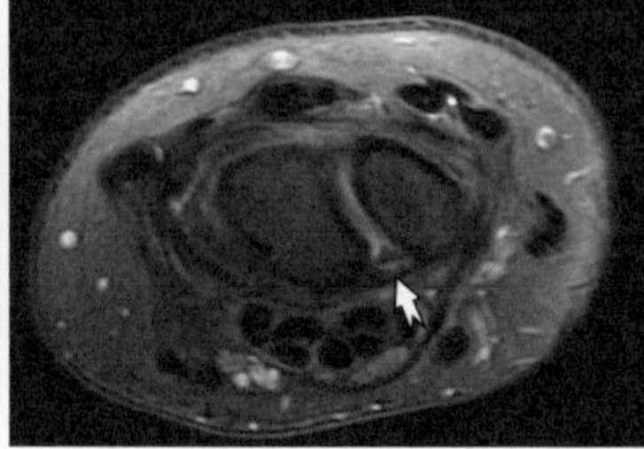 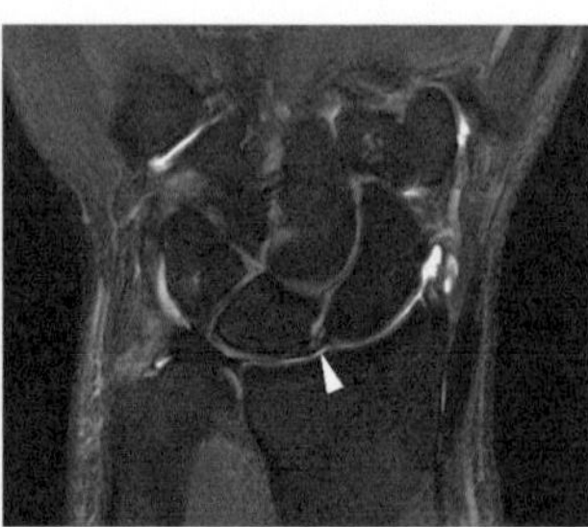

Axial T2 fat saturated   Axial T2 fat saturated   Coronal T2 fat saturated

Normal appearance of the scapholunate ligament, showing the dorsal (arrow), volar (notched arrow), and membranous (arrowhead) components

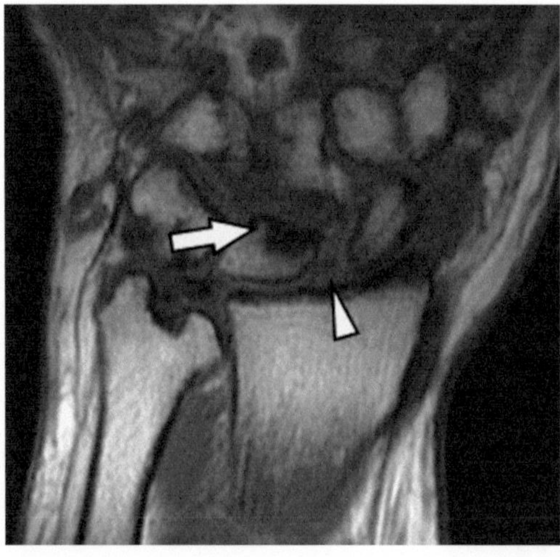 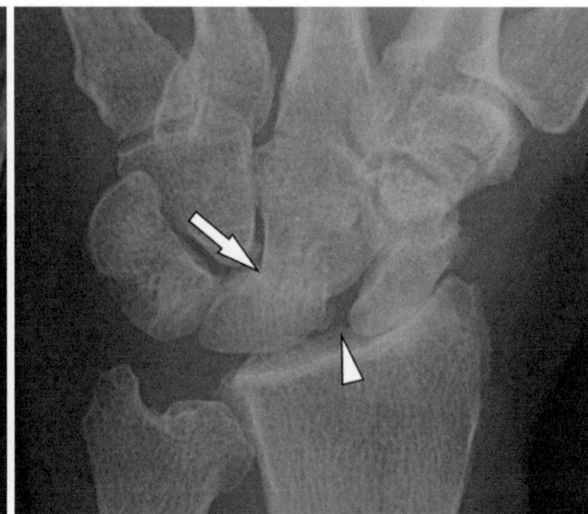

Coronal T1

SLAC wrist in a 76-year-old man with chronic wrist pain. On the MR and radiograph images, there is abnormal widening of the scapholunate interval and non-visualization of the scapholunate ligament (arrowheads) consistent with complete tear. There is sclerosis of the distal lunate subchondral surface (arrow). The radiograph nicely shows complete loss of the joint space between the capitate and lunate

Report checklist

1. Is the scapholunate ligament sprained or torn?
2. If there is a tear, is it partial thickness or full thickness?
3. Which component(s) of the ligament are involved (dorsal, central, or volar band)?
4. Is there an associated osseous fracture?
5. If the study is an MR arthrography, is there abnormal extension of intra-articular contrast from the radiocarpal joint to the midcarpal compartment indicating a full- thickness ligament tear?
6. Is there widening of the scapholunate interval?
7. Assess integrity of the lunotriquetral ligament
8. Is there proximal migration of the capitate (SLAC wrist)? And is there secondary radioscaphoid osteoarthritis?

Suggested Reading

Bateni CP, Bartolotta RJ, Richardson ML, Mulcahy H, Allan CH. Imaging key wrist ligaments: what the surgeon needs the radiologist to know. AJR Am J Roentgenol. 2013;200:1089–95.

Spaans AJ, Minnen Pv, Prins HJ, Korteweg MA, Schuurman AH. The value of 3.0-tesla MRI in diagnosing scapholunate ligament injury. J Wrist Surg. 2013;2:69–72.

Case 3.3

Indication   A 48-year-old female with ulnar-sided wrist pain. Assess TFCC.

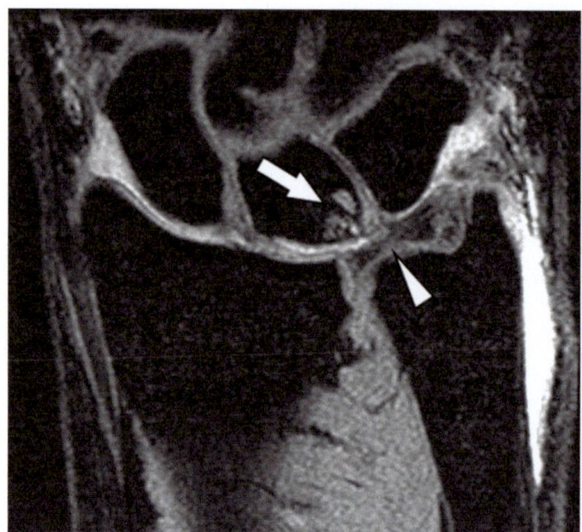

Coronal GRE T2

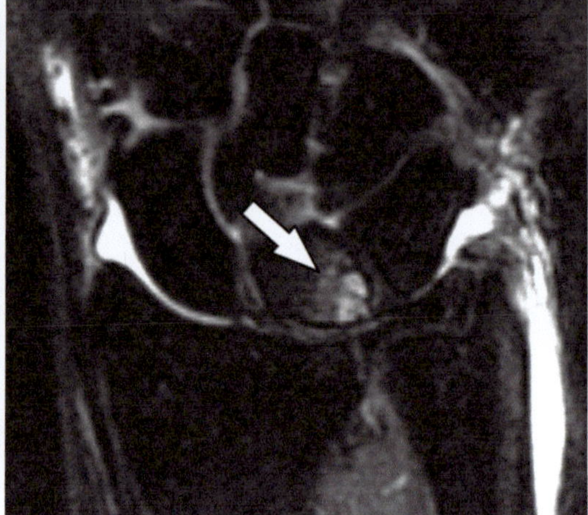

Coronal T2 fat saturated

Findings

There is focal chondrosis (loss of articular cartilage) at the proximal lunate articular surface with subchondral cystic changes and bone marrow edema at the ulnar aspect of the lunate (arrows). There is also a small focal central perforation of the central triangular fibrocartilage (arrowhead), best seen on the gradient echo sequences. There is neutral ulnar variance.

Impression/Recommendation

Ulnar impaction syndrome with associated central TFC tear.

Discussion: Ulnar Impaction Syndrome

Ulnar variance is best assessed on posterior-anterior radiographs taken while the patient's forearm is in neutral position (shoulder abducted 90° and elbow in 90° flexion); however, MRI can give a good estimate on variance as well. If the patient is in the prone position with the hand extended above the head with elbow extension, the palm of the hand should be resting on the scanner table. Patients with ulnar positive variance are predisposed to excessive loading and abutment between the ulnar head and the adjacent lunate known as ulnar impaction syndrome or ulnolunate abutment. This results in subsequent degeneration of the triangular fibrocartilage complex (TFCC); chondromalacia of the articular surfaces of the lunate, triquetrum, and ulna; and disturbance of the lunotriquetral ligament leading to secondary ulnocarpal osteoarthritis. It is important to know that positive ulnar variance is not required for diagnosis of ulnar impaction syndrome.

MRI allows for detection of earlier signs of abutment which include chondral fissures at the ulnar aspect of the lunate articular surface and distal ulna which is the hallmark of this disease. It eventually leads to full-thickness chondral defects with subchondral bone marrow edema and cystic changes. With time, degeneration and central perforation of the TFC can occur. Sclerotic changes are seen with further progression as areas of low signal intensity on both T1- and T2-weighted images. In patients with radiographic evidence of ulnar impaction syndrome, there can be a need to assess the integrity of the TFCC and lunotriquetral ligament by MR imaging.

The differential diagnosis on MR imaging include Kienbock's disease. The bone marrow edema and cystic changes in Kienbock's disease are usually localized to the lunate and affect the radial aspect of the lunate bone *(please refer to Case 3.5 for discussion on Kienbock's disease)*. However, in ulnar impaction, the ulnar aspect of the lunate bone is involved, and there is typically ulnar positive variance.

Treatment options may include conservative treatment or ulnar shortening procedures with debridement of the TFC.

> **Report checklist**
> 1. Is there ulnar variance (positive, neutral, or negative)?
> 2. Are there cartilage abnormalities at the lunate and ulnar articular surfaces? If so, are there bone marrow edema or subchondral cystic changes?
> 3. How is the TFC (tear, degenerative signal)?
> 4. How is the integrity of the lunotriquetral ligament?

Suggested Reading

Cerezal L, del Piñal F, Abascal F, García-Valtuille R, Pereda T, Canga A. Imaging findings in ulnar-sided wrist impaction syndromes. Radiographics. 2002;22:105–21.

Squires JH, England E, Mehta K, Wissman RD. The role of imaging in diagnosing diseases of the distal radioulnar joint, triangular fibrocartilage complex, and distal ulna. AJR Am J Roentgenol. 2014;203:146–53.

Case 3.4a

Indication A 16-year-old female with ulnar-sided pain after a fall, MR arthrogram to assess TFCC.

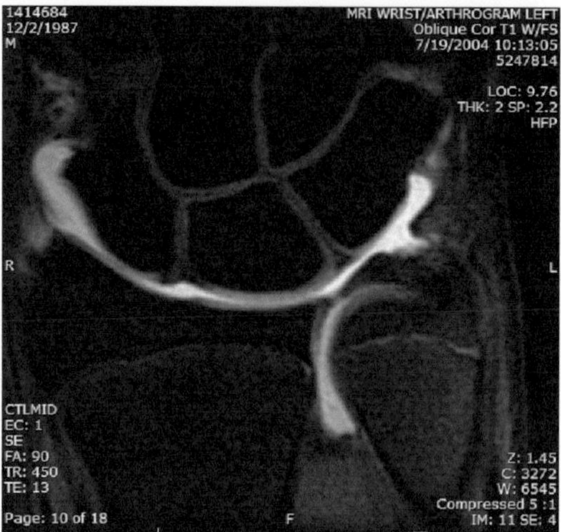

Coronal T1 fat saturated (MR arthrogram)

Findings

MR arthrogram shows a small slit-like 2 mm perforation within the central portion of the articular disc (arrow) with intra-articular contrast extending through the defect and into the DRUJ (arrowhead). The peripheral ulnar attachments of the TFC are intact (notched arrow). The articular cartilage and lunotriquetral ligament are normal.

Case 3.4b

Indication A 28-year-old male with fall 2 weeks ago, MR arthrogram to assess TFCC.

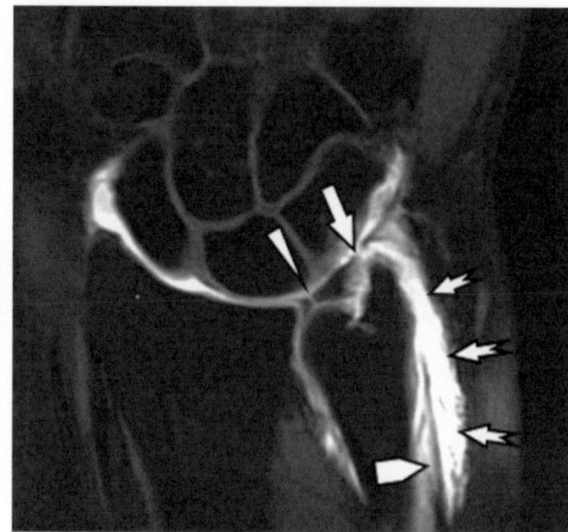

Coronal T1 fat saturated (MR arthrogram)

Findings

MR arthrogram shows a full-thickness tear of the peripheral TFC at its ulnar styloid attachments (arrow) with intra-articular contrast extending through the defect into the DRUJ. There is a small slit-like central TFC perforation (arrowhead). There is also a prominent amount of contrast around the proximal ulna (notched arrows) surrounding the extensor carpi ulnaris (ECU) tendon (block arrow) indicating injury of the ECU tendon subsheath.

Impression/Recommendation
- **Case 3.4a:** Central perforation of the TFC articular disc.
- **Case 3.4b:** Full-thickness tear of the peripheral TFC at its ulnar styloid attachment. Central TFC perforation. Tear of the ECU subsheath with contrast extending into the ECU tendon sheath.

Discussion: TFCC Tear

The distal radioulnar joint is primarily stabilized by the triangular fibrocartilage complex (TFCC) and separates the distal radioulnar joint (DRUJ) from the radiocarpal joint. This complex is present at the distal end of the ulna and consists of several interlinked components: (1) the triangular fibrocartilage (TFC) articular disc, (2) the palmar and dorsal radioulnar ligaments, (3) the meniscal homologue, (4) the lunotriquetral (LT) ligament, and (5) the sheath of the extensor carpi ulnaris tendon. Although all components are vital for proper function of the wrist, the most essential components for clinical purposes are the TFC articular disc and the radioulnar ligaments. The central portion of the articular disc is a thin 1–2 mm avascular fibrocartilage that forms the central component of the TFCC. On the radial side, the articular disc is affixed to the distal radial articular cartilage at the level of the sigmoid notch. On the ulnar side, the TFC is more vascular and fans out becoming thicker attaching to both the ulnar fovea and ulnar styloid process. The palmar and dorsal radioulnar ligaments merge with the TFC on its palmar and dorsal aspects.

On a normal wrist MRI, the central TFC disc shows homogenous low signal intensity on all pulse sequences. This disc appears as a biconcave bowtie on coronal images, a discoid structure on sagittal images with thicker peripheral margins, and triangular on axial images with its apex at the ulnar styloid. At the ulnar attachment, it is normal for the TFC to have a striated appearance with areas of high signal due to the presence of loose connective tissue. This can sometimes mimic a partial tear or sprain. The palmar and dorsal radioulnar ligaments are most easily noted on sagittal or axial images and represent the thickest portions at the volar and dorsal margins of the TFC disc, respectively.

Abnormalities of the TFCC are a common cause of ulnar-sided pain and are divided into type 1 (traumatic) and type 2 (degenerative) as per the Palmer classification. The importance of this classification system is to appropriately describe either the location of a traumatic tear or extent of degeneration in degenerative tears and hence help guide clinical management.

Type I: traumatic injury

- IA: central perforation
- IB: ulnar avulsion with/without ulnar styloid fracture
- IC: distal avulsion from the carpal attachment to the lunate or triquetrum
- ID: radial avulsion with/without sigmoid notch fracture

Type II: degenerative injury

- IIA: TFC thinning and degeneration, predominantly on the ulnar side
- IIB: TFC thinning and degeneration with lunate or ulnar chondromalacia
- IIC: TFC perforation with lunate or ulnar chondromalacia
- IID: TFC perforation with lunate or ulnar chondromalacia and LT ligament rupture
- IIE: TFC perforation with lunate or ulnar chondromalacia, LT ligament rupture, and osteoarthritis

On MRI, tears of the central TFC are more commonly on the radial side of the disc and are best visualized on coronal images, where there will be a small slit-like discontinuity with fluid signal traversing the TFC defect. MR arthrography has greater sensitivity and specificity for detecting small TFC tears which will be demonstrated as hyperintense fluid within the tear on the T1 fat-suppressed sequences with contrast extending into the DRUJ after radiocarpal injection of intra-articular contrast. Traumatic tears of the peripheral TFC at its ulnar attachment are more difficult to detect, and careful evaluation of the foveal and ulnar styloid attachments should be scrutinized for either excessive fluid or change in the normal striated morphology. Indirect clues of a peripheral tear include bone edema at the ulnar styloid and focal synovitis in the area. Again, MR arthrography performs better in detecting small tears.

Degenerative changes of the central TFC is a common finding in older individuals demonstrated by increased signal intensity and fraying of the disc. These are usually asymptomatic; however, with worsening degeneration, a central perforation will be seen which will then lead to chondrosis at the lunate and ulna. Lastly, tears of the LT ligament and osteoarthritis can occur. In these situations, it is important to assess the dorsal and palmar radioulnar ligaments, as tears of these structures can lead to DRUJ instability. It is also important to comment on whether there is negative or positive ulnar variance.

Peripheral TFC tears can be treated surgically by suturing; however, tears of the central disc are usually treated with debridement.

Report checklist

1. Where is the tear located (central articular disc, peripheral at its radial, or ulnar attachments)?
2. Is it a partial-thickness tear or full-thickness tear/perforation? What is the size of the defect?
3. What is the integrity of the palmar and dorsal radioulnar ligaments? Integrity of the lunotriquetral ligament?
4. Are there any bony avulsion fractures?
5. Is there a DRUJ effusion or contrast? Contrast extension would indicate a full-thickness TFC tear (assuming injection from the radiocarpal joint).
6. Are there degenerative changes of the radiocarpal joint?
7. Is there ulnar variance? Positive ulnar variance can predispose to TFC tear.

Suggested Reading

Ng AWH, Griffith JF, Fung CSY, Lee RKL, Tong CSL, Wong CWY, Tse WL, Ho PC. MR imaging of the traumatic triangular fibrocartilaginous complex tear. Quant Imaging Med Surg. 2017;7:443–60.

Rüegger C, Schmid MR, Pfirrmann CW, Nagy L, Gilula LA, Zanetti M. Peripheral tear of the triangular fibrocartilage: depiction with MR arthrography of the distal radioulnar joint. AJR Am J Roentgenol. 2007;188:187–92.

Case 3.5

Indication   A 54-year-old female with wrist pain for 1 year. Radiographs show sclerosis of the lunate.

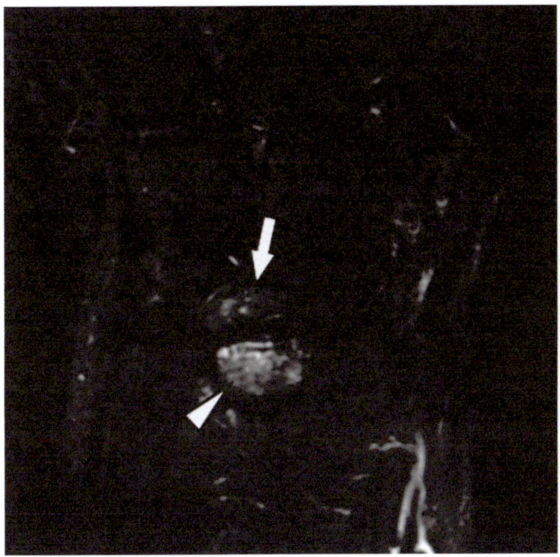

Coronal T2 fat saturated

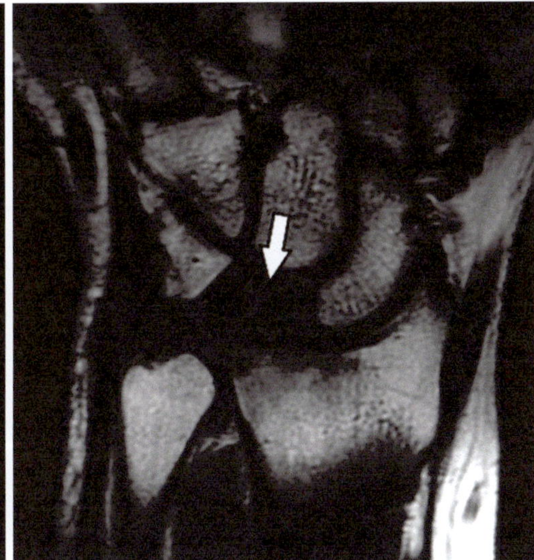

Coronal T1

Findings

There is extensive bone marrow edema and mixed heterogeneous T2 signal within the lunate bone and cortical collapse of the proximal articular surface (arrows). There is also mild bone edema at the distal radius (arrowhead) indicating secondary radiocarpal degenerative changes.

Impression/Recommendation

Avascular necrosis of the lunate, also known as Kienböck's disease.

Discussion: Kienböck's Disease

The lunate bone is situated in the center of the proximal carpal row and helps with axial loading across the wrist. The lunate's vascularity is supplied by the palmar and dorsal intercarpal and radiocarpal arches; however, only terminal branches reach its proximal pole, where avascular necrosis likely begins. Kienböck's disease is a condition where the blood supply to the lunate is disrupted leading to avascular necrosis of the bone. The precise etiology of this disease remains unclear but is thought to result from chronic repetitive trauma and is frequently associated with ulnar negative variance. The disease is progressive which can result in carpal instability and destruction if untreated; therefore, early diagnosis and treatment is important.

Early in the disease, there will be bone marrow edema evident by high signal intensity on the T2-weighted fat-suppressed images and low signal on the T1-weighted images. This usually starts at the proximal pole, commonly along its radial aspect. The use of intravenous gadolinium to assess blood flow to the lunate has been advocated by some which would indicate potential viability of the bone. As the disease progresses, necrosis of the lunate would be seen as diffuse low signal intensity on both the T1- and T2-weighted images with lack of enhancement on the post-contrast images. If left untreated, this will lead to microfractures and collapse of the articular surfaces with secondary fragmentation. As carpal instability ensues, there can be malalignment with adjacent carpal bones and secondary osteoarthritic changes in the form of subchondral sclerosis and cystic changes.

An important differential diagnosis for abnormal appearance of the lunate on MRI is ulnar impaction syndrome which is seen as bone marrow edema and sclerosis localized to the proximal ulnar aspect of the lunate as opposed to the radial aspect in Kienböck's disease *(please refer to Case 3.3 for discussion on ulnar impaction syndrome)*.

Treatment for Kienböck's disease depends upon the stage and severity. In the early stages, treatment is with immobilization. For more advanced stages, surgery is performed.

Report checklist
1. Is there marrow edema in the lunate? (Diffuse edema is more consistent with Kienböck's disease, whereas subchondral edema near the ulnar articulation is suggestive of ulnar impaction syndrome)
2. Is there bone osteonecrosis evident by low signal on both T1- and T2-weighted images?
3. Is there subchondral collapse of the articular surface and/or fragmentation?
4. Is there malalignment and osteoarthritis with adjacent carpal articulations?
5. Is there ulnar negative variance?

Suggested Reading

Arnaiz J, Piedra T, Cerezal L, Ward J, Thompson A, Vidal JA, Canga A. Imaging of Kienböck disease. AJR Am J Roentgenol. 2014;203:131–9.

Chen WS. Kienböck disease and negative ulnar variance. J Bone Joint Surg Am. 2000;82:143–4.

Case 3.6

Indication A 27-year-old female with radial-sided wrist pain for 6 weeks. Assess for tendon tear.

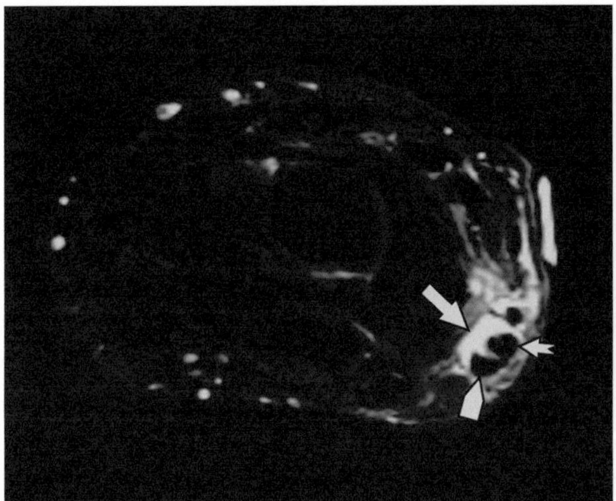

Axial T2 fat saturated

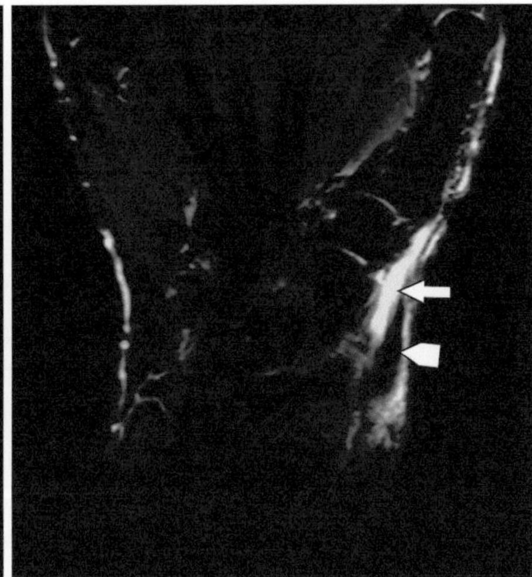

Coronal T2 fat saturated

Findings

There is a moderate amount of fluid in the tendon sheath (arrow) of both the abductor pollicis longus (block arrow) and extensor pollicis brevis (notched arrow) tendons consistent with tenosynovitis. There is also mild increase T2 signal in both tendons compatible with tendinosis.

Impression/Recommendation

Moderate tendinosis and tenosynovitis of the abductor pollicis longus and extensor pollicis brevis tendons (De Quervain's tenosynovitis)

Discussion: De Quervain's Tenosynovitis

The first extensor (dorsal) tendon compartment of the wrist is comprised of the extensor pollicis brevis (EPB) and the abductor pollicis longus (APL) tendons. The EPB and APL tendons are firmly held against the radial styloid by the covering retinaculum which creates a fibro-osseous tunnel. On normal MR imaging, these tendons are discrete black structures on all pulse sequences.

Tendinopathy and tenosynovial inflammation of the first extensor tendon compartment of the wrist is known as De Quervain's tenosynovitis. It is thought to be related to repetitive chronic overuse that can cause thickening and edema of the tendons and its associated retinaculum which restrains normal gliding within the sheath. This results in inflammation and additional edematous thickening of the tendons aggravating the local stenosing effect. Patients may be predisposed to De Quervain's tenosynovitis by an anatomical variation where there is a thin septum within the 1st extensor compartment that leads to two tunnels *(see supplementary images)*. De Quervain's tenosynovitis is usually diagnosed clinically in patients presenting with localized swelling and pain at the level of the radial styloid, and MRI is obtained to assess the underlying severity as well as evaluate for focal tears of the involved tendons. Findings on MRI include:

1. Tendinosis – is demonstrated by diffuse enlargement of the tendons as well as slightly increased intertendinous T1 and T2 signal compared to other tendons which should be uniformly dark. In more severe cases, linear high signal intensity within the tendon substance reaching fluid

signal should be considered a longitudinal split tear, and it is important to give an approximate percentage of involvement relative to the cross-sectional area of the tendon.

2. Tenosynovitis – has high T2 and low-intermediate T1 fluid in the tendon sheath. Intermediate T1 signal may also be seen which signifies debris within the sheath. Other MRI findings include peritendinous soft tissue edema, thickened edematous retinaculum, and reactive bone marrow edema in the adjacent radial styloid.

Evaluation for a small septum between the EPB and APL tendons within the tendon sheath should be sought out for, representing two tunnels and described in the report as this is important for presurgical planning.

It is important to consider other causes of tenosynovitis such as rheumatoid arthritis, and other inflammatory arthropathies, when the clinical presentation is atypical. Intersection syndrome, which occurs more proximally in the distal forearm, should also be considered. This condition occurs from peritendinous inflammatory changes at the site of intersection of the 1st and 2nd extensor tendon compartments about 4–6 cm proximal to the radiocarpal joint. Note should be made that this region is not always included in the field of view in routine wrist MRI, and if clinically suspected, imaging more proximally is needed to visualize this region which would demonstrate tendinosis and tenosynovitis at the region of crossing between the tendon compartments. Another differential diagnosis is an occult fracture of the scaphoid or distal radius if there is recent history of trauma.

MRI aids in guiding management by revealing the severity of individual tendon pathology, number of slips of each tendon, and presence of an intervening septum which aids in deciding the best treatment course. Conservative treatment includes rest, immobilization in a thumb spica brace, and nonsteroidal anti-inflammatory drugs. Ultrasound-guided injection with steroids can be performed. Surgery is usually reserved for cases that have failed conservative treatment.

Supplementary Images

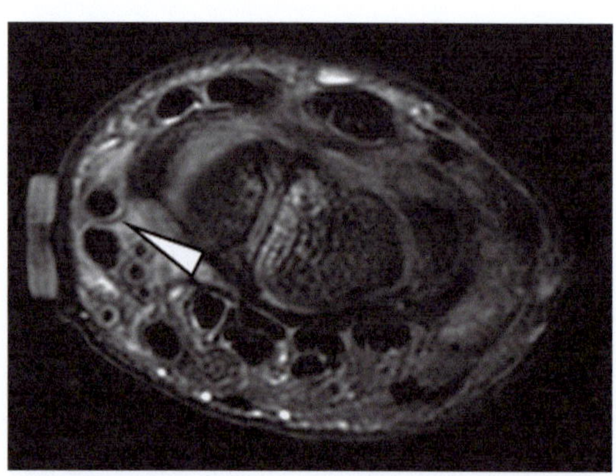

Axial T2 fat saturated

Thin septum (arrowhead) is seen between the extensor pollicis brevis (EPB) and abductor pollicis longus (APL) in the first extensor compartment. This anatomic variant can predispose patients to De Quervain's tenosynovitis

Report checklist

1. What is the degree of tendinosis of both tendons (extensor pollicis brevis (EPB) and abductor pollicis longus (APL)) as well as craniocaudal length of involvement?
2. Presence or absence of tenosynovitis and degree.
3. Is there is a longitudinal tendon split tear?
4. Is a thin septum in the tendon sheath between the two tendons visualized?
5. Is there reactive bone marrow edema within the adjacent radial styloid?

Suggested Reading

Anderson SE, Steinbach LS, De Monaco D, Bonel HM, Hurtienne Y, Voegelin E. "Baby wrist": MRI of an overuse syndrome in mothers. AJR Am J Roentgenol. 2004;182:719–24.

Meraj S, Gyftopoulos S, Nellans K, Walz D, Brown MS. MRI of the Extensor Tendons of the Wrist. AJR Am J Roentgenol. 2017;209:1093–102.

Case 3.7a

Indication A 38-year-old female presenting with volar-sided wrist mass.

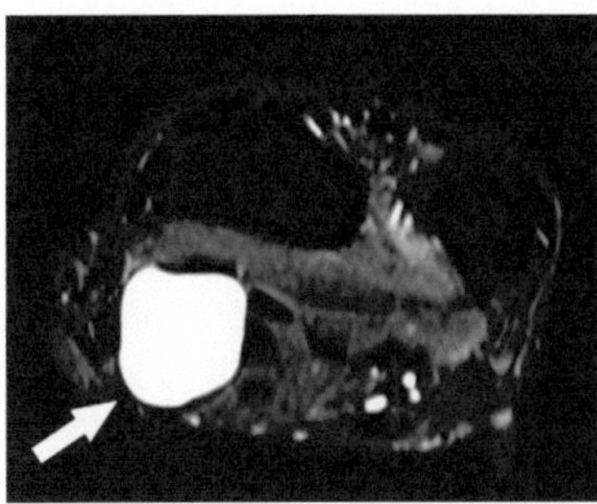
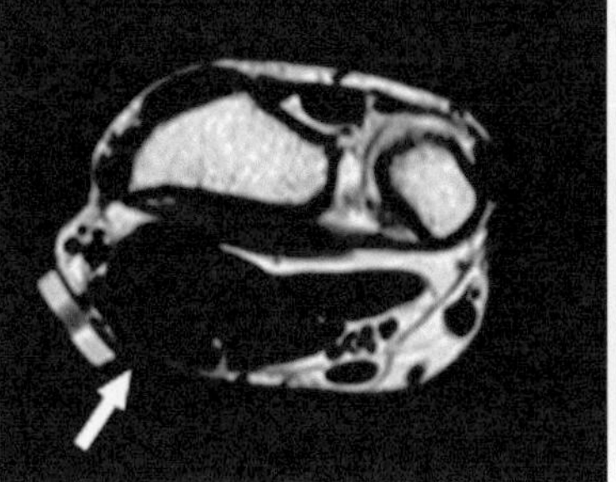
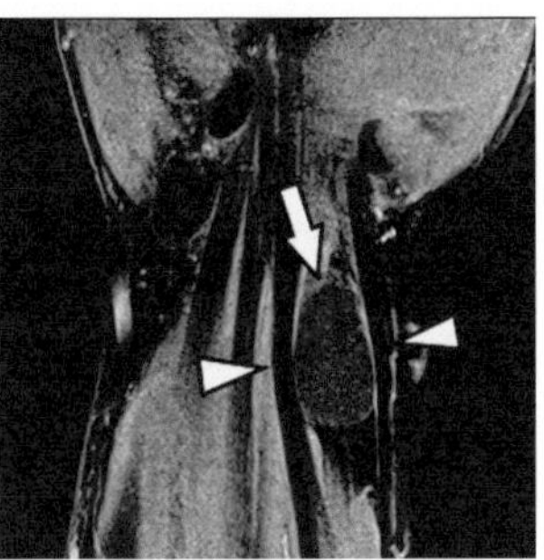

Axial T2 fat saturated

Axial T1

Coronal T1 fat saturated
post contrast

Findings
There is a 2.5 × 2.4 × 2.9 cm well-defined uni-locular cystic mass (arrows) at the radial aspect of the volar wrist demonstrating homogeneous hypointense signal on the T1- weighted images and high signal on the T2-weighted images. There is thin peripheral enhancement on the post-contrast images compatible with a cystic mass. The mass displaces the adjacent flexor tendons (arrowheads).

Case 3.7b

Indication A 52-year-old male with chronic dorsal wrist pain and swelling.

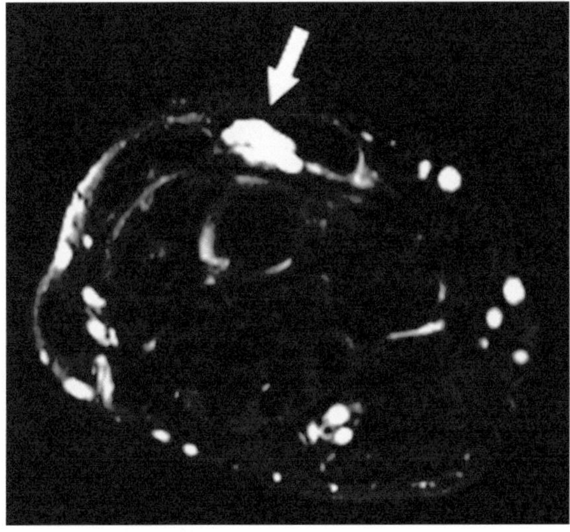
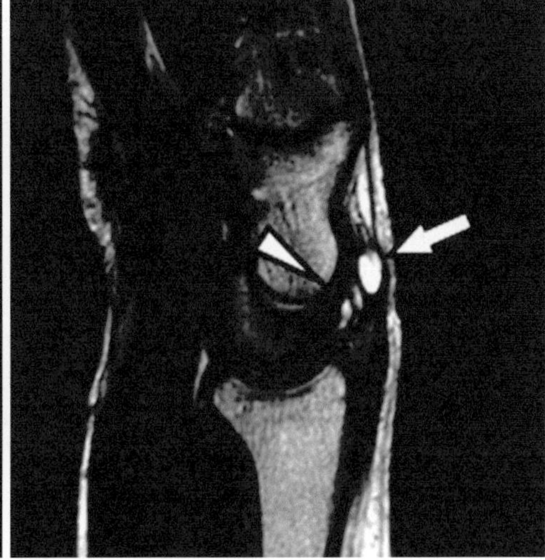

Axial T2 fat saturated

Sagittal T2

Findings

There is a small $0.9 \times 0.5 \times 1.2$ cm multiloculated cystic mass arising from the dorsal aspect of the wrist (arrows) demonstrating homogenous high signal on the T2- weighted images with a small neck extending to the dorsal scapholunate ligament (arrowhead).

Impression/Recommendation

- **Case 3.7a:** Ganglion cyst
- **Case 3.7b:** Ganglion cyst

Discussion: Ganglion Cyst

Ganglion cyst is the most common soft tissue mass in the hand and wrist. It is a nonneoplastic synovial lined cystic mass that results from mucoid degeneration of the adjacent tendon sheath, ligament, or joint capsule, where they commonly originate. They can occur in any location containing synovial tissue, but commonly occur at the dorsal aspect of the wrist and hand (60–70%), often near the scapholunate ligament. They are often seen incidentally on routine MRI examinations and are usually small and asymptomatic. However, patients can present with a palpable mass that can be painful or symptoms of nerve compression.

On MRI, ganglion cysts present as multilocular or unilocular lobular fluid signal masses with variable size. An important clue for its diagnosis is visualizing a small stalk arising from an adjacent tendon sheath, ligament, or joint capsule. Although ultrasound is very accurate in diagnosing superficial ganglion cysts, MRI is more helpful in evaluating deep ganglia as well as differentiating them from other soft tissue masses. Ganglia often contain proteinaceous material or internal hemorrhage resulting in isointense or hyperintense signal on the T1-weighted images. Also, they can be complicated by rupture, which results in soft tissue edema around an unevenly delineated cyst. After the administration of intravenous contrast, the ganglion should have a thin peripheral enhanc-

ing wall but may have internal septations. Giant cell tumor of the tendon sheath is a common lesion in the differential diagnosis, which would appear more solid in nature, often with hypointense T2 signal, and with heterogeneous enhancement. A small effusion may simulate a ganglion; however, the hint to diagnosis of a ganglion is the lack of fluid in the remainder of the joint and its focal nature.

It is important to properly describe the precise location of the cyst in your report for preoperative planning mainly in relation to adjacent anatomic landmarks as well as relation to adjacent structures. Beware of cyst-like neoplasms such as myxomas and peripheral nerve sheath tumors. When in doubt, contrast administration can be very helpful to show the peripheral/rim enhancement of a ganglion cyst.

More than half of ganglion cysts resolve without any treatment. Ultrasound-guided aspiration and steroid injection can be performed, but there is a high chance for recurrence. Surgical resection may be considered in severe cases especially with neurovascular manifestations.

Report checklist

1. What is the size and precise location of the ganglion cyst in relation to anatomic landmarks?
2. Is the ganglion cyst unilocular or multilocular?
3. Is there internal hemorrhage or rupture?
4. Is there a stalk seen to indicate its origin?
5. Is there mass effect on adjacent neurovascular structures?
6. Could this be a cystic-like neoplasm? If possible, consider giving intravenous contrast.

Suggested Reading

Freire V, Guérini H, Campagna R, Moutounet L, Dumontier C, Feydy A, Drapé JL. Imaging of hand and wrist cysts: a clinical approach. AJR Am J Roentgenol. 2012;199:W618–28.

Neto N, Nunnes P. Spectrum of MRI features of ganglion and synovial cysts. Insights Imaging. 2016;7(2):179–86.

Case 3.8

Indication A 44-year-old female with wrist pain and swelling for 3 months. MRI to assess for flexor tenosynovitis.

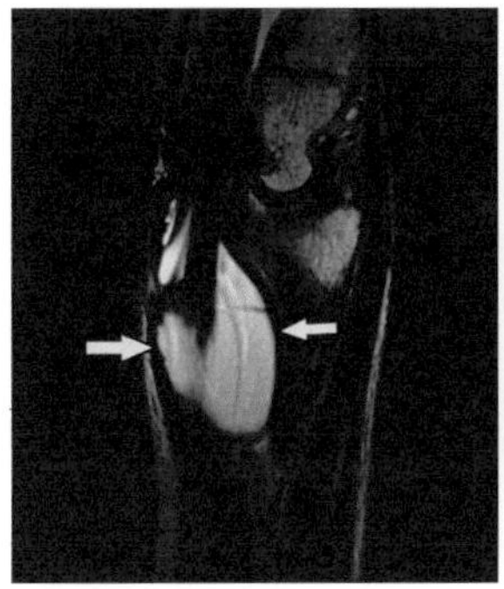 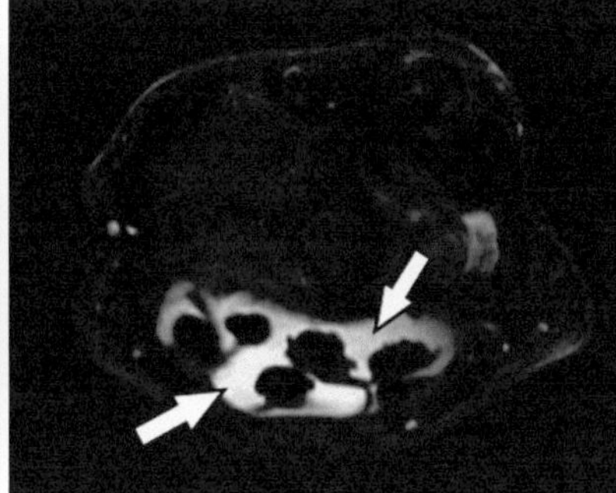 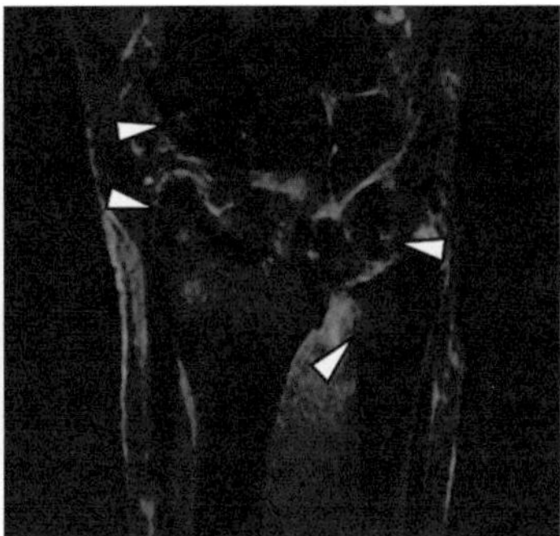

Sagittal T2   Axial T2 fat saturated   Coronal T2 fat saturated

Findings

There is severe distention of the flexor tendon sheath within and just proximal to the carpal tunnel with fluid compatible with severe tenosynovitis (arrows). The underlying flexor tendons are intact without tendinosis or focal tear. There is also bone marrow edema and erosions (arrowheads) along the distal radius and ulna as well as the bones of the proximal carpal row, consistent with an inflammatory arthritis.

Impression/Recommendation

Severe flexor tenosynovitis secondary to an inflammatory arthritis (rheumatoid arthritis)

Discussion: Flexor Tenosynovitis

The flexor tendons of the wrist and hand are terminal functional units of the forearm muscles. They arise from the medial humeral epicondyle, and at the level of the wrist, divide into two groups. Some travel within and others outside of the carpal tunnel. The nine tendons within the carpal tunnel include the flexor pollicis longus (FPL) tendon to the thumb, four tendons of the flexor digitorum profundus (FDP) which insert at the base of the distal phalanges, and four tendons of the flexor digitorum superficialis (FDS) which insert at the base of the middle phalanges. The three tendons that do not traverse the carpal tunnel include the palmaris longus, the flexor carpi radialis (FCR), and flexor carpi ulnaris (FCU) tendons. Within the carpal tunnel, the flexor tendons are enveloped in two bursae which extend from the level of the distal radius to the mid-palm distally. The FPL is surrounded by the smaller radial bursa, while the larger ulnar bursa surrounds the remaining eight flexor digitorum tendons. These bursae are not visible on MRI unless distended by fluid. In general, bursae do not connect to the joint space but can have synovial tissue.

On a normal MRI of the hand, flexor tendons are easily viewed on axial images. They can be noted as distinct black bundles on both the T1- and T2-weighted sequences. The tenosynovial fluid surrounding them is more apparent on fluid-sensitive sequences.

Inflammation of the synovial sheath surrounding a flexor tendon is referred to as tenosynovitis. This typically presents with pain, swelling, and stiffness either at the wrist or of the affected digit. Typically, greater than 50% of the circumference of the tendon sheath should contain fluid before tenosynovitis is reported. The causes of flexor tenosynovitis can be broadly divided into infectious and noninfectious etiologies. Noninfectious tenosynovitis usually occurs from repeated microtrauma or from an inflammatory arthropathy like rheumatoid arthritis. Infection of the synovial sheath is often bacterial in origin, caused by trauma or via systemic spread, or less commonly due to mycobacterium. The synovium is often thickened, and there can be associated cellulitis.

On MRI, flexor tenosynovitis is classically seen as increased fluid signal intensity in the tendon sheath with distention and synovial proliferation. The underlying tendons are usually normal, but there can be tendinosis, and in severe cases, they can have interstitial tears. It is often difficult to identify the underlying etiology based on MRI findings alone, and correlation with patient's clinical presentation is often required. Scarring or fibrosis within the tendon sheath identified as focal areas of low signal septa or nodules, suggesting stenosing tenosynovitis. Interestingly, tenosynovitis of the FCR is frequently associated with osteoarthritis of the triscaphe joint given their intimate anatomic relationship.

Treatment of infectious flexor tenosynovitis involves antibiotic therapy and minimally invasive irrigation procedures. Noninfectious flexor tenosynovitis is usually managed with nonsteroidal anti-inflammatory drugs along with corticosteroid injections.

Report checklist
1. Which tendon sheath is involved?
2. What is the craniocaudal extent of involvement?
3. Is there tendinosis or tearing of the underlying tendon?
4. Is there distention of the radial and ulnar palmar bursae?
5. Could this be infectious tenosynovitis? Is there synovial thickening and associated soft tissue swelling?
6. Could this be the initial presentation of an inflammatory arthritis like rheumatoid arthritis?

Suggested Reading

Plotkin B, Sampath SC, Sampath SC, Motamedi K. MR Imaging and US of the Wrist Tendons. Radiographics. 2016;36:1688–700.

Ragheb D, Stanley A, Gentili A, Hughes T, Chung CB. MR imaging of the finger tendons: normal anatomy and commonly encountered pathology. Eur J Radiol. 2005;56:296–306.

Case 3.9

Indication A 22-year-old male with ulnar-sided thumb pain after trauma. Evaluate ulnar collateral ligament.

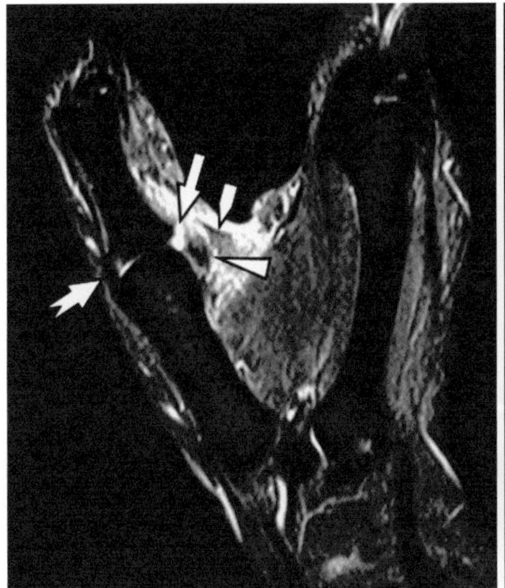

Coronal T2 fat saturated

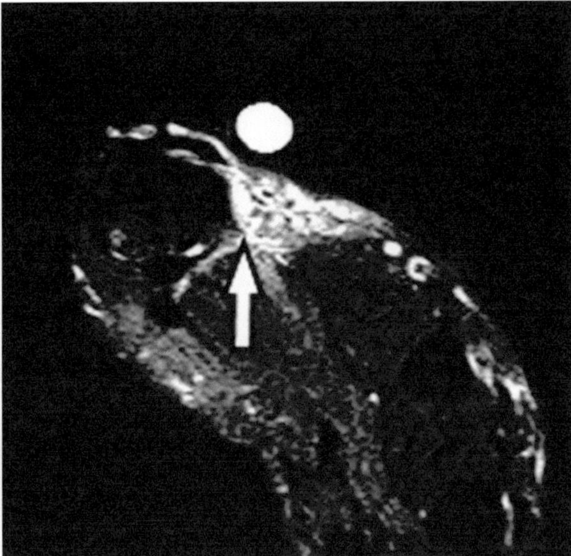

Axial T2 fat saturated

Findings

There is a full-thickness tear of the 1st MCP joint ulnar collateral ligament (UCL). The UCL (arrowhead) is thickened and retracted proximally by 2 mm, and there is fluid (arrows) at its expected distal attachment onto the first proximal phalanx base. There is adjacent soft tissue edema. The UCL is normally positioned deep to the adductor aponeurosis (block arrow). The radial collateral ligament (notched arrow) is normal. There is no associated cortical bony avulsion or a Stener lesion.

Impression/Recommendation

Full-thickness tear of the ulnar collateral ligament at the MCP joint of the thumb (Gamekeeper's thumb). No Stener lesion is seen.

Discussion: Gamekeeper's Thumb

Dynamic and static stabilizers support the metacarpophalangeal joint of the thumb. The dynamic stabilizers are the extrinsic muscles of the thumb.

The static restraints include the volar plate, the dorsal capsule, and the radial and ulnar collateral ligaments. The ulnar collateral ligament originates from the head of the 1st metacarpal bone and insert on the volar side of the proximal phalanx. On MRI, the normal UCL appears as a thick, homogenously hypointense band. The aponeurosis of the adductor pollicis muscle is seen as a thin hypointense band lying superficial to the UCL.

Tear of the UCL can occur from excessive valgus force resulting in a lesion known as "gamekeeper's thumb" or "skier's thumb." Proper MRI imaging technique is important for optimal visualization of the UCL. First a small field of view centered at the thumb will improve spatial resolution. Also the imaging planes must be performed coronal and sagittal to the thumb rather than the hand. This is especially important for the coronal plane, where UCL tears are best seen.

Injuries to the UCL may be a sprain, partial thickness, or full-thickness tears. In a low-grade sprain, there will be edema and thickening of the ligament, but the ligament is otherwise still intact. Partial-thickness tears show thinning and fluid signal intensity within the ligament, but some fibers should still be visualized. Full-thickness tears usually involve the distal attachment of the ligament, which would be seen as complete disruption of the fibers with fluid signal intensity interposed at the site of tear. The UCL typically remains deep to the adductor aponeurosis without significant retraction. However, not uncommonly, the torn UCL retracts proximally and folds back on itself, lying superficial to the adductor aponeu-

rosis termed a "Stener lesion." The retracted ligament would appear rounded which has been called the "yo-yo on a string" sign, with the string representing the adductor aponeurosis and yo-yo representing the rounded and proximally retracted UCL *(see supplementary images)*.

At times, a small avulsion bony fragment can be seen at the distal attachment of the UCL on the proximal phalanx.

Partial and non-displaced full-thickness tears are treated by immobilization, while both bony avulsions and Stener lesions require surgical repair.

Supplementary Images

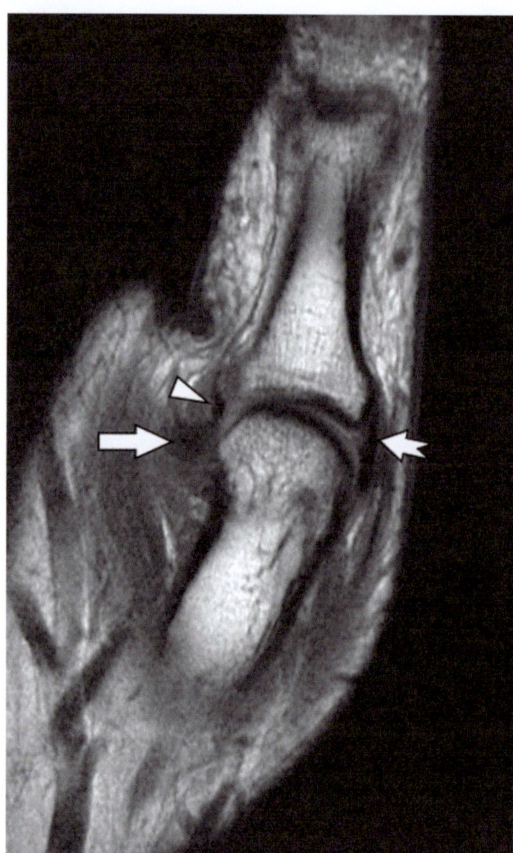

Coronal T1

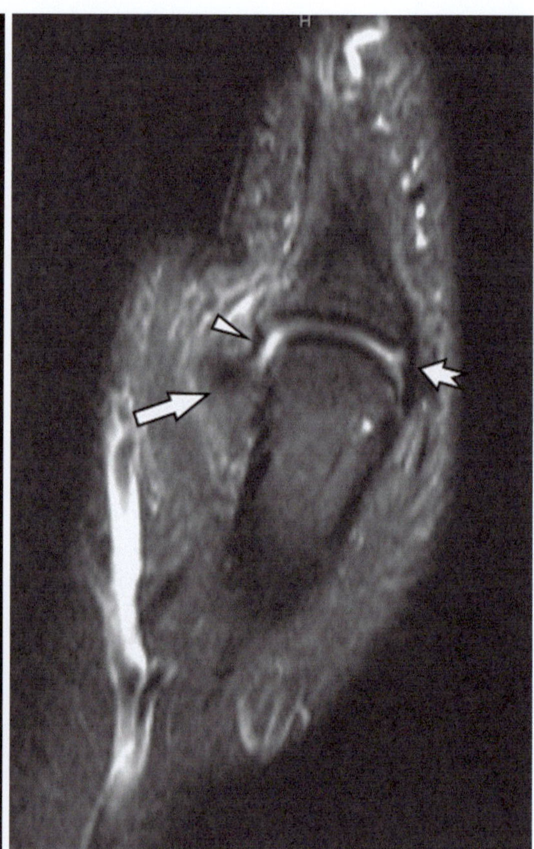

Coronal T2 fat saturated

UCL tear with Stener lesion. There is marked thickening and intermediate signal of the torn and retracted UCL (arrows). The adductor aponeurosis (arrowheads) is seen as a linear low signal structure interposed between the base of the proximal phalanx and the retracted UCL, compatible with a Stener lesion. This has been called the "yo-yo on a string" sign. The adductor aponeurosis should normally lie superficial to the UCL. The radial collateral ligament (notched arrows) is intact. (Case is courtesy of Dr. Andrew Haims)

Report checklist

1. Is there an injury to the UCL (sprain, partial tear, full-thickness tear)?
2. Describe the location of the tear (proximal, midsubstance, or distal)?
3. Is there a bony avulsion fragment?
4. Is there retraction of the UCL and is it entrapped superficial to the adductor aponeurosis (Stener lesion)?

Suggested Reading

Hirschmann A, Sutter R, Schweizer A, Pfirrmann CW. MRI of the thumb: anatomy and spectrum of findings in asymptomatic volunteers. AJR Am J Roentgenol. 2014;202:819–27.

Milner CS, Manon-Matos Y, Thirkannad SM. Gamekeeper's thumb – a treatment-oriented magnetic resonance imaging classification. Send to J Hand Surg Am. 201540(1):90–5.

Case 3.10

Indication A 22-year-old male with decreased range of motion and pain at the ring finger after a laceration 5 weeks ago. Evaluate extensor tendon.

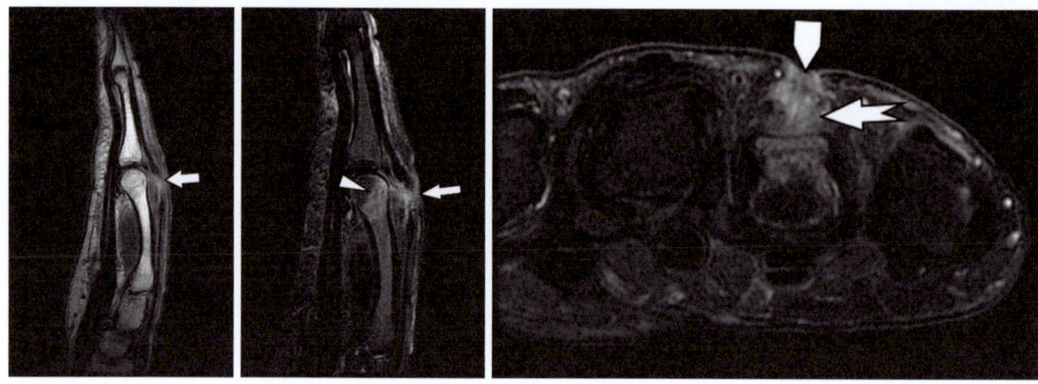

Sagittal T2   Sagittal T2 fat saturated   Axial T2 fat saturated

Findings

There is a complete tear of the ring finger extensor digitorum tendon at the level of the metacarpal head with a tendon gap of approximately 1 cm (arrow). There is associated soft tissue edema (notched arrow) and a soft tissue defect (block arrow). Minimal bone marrow edema at the metacarpal head (arrowhead) is likely related to a contusion.

Impression/Recommendation

Complete tear of the extensor digitorum tendon of the ring finger.

Discussion: Extensor Tendon Injury

Each digit has a single extensor tendon which attaches at the dorsal aspect of the joint capsule at the level of the metacarpophalangeal (MCP), proximal interphalangeal (PIP), and distal interphalangeal (DIP) joints. An adequately performed, small field of view MRI in the axial and sagittal planes of the involved finger is crucial for adequate visualization and assessment of the tendons which are uniformly low signal intensity on all pulse sequences. At the level of the MCP joint, the extensor tendon is stabilized by the sagittal bands which are major components of the extensor hood. The sagittal band is best seen on the axial plane and appears as a thin low signal intensity structure extending from the palmar aspect of the volar plate of the MCP joint to the dorsal aspect of the extensor tendon. Distal to the MCP joint, the extensor tendon splits into two lateral bands and a central slip. The central slip attaches at the base of the middle phalanx, while the lateral bands fuse with fibers from the intrinsic tendons that distally converge to form the terminal tendon which inserts at the base of the distal phalanx.

Injury to the extensor tendon can range from tendinosis, tenosynovitis, partial tears, and ultimately full-thickness tears and can be divided into either open or closed injuries. Open injuries can be caused by penetrating trauma or laceration. The presence of increased fluid signal intensity on T2-weighted images within the tendon substance suggests a partial tear, while complete disruption of the tendon with retraction of the torn tendon fibers suggests a complete tear. It is important to describe whether the tear is partial or full thickness as well as describe the length of the tendon gap. In closed injuries, a tear of the extensor tendon at the level of the DIP joint results in a mallet finger which may or may not be associated with a small avulsion fracture from the dorsal base of distal phalanx. A tear of the central slip tendon from its middle phalangeal base insertion at the level of the PIP joint leads to a boutonniere deformity. These tears are usually full thickness, and the amount of tendon retraction as well as the presence of bony avulsion should be documented.

Tear of the sagittal bands of the extensor hood can cause dislocation of the extensor tendon at the MCP joint, most commonly to the ulnar aspect. This is best visualized on the axial plane which would show disruption of the normal low signal intensity sagittal band either on one or both sides of the MCP joint with surrounding soft tissue edema.

Treatment broadly depends on the site and nature of the injury. It can either be immobilized by splinting or surgically repaired.

Report checklist
1. Location of the tendon tear
2. Is it a partial- or full-thickness tear?
3. The length of the tendon gap
4. Is there an associated bony avulsion and what is its size?
5. Is the sagittal band intact or torn?
6. Is there dislocation of the tendon to the radial or ulnar aspect of the digit?

Suggested Reading

Clavero JA, Alomar X, Monill JM, Esplugas M, Golanó P, Mendoza M, Salvador A. MR imaging of ligament and tendon injuries of the fingers. Radiographics. 2002;22:237–56.

Gupta P, Lenchik L, Wuertzer SD, Pacholke DA. High-resolution 3-T MRI of the fingers: review of anatomy and common tendon and ligament injuries. AJR Am J Roentgenol. 2015;204:W314–23.

Case 3.11

Indication A 28-year-old male with flexion deformity and pain at the ring finger after a rock climbing injury 5 days prior.

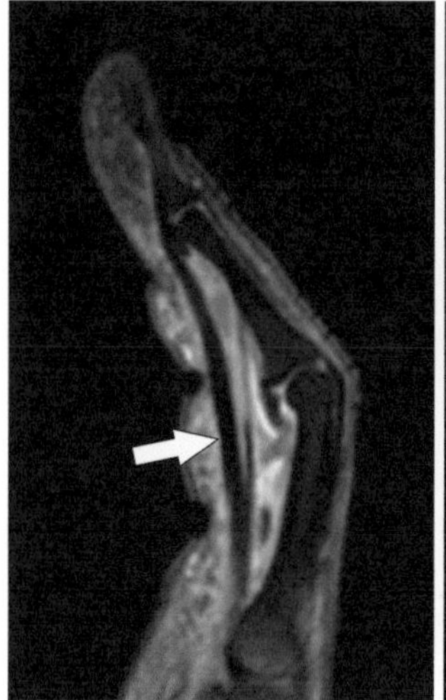
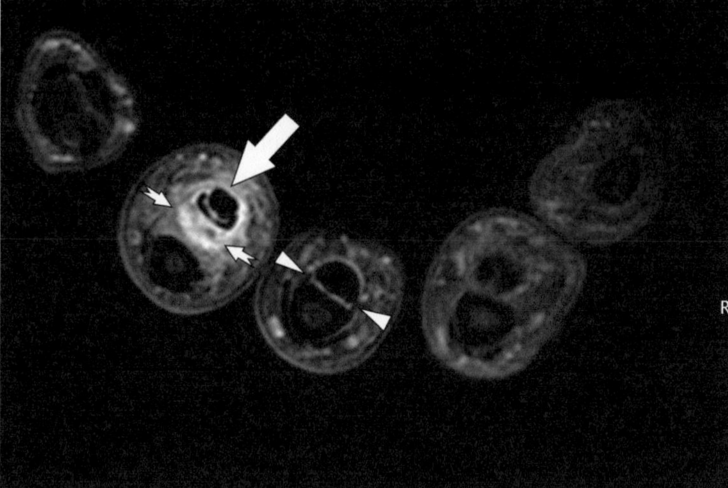

Sagittal T2 fat saturated   Axial T2 fat saturated

Findings
There is complete tear of the A2, A3, and A4 pulleys with displacement of the flexor tendon (arrows) from the underlying bones (bowstringing sign). This is associated with soft tissue edema between the flexor tendon and underlying bone (notched arrows). The flexor tendon is otherwise still intact. The other digits are intact. (Note the normal A2 tendon pulley (arrowheads) of the long finger).

Impression/Recommendation
Complete tear of A2, A3, and A4 pulleys at the ring finger.

Discussion: Flexor pulley injury
The flexor tendon pulley system is a fibro-osseous tunnel on the palmar aspect of each digit, through which the deep and superficial flexor tendons pass and represent focal condensations of the tendon sheath. This pulley system maintains proper position of the flexor tendons against the phalanges, thus preventing bowstringing during flexion. In the thumb, the flexor tendon pulley system is composed of two annular pulleys (A pulleys) and a single oblique pulley. In the remaining digits, there are five A pulleys and three cruciate pulleys. The narrow A pulleys (A1, A3, and A5) overlie the palmar aspect of the metacarpophalangeal, proximal interphalangeal, and distal interphalangeal joints, respectively. The broad A pulleys (A2 and A4) are located between joints. The A2 and A4 pulleys are the strongest and functionally most important. On a normal MRI of the hand, the pulleys appear as focal thickenings of low signal intensity and are best appreciated on T1 imaging without fat saturation. The A2 and A4 pulleys are almost always visible, while the other pulleys are not routinely visualized on conventional MRI.

The flexor tendon pulleys may rupture, usually in a flexed finger that is forcibly extended. Such injuries are seen in activities such as rock climbing, in which extreme stress may be inflicted upon the pulley system. In comparison to other segments, the A2 segment is most commonly affected, and its injury is also associated with the most morbidity. This can then extend in a predictable sequence to involve the A3 and A4 pulleys. The A1 pulley is rarely injured.

MRI is highly accurate in diagnosing a pulley rupture and is especially useful in the acute phase, where pain and soft tissue swelling may make clinical examination difficult. Axial imaging is the main imaging plane for evaluating the pulleys, and an injury is indicated when there is an attenuated or ruptured sheath with surrounding soft tissue edema. Axial imaging is mainly used for evaluating the integrity of the lateral attachments of the pulleys. The sagittal plane can also be helpful where there will be non-visualization of the normal focal thickening anterior to the flexor tendon. Another method for evaluating the integrity of the pulley system involves obtaining two sets of sagittal images of the affected finger: one with the finger in full extension and another one at approximately 45 degrees of flexion. The position of the flexor tendons is noted in each case. If a pulley rupture is present, the flexor tendons will be markedly separated from the underlying bone when the digit is flexed "bowstring sign." Other secondary findings would be soft tissue edema between the flexor tendon and adjacent bone as well as tenosynovitis of the affected tendon sheath.

Treatment depends on the type of rupture; all complete A2 and A4 pulley ruptures require surgical intervention. Ruptures of A1, A3, and A5 may be managed conservatively.

Report checklist
1. Which pulley is involved?
2. Is the pulley sprained or completely disrupted?
3. Is there bowstringing of the flexor tendon?
4. Is there associated tenosynovitis of the flexor tendon sheath?

Suggested Reading

Gupta P, Lenchik L, Wuertzer SD, Pacholke DA. High-resolution 3-T MRI of the fingers: review of anatomy and common tendon and ligament injuries. AJR Am J Roentgenol. 2015;204:W314–23.

Hoff MN, Greenberg TD. MRI sport-specific pulley imaging. Skeletal Radiol. 2018;47: 989–92.

Case 4.1

Indication A 29-year-old soccer player with right hip pain and clicking sensation. Assess for labral tear.

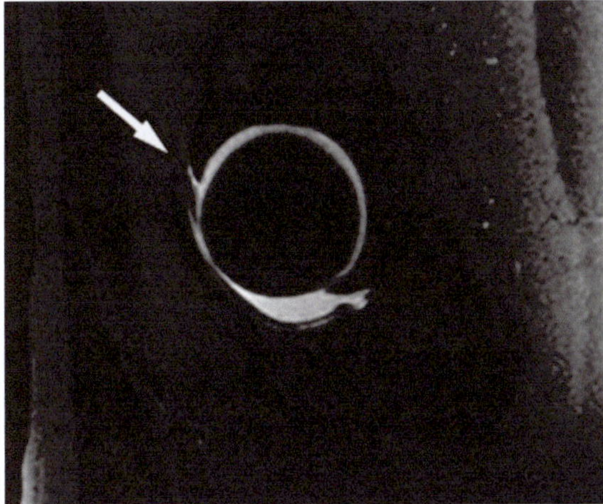

Sagittal T1 fat saturated (MR arthrogram)

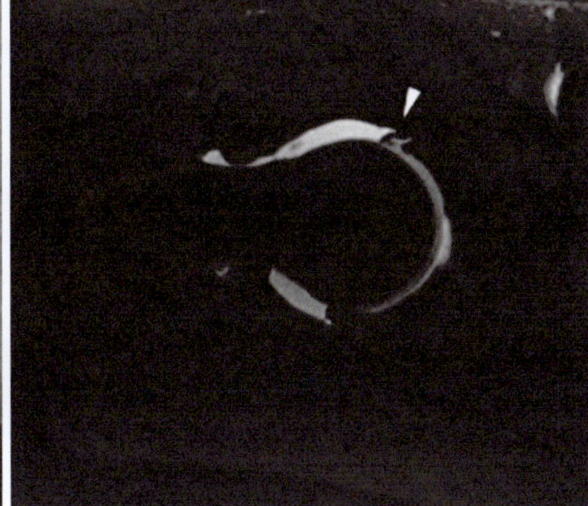

Axial oblique T1 fat saturated (MR arthrogram)

Findings
There is abnormal extension of intra-articular contrast between the base of the labrum and acetabular rim (arrow) at the anterosuperior quadrant (2 o'clock position) with extension into the anterior labral substance at the 3 o'clock position (arrowhead). Findings are compatible with a detached labral tear. There is no displaced labral fragment. The adjacent cartilage surface is intact without chondral loss. There is no paralabral cyst.

Impression/Recommendation
Full-thickness labral detachment and intrasubstance tear.

Discussion: Acetabular Labrum Tear
The fibrocartilaginous labrum attaches to the acetabulum which deepens the acetabular fossa making the hip more stable. The labrum extends 270° around the acetabulum being incomplete inferiorly. At its inferior aspect, the transverse liga-

© Springer Nature Switzerland AG 2020

T. M. Hegazi, J. S. Wu, *Musculoskeletal MRI*, https://doi.org/10.1007/978-3-030-26777-3_4

ment extends between the anteroinferior and posteroinferior acetabular notches. On MRI, the normal labrum appears triangular and homogeneously hypointense on all pulse sequences *(see supplementary images)*.

A few normal variants at the hip joint can be mistaken for labral injuries, and hence knowledge of these variants is essential. The hip joint capsule attaches to the acetabular rim, and a small amount of joint fluid may extend between the labrum and the capsule, called a perilabral sulcus. This should not be misinterpreted as a labral tear or paralabral cyst. This is commonly seen on the coronal images between the superior labrum and joint capsule. There are normal sublabral sulci at the chondrolabral junction. They can occur in any quadrant, however more commonly at the posterosuperior and posterior quadrants *(see supplementary images)*. There is debate in the literature on the presence of sulci at the anterior and anterosuperior quadrants. Nevertheless, to differentiate between a normal sulcus and a labral tear, any high signal intensity extending into the labral substance should be linear and smooth in a sulcus, but is irregular in a labral tear. Also, the high signal intensity in normal sublabral sulcus should extend by less than 50% of the depth of the labrum, while a labral tear should be called when it extends by more than 50% of the depth. Any abnormal signal extending into the labral substance should be considered a tear (intrasubstance tear) and not a sulcus. The labrum may have a slightly irregular or rounded morphology in older patients, representing normal degeneration. In fact, labral abnormalities are commonly found in 30% of asymptomatic patients.

Labral injuries include degeneration and fibrillation, labral detachment at the chondrolabral junction, or intrasubstance labral tears. Labral injuries can be post-traumatic, degenerative, or impingement related. Conventional MRI utilizing small field of view and high-resolution imaging can visualize labral tears; however, MR arthrography is usually recommended for better detection and evaluation of labral injuries with higher accuracy.

Intrasubstance degeneration is usually seen as intermediate signal within the labral substance but does not extend to the labral surface. Labral tears manifest as linear high signal intensity or extension of intra-articular contrast to the articular surface of the labrum. Labral detachment is seen as separation at the base of the labrum. Labral detachment or tears associated with femoroacetabular impingement are usually located at the anterosuperior quadrant in cam-type impingement and the posterosuperior quadrant in pincer-type impingement *(please refer to case 4.4 for further discussion on femoroacetabular impingement)*. Traumatic tears are usually located in the anterior quadrant. When describing labral injuries, first describe if the injury is labral degeneration, labral tear, or labral detachment. Then describe the location and extent of the labral injury in terms of four quadrants: anterior, anterosuperior, posterosuperior, or posterior quadrant as well as in terms of a clock face, with the anterior aspect at 3:00 and the superior aspect at 12:00 positions. Anterior labral tears are best visualized on axial and sagittal planes, while superior labral tears are best seen on the coronal and sagittal planes.

Labral tears may be associated with a paralabral cyst which is seen adjacent to the labral tear and usually 1–2 cm in size *(see supplementary images)*. They can be multiloculated with internal septations. Not uncommonly, paralabral cysts can be quite large (4–5 cm) and can also erode into the adjacent bone. In approximately 30% of patients with labral tears, there are associated chondral lesions and most commonly located within the anterosuperior quadrant adjacent to the labral tear. Description of associated chondral abnormalities is important. This includes the location and size of the chondral loss, partial thickness or full thickness, and the presence of subchondral cystic changes and marginal osteophytes indicating hip joint osteoarthritis. Lastly, there may be an associated reactive joint effusion and intra-articular loose bodies.

Treatment of labral injuries is initially conservative with activity modification, anti-inflammatory medications, and intra-articular steroid injections. Surgery includes labral debridement or repair.

Supplementary Images

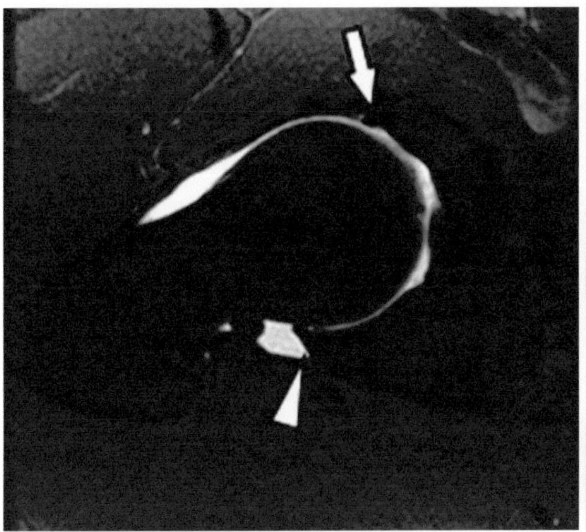

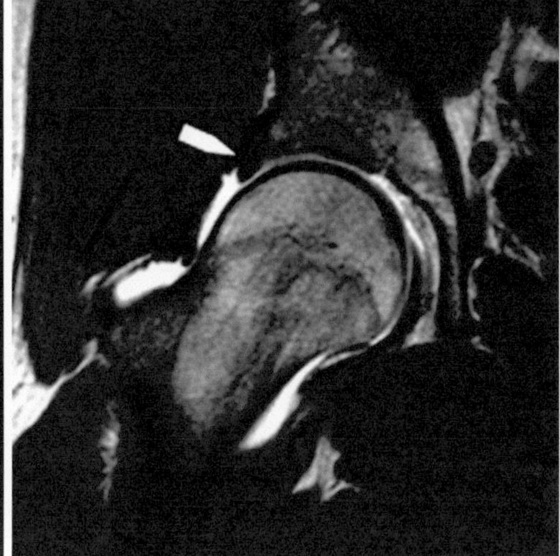

Oblique axial T1 fat saturated (MR arthrogram)   Coronal T1 (MR arthrogram)

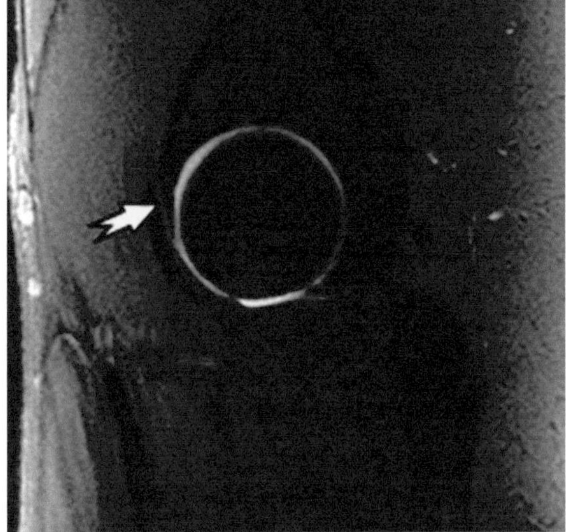

Sagittal T1 fat saturated (MR arthrogram)

Normal appearance of the hip labrum. Axial plane shows the anterior (arrow) and posterior labrum (arrowhead), coronal plane shows the anterosuperior labrum (block arrow), and sagittal plane shows the anterior labrum (notched arrow). Note that the labrum has a triangular appearance in all planes

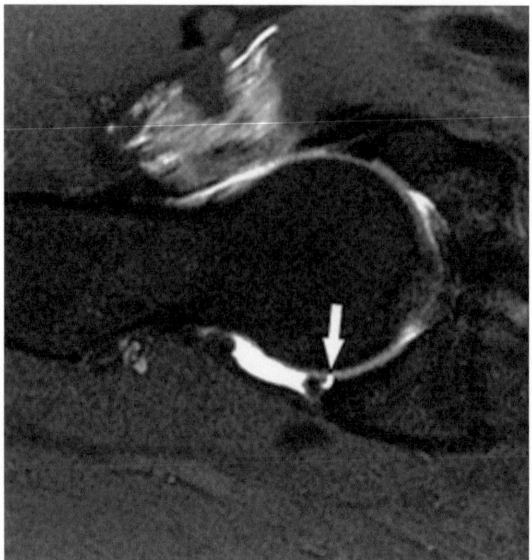

Axial oblique T1 fat saturated (MR arthrogram)

Intra-articular contrast undermines the posterior labrum demonstrating smooth rounded contours extending less than 50% of the depth of the labrum (arrow) most compatible with a sublabral sulcus

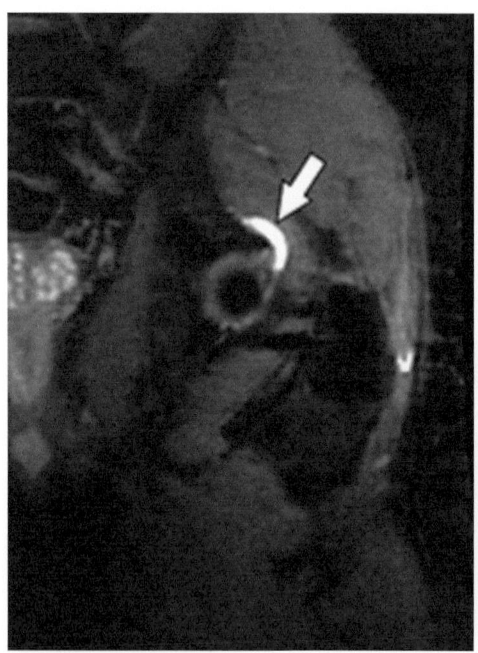

Coronal T2 fat saturated

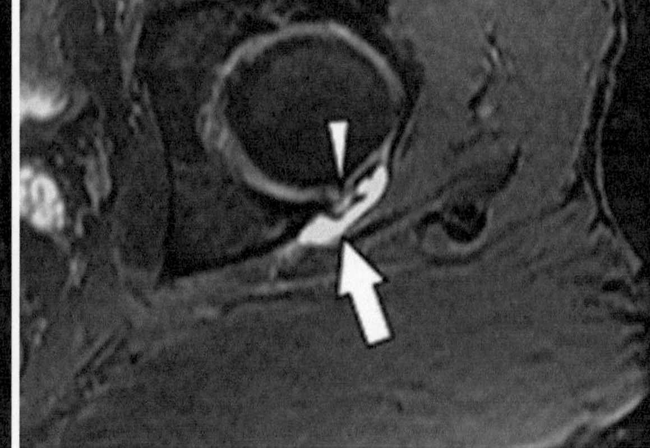

Axial T2 fat saturated

Paralabral cyst in a 45-year-old man with hip pain. There is a 2.0 × 0.4 cm T2 hyperintense lesion (arrows) along the posterior aspect of the hip joint. There is hyperintense signal within the posterior labrum consistent with an intrasubstance tear (arrowhead)

Report checklist

1. Is there labral degeneration, labral detachment, or an intrasubstance labral tear?
2. Where is the labral injury located? (Use quadrant and/or clock face position)
3. Is there a displaced labral fragment?
4. Is there associated cartilage loss and subchondral cystic changes?
5. Is there a paralabral cyst?
6. Is there a joint effusion (if non-arthrogram MR study)?

Suggested Reading

Rakhra KS. Magnetic resonance imaging of acetabular labral tears. J Bone Joint Surg Am. 2011;93 Suppl 2:28–34.

Toomayan GA, Holman WR, Major NM, Kozlowicz SM, Vail TP. Sensitivity of MR arthrography in the evaluation of acetabular labral tears. AJR Am J Roentgenol. 2006;186(2):449–53.

Case 4.2

Indication A 44-year-old female with left hip pain for 2 weeks. Plain radiographs were normal. MRI performed to rule out a femoral neck fracture.

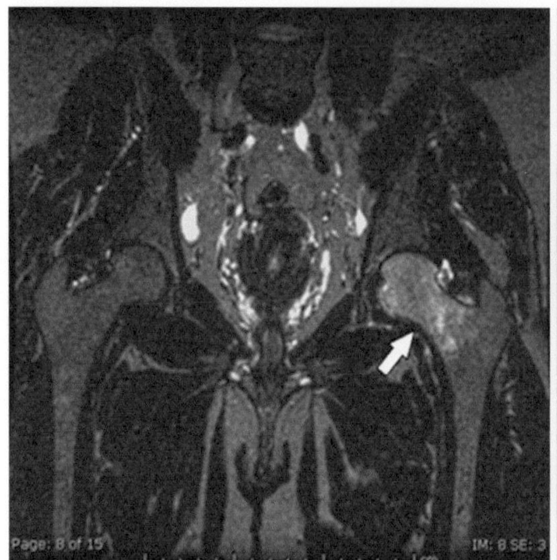

Coronal STIR

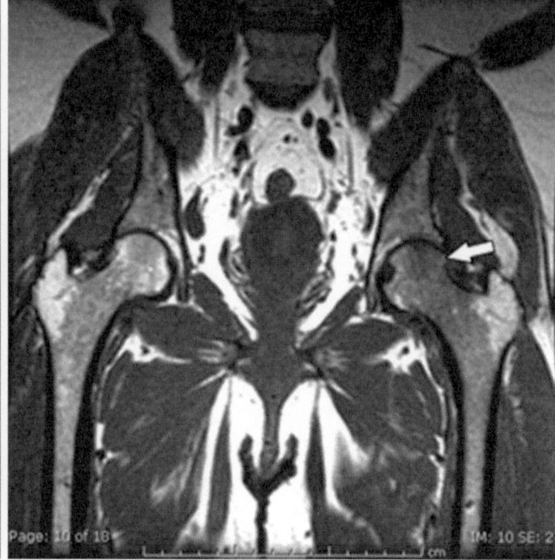

Coronal T1

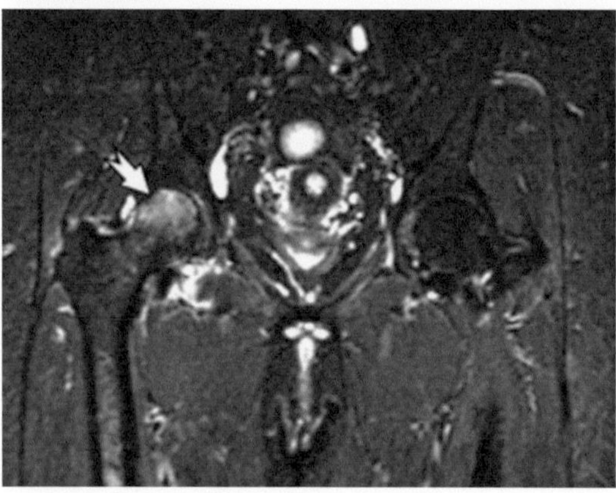

Coronal STIR (4 months prior)

Findings

Since the prior study from October 3, 2018 (4 months prior), there has been resolution of the marrow edema in the right femoral head. There is now new moderate bone marrow edema in the left femoral head and neck (arrow) on the T2-weighted images without a fracture line. There is corresponding hypointense signal in the left proximal femur (arrow) on the T1-weighted images. There is no collapse of the articular surface, and the overlying articular surface is intact. The left acetabulum is normal. There is no hip joint effusion.

Impression/Recommendation

Transient osteoporosis of the left hip. Rest and limited weight-bearing are recommended.

Discussion: Transient Osteoporosis of the Hip (TOH)

Transient osteoporosis of the hip is an idiopathic, self-limited bone marrow edema of the femoral head and neck. The exact cause is unknown; however, it is thought to represent an occult subchondral insufficiency fracture that is not seen on MRI. Clinically, patients usually present with sudden onset of hip pain without a preceding traumatic event. It was first described in pregnant women in the third trimester but is more commonly seen in men in the fourth to sixth decades. Although transient osteoporosis can affect any joint of the lower extremity, it is more commonly seen in the hip. It is commonly misinterpreted by radiologists as early avascular necrosis of the femoral head; however, these conditions should be differentiated since the treatment is different. TOH is usually treated by rest, NSAIDs, and limiting weight-bearing.

On MRI, TOH appears as diffuse bone marrow edema (diffuse high signal intensity on T2 fat-suppressed or STIR sequences and low signal intensity on T1-weighted images) of the femoral head which can extend to the femoral neck and intertrochanteric region. Most cases have an associated small to moderate hip joint effusion. A small hypointense crescentic fracture line that is parallel to the subchondral plate can be seen in many of the cases; however, this usually requires high resolution, small field of view imaging of the hip to be appropriately seen.

If a clear subchondral fracture line is seen at the femoral head, then this can be confidently diagnosed as a subchondral insufficiency fracture. If no clear fracture line is seen, then this can be diagnosed as TOH. A comment should also be made on the articular surface contour, if there is collapse or still preserved. To differentiate these two conditions from avascular necrosis (AVN) of the femoral head, few points need to be addressed. AVN usually does not have as much bone marrow edema as TOH or possess a subchondral insufficiency fracture. Moreover, if there is bone marrow edema in AVN, then this is usually localized to the femoral head. Also, TOH lacks the typical serpiginous "double line sign" seen in osteonecrosis. There is preservation of the normal spherical contour of the femoral head in TOH, while in more advanced AVN, there can be collapse of the articular surface with underlying subchondral cystic changes. In atypical cases, dynamic contrast-enhanced MRI can be performed which will show early hyperenhancement in TOH due to the hyperemia, while there is no enhancement in early avascular necrosis (*please refer to case 4.3 for further discussion on femoral head AVN*).

TOH typically resolves both clinically and on MRI within 6–8 months with rest and limited weight-bearing.

Report checklist
1. Describe the location and extent of the bone marrow edema.
2. Is there any linear hypointense signal parallel to the subchondral plate to indicate a subchondral insufficiency fracture?
3. Is there collapse of the femoral head articular surface?
4. Is there associated cartilage loss and/or subchondral cystic changes?
5. Is there bone marrow edema in the acetabulum or is it spared?
6. Is there a joint effusion?

Suggested Reading

Hayes CW, Conway WF, Daniel WW. MR imaging of bone marrow edema pattern: transient osteoporosis, transient bone marrow edema syndrome, or osteonecrosis. Radiographics. 1993;13(5):1001–11.

Szwedowski D, Nitek Z, Walecki J. Evaluation of transient osteoporosis of the hip in magnetic resonance imaging. Pol J Radiol. 2014;79:36–8.

Case 4.3

Indication A 28-year-old man with known sickle cell disease with worsening left hip pain. MRI performed to assess for avascular necrosis.

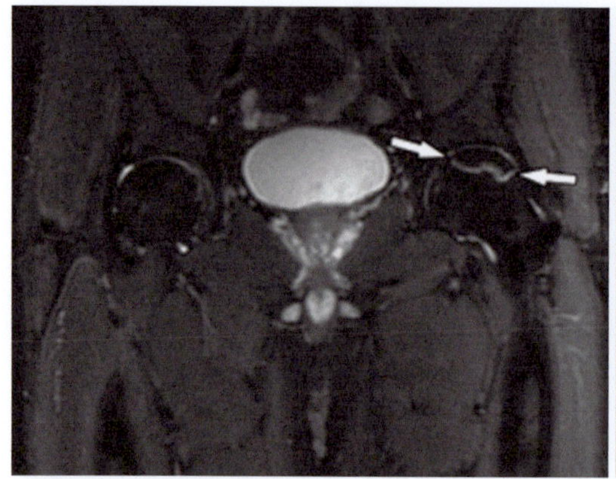

Coronal \T2 fat saturated

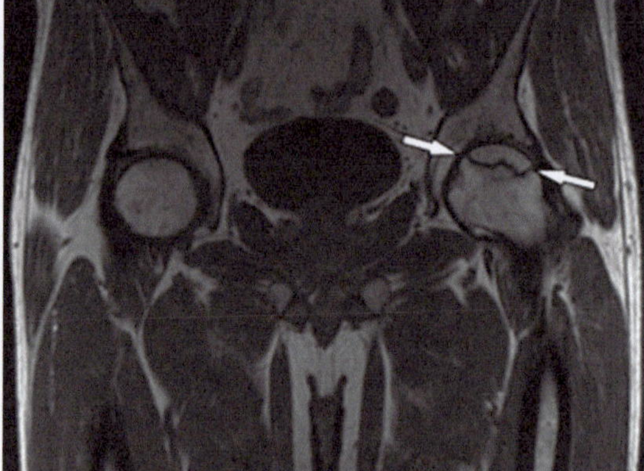

Coronal T1

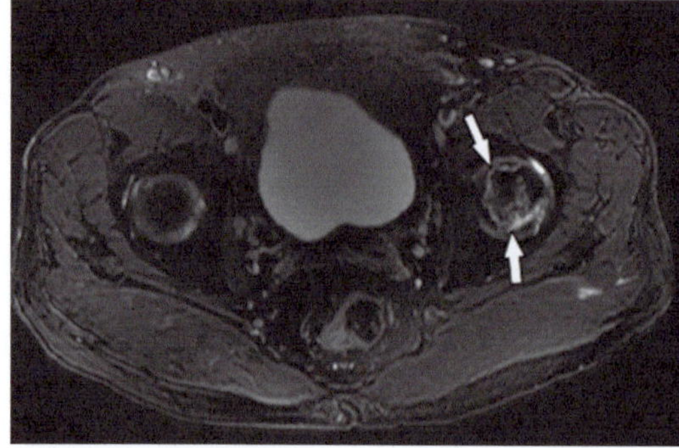

Axial T2 fat saturated

Findings

There is a geographic area in the superolateral aspect of the left femoral head demarcated by a hypointense T1 and hyperintense T2 serpiginous line compatible with avascular necrosis (arrows). It involves approximately 50% of the articular surface. There is no articular collapse, and there are no secondary signs of osteoarthritis. There is no hip joint effusion. The right femoral head is normal.

Impression/Recommendation

Avascular necrosis of the left femoral head without collapse of the articular surface or secondary hip joint osteoarthritis.

Discussion: Avascular Necrosis (AVN) of the Femoral Head

Osteonecrosis is a general term that represents bone cell death resulting from an ischemic injury. Avascular necrosis (AVN) is used to describe osteonecrosis when they occur at the bone epiphysis, while the term "bone infarct" is used when osteonecrosis involves the metaphyseal or diaphyseal bone and does not contact the articular surface. The most common cause of femoral head AVN is trauma, either from a femoral neck fracture or dislocation. Nontraumatic causes are many and include hemoglobinopathies, SLE, alcoholism, and corticosteroid use and are more commonly bilateral. Patients with AVN are initially asymptomatic; however, as the disease progresses, patients can present with groin pain that worsens with weight-bearing. The disease has a predictive pattern if left untreated which leads to collapse of the femoral head and eventually hip joint osteoarthritis. Early diagnosis is therefore crucial in the workup of these patients as cessation of the causative agent can salvage the femoral head before it collapses.

In the early stages of AVN when radiographs are normal, MRI usually demonstrates nonspecific diffuse bone marrow edema of the femoral head. The differential diagnosis at this stage includes AVN, transient osteoporosis of the hip (TOH), subchondral insufficiency fracture (SIF), and neoplasm. It is important to differentiate between these causes as the treatment of these diagnoses is different *(please refer to case 4.2 for further discussion on TOH and SIF)*. The hallmark finding of AVN is a demarcation of a geographic subchondral fragment in the femoral head surrounded by a "double line sign" on T2-weighted fat-suppressed images which comprises both an inner high signal intensity line and an outer hypointense line which represents the interface between dead and living bone with a rim of hypervascular granulation tissue. The geographic regions will have internal fatty signal which is helpful for distinguishing from neoplasms.

There are numerous classification systems for grading AVN, the most common being the classification system of Ficat and Arlet; however, these systems are sometimes misleading and are not used by all referring physicians. It is, therefore, more important to be descriptive in the report rather than list the stage. Four essential questions need to be answered when confronted with a case suggestive of AVN:

1. Is the signal abnormality and area of demarcation in the femoral head suggestive of AVN?
2. If yes, then where is it located within the femoral head (e.g., anterosuperior) and how much of the articular surface is involved?
3. Is there collapse of the articular surface?
4. Are there signs of secondary joint osteoarthritis?

The extent of osteonecrosis determines the likelihood of femoral head articular collapse. Involvement of less than 30% of the articular surface of the femoral head usually suggests a good prognosis, while involvement of more than 60% suggests a bad prognosis. Evaluation of the normal spherical contour of the femoral head should be looked for as any irregularity would suggest early collapse. The presence of a crescent sign, which is related to separation of the subchondral plate from the underlying necrotic bone with surrounding bone marrow edema also suggests impending articular surface collapse.

Once the femoral head surface collapses, then evaluation of secondary signs of osteoarthritis should be assessed, including the degree of cartilage loss, marginal osteophytes, and intra-articular loose bodies. Given that approximately 60% of patients with AVN have bilateral involvement, large field of view imaging of the pelvis to include both hip joints should be included in the protocol to assess the contralateral femoral head.

Treatment options depend on whether there is articular surface collapse or not. Early on in the disease, conservative measures include observation and limited weight-bearing. However, given the high rate of progression of the disease, many surgeons recommend early surgical intervention as core decompression and osteotomy. Once there is articular surface collapse, then follow-up imaging with radiographs can be performed till they require a hip replacement.

Report checklist

1. Is there bone marrow edema in the femoral head to suggest AVN?
2. Where is the location of the AVN? And how much of the articular surface is involved (estimate percentage)?
3. Is there collapse of the femoral head articular surface?
4. Are there secondary signs of osteoarthritis including cartilage loss, subchondral cystic changes, marginal osteophytes, and intra-articular loose bodies?
5. Is there a joint effusion?
6. Is there involvement of the contralateral femoral head?

Suggested Reading

Choi HR, Steinberg ME, Y Cheng E. Osteonecrosis of the femoral head: diagnosis and classification systems. Curr Rev. Musculoskelet Med. 2015;8:210–20.

Zibis AH, Karantanas AH, Roidis NT, Hantes ME, Argiri P, Moraitis T, Malizos KN. The role of MR imaging in staging femoral head osteonecrosis. Eur J Radiol. 2007;63:3–9.

Case 4.4

Indication A 31-year-old male athlete with chronic right hip pain that worsens with hip flexion. MR arthrogram performed to assess for labral tear.

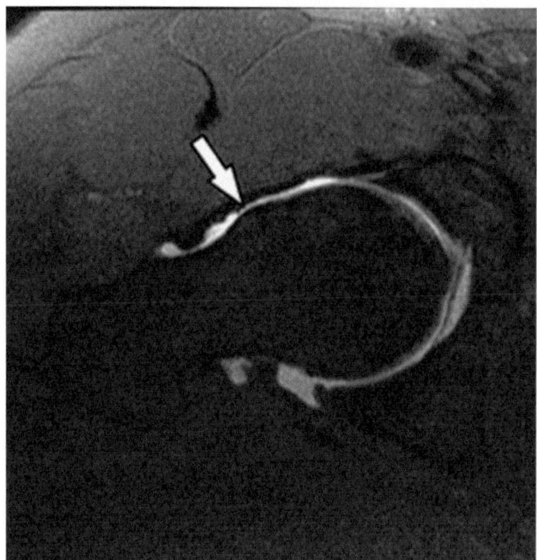

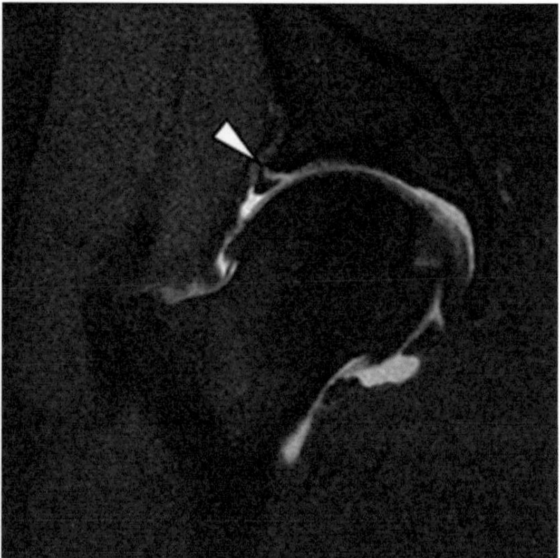

Axial oblique T1 fat saturated (MR arthrogram)   Coronal T1 fat saturated (MR arthrogram)

Findings

There is an osseous protuberance at the anterosuperior femoral head-neck junction (arrow) resulting in an increased alpha angle measuring 67° suggesting cam-type femoroacetabular impingement morphology. In addition, there is labral detachment at the superior aspect of the acetabulum (arrowhead). Osteophytic spurs are seen of the femoral head, and there are partial-thickness articular cartilage defects on both sides of the superior hip joint. There is no acetabular retroversion or intra-articular loose bodies.

Impression/Recommendation

Cam-type femoroacetabular impingement with anterosuperior labral detachment and osteoarthritis.

Discussion: Femoroacetabular Impingement (FAI)

Femoroacetabular impingement (FAI) occurs as a result of abnormal abutment between the proximal femur and the acetabulum. Overtime this can lead to degeneration of the articular cartilage as well as labral tears which can lead to early hip

osteoarthritis. Early diagnosis is therefore important to prevent or delay degeneration of the hip. There are two main types of FAI: cam type (due to femoral causes) and pincer type (due to acetabular causes); however, it is also common to have mixed cam- and pincer-type impingement. Pincer-type impingement is due to over coverage of the acetabulum as seen in protrusio acetabuli, coxa profunda, or acetabular retroversion. Cam-type impingement is due to abnormal prominence of the anterosuperior femoral head-neck junction. Patients with FAI are usually young and athletic and present with hip pain that worsens with hip flexion and internal rotation. It is however important to note that FAI-like appearance on imaging can be seen in asymptomatic individuals.

When assessing an MRI of the hip for suspected cam-type FAI, assessment begins at the femur for prominence at the anterior aspect of the femoral head-neck junction. This can be visualized as a focal osseous bump anteriorly, best seen on an axial oblique plane *(see supplementary images)* which is prescribed from a parallel line along the long axis of the femoral neck in the coronal plane and hence suggest cam-type impingement. This can also be quantified by measuring an alpha angle on the axial oblique plane. To measure the alpha angle, the femoral head is first outlined by a best fit circle, then an angle is calculated from two intersecting lines: one drawn along the central axis of the femoral neck and another line drawn from the center of the femoral head to a point where the femoral head-neck contour deviates from the circle *(see supplementary images)*. A cam-type impingement is present when the angle is >55°; however, some investigators consider an angle >60° in order to prevent a false-positive diagnosis. There is debate in the literature on the use of alpha angles in clinical practice given its low reproducibility and large variation limit, and it is likely that its clinical relevance will decline. Acetabular retroversion is present when the anterior acetabular rim is neutral or lateral to the posterior wall when assessed on the true axial plane through the most superior aspect of the femoral head, which can suggest pincer-type impingement.

As the femoral head-neck junction abuts the acetabular rim, this can cause a delamination of the articular cartilage at the labral-chondral transition zone which most commonly occurs at the anterosuperior and anterior quadrants of the acetabulum. Over time, this can then lead to tearing and detachment of the anterosuperior labrum. In pincer-type impingement, there can also be smaller focal chondromalacia changes at the posteroinferior aspect of the acetabulum. Labral tears and chondral injuries are best detected on MR arthrography. Os acetabuli has been suggested to represent either acetabular rim fractures or ossification of a degenerated lateral labrum from repeated microtrauma. Lastly, assessment for a joint effusion and intra-articular loose bodies should be performed.

Treatment of FAI includes conservative measures with activity modification, anti-inflammatory medications, and intra-articular steroid injections. Surgery can be performed in patients who fail conservative treatment, which includes osteotomy to allow for sufficient impingement free range of motion. In addition, labral and chondral debridement can be performed.

Supplementary Images

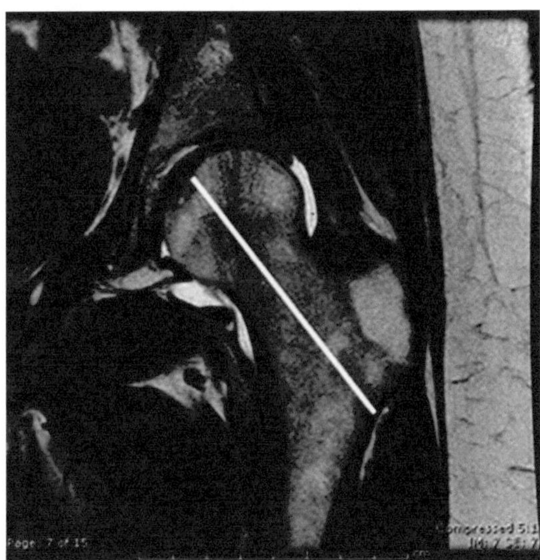

Coronal T1 (MR arthrogram)

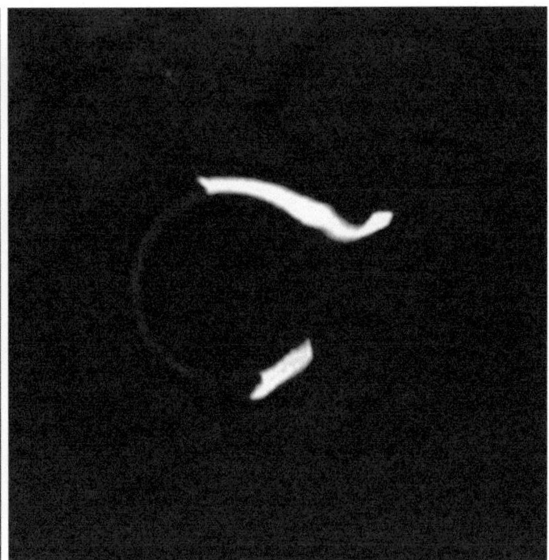

Axial oblique T1 fat saturated (MR arthrogram)

The axial oblique images are obtained from a reference line (white line) prescribed along the long axis of the femoral neck in the coronal plane

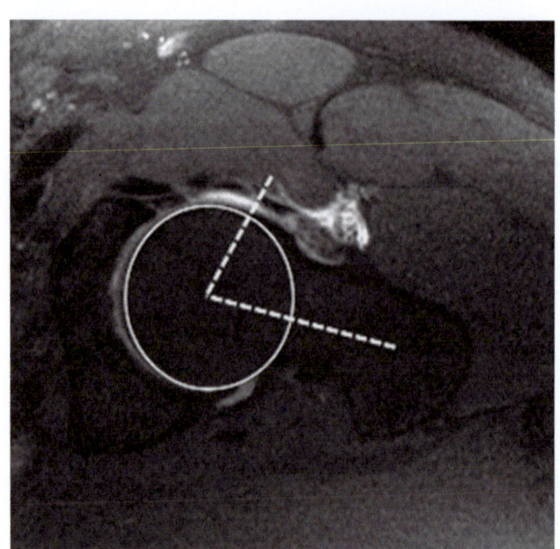

Axial oblique T1 fat saturated (MR arthrogram)

Alpha angle measures 67°, measured from an axial oblique MR arthrogram

Report checklist
1. Is there prominence of the anterosuperior femoral head-neck junction on the axial oblique images?
2. Is there acetabular retroversion?
3. Measure alpha angle from the axial oblique plane? (Normal is ≤55°)
4. Is there a labral tear?
5. Are there associated cartilage loss and subchondral cystic changes?
6. Is there a joint effusion (if non-arthrogram MRI)?

Suggested Reading

James SLJ, Ali K, Malara F, Young D, O'Donnell J, Connell DA. MRI findings of femoroacetabular impingement. AJR Am J Roentgenol. 2006;187:1412–9.

Pfirrmann CWA, Mengiardi B, Dora C, Kalberer F, Zanetti M, Hodler J. Cam and pincer Femoroacetabular impingement: characteristic MR arthrographic findings in 50 patients. Radiology. 2006;240:778–85.

Case 4.5

Indication A 24-year-old female jogger with acute on subacute right hip pain. Radiographs are normal. Assess for occult fracture

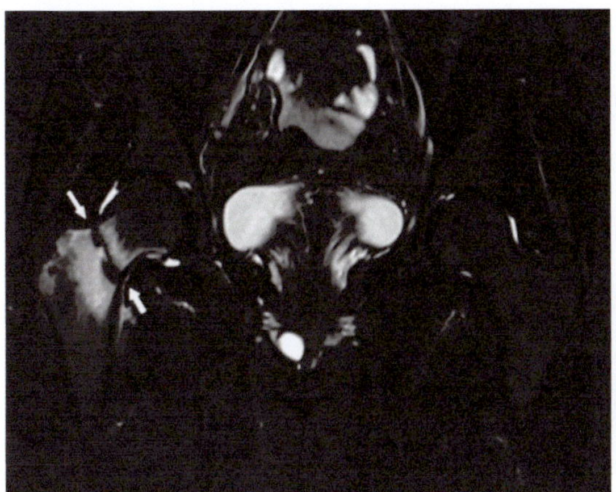

Coronal STIR

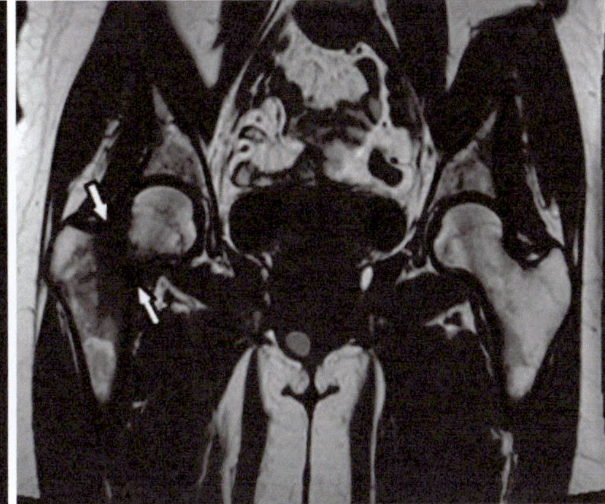

Coronal T1

Findings
There is a linear hypointense fracture line through the right femoral neck with surrounding bone marrow edema (arrows) on both the STIR and T1-weighted images. There is no fracture displacement. There is no avascular necrosis of the femoral head and no hip joint effusion.

Impression/Recommendation
Femoral neck stress fracture. Limited weight-bearing is recommended.

Discussion: Femoral Neck Stress Fracture
Stress fractures result from ongoing mechanical stress to bone leading to microfracture, incomplete fracture and finally progression to a complete fracture. Stress fractures are categorized into two categories: fatigue fractures (abnormal stress to normal bone) and insufficiency fractures (normal stress to abnormal bone). Fatigue fractures are seen in young adults, usually in the setting of increased physical activity, such as long-distance runners and military recruits. Insufficiency fractures are more commonly seen in elderly patients as a result of osteoporosis.

Femoral neck stress fractures tend to occur more commonly at the base of the medial femoral neck (compressive type) and are more common in younger patients. Fractures in this location tend to have a better prognosis for healing. Femoral neck fractures can also occur along the superolateral aspect of the femoral neck (tension-type); however, they are less frequent *(see supplementary images)*. These types of fractures are more unstable as normal weight-bearing will tend to widen the fracture site. Tension fractures are at higher risk of displacement than compressive fractures and can be prophylactically treated with pin fixation.

Radiographs are the initial study of choice; however, they have low sensitivity. MRI is the best imaging test, and one should perform T2-weighted fat-suppressed or STIR sequences or both to highlight areas of marrow edema which is the primary finding of osseous stress injury. A discrete fracture line may or may not be evident depending on the injury time frame. If a fracture line is seen, then the extent of the fracture line across the width of the bone needs to be commented on as this may influence clinical management. One should also search for other sites of stress fracture, such as the contralateral femur, sacrum, or pubic rami.

Most cases of femoral neck fractures, mainly the compressive type, are treated with limited weight-bearing and cessation of activities until symptoms resolve. Tension-type fractures may need to be treated operatively with pin fixation.

Supplementary Images

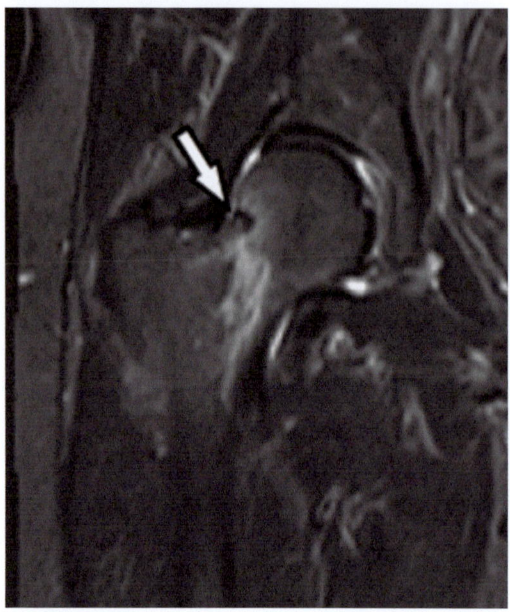

Coronal STIR

A hypointense fracture line (arrow) is seen at the superolateral aspect of the femoral neck with surrounding bone marrow edema, most compatible with a tension-type stress fracture

Report checklist

1. What is the location and extent of bone marrow edema?
2. Is there a hypointense signal line to indicate a discrete fracture?
3. Is the fracture line along the medial cortex (compressive type) or superolateral (tension type) aspect of the femoral neck?
4. How much of the bone width does the fracture line involve?
5. Is there displacement of the fracture?
6. Are there other fractures (i.e., contralateral femur, sacrum, pubic rami)?

Suggested Reading

Rohena-Quinquilla IR, Rohena-Quinquilla FJ, Scully WF, Evanson JRL. Femoral neck stress injuries: analysis of 156 cases in a U.S. military population and proposal of a new MRI classification system. AJR Am J Roentgenol. 2018;210:601–7.

Sheehan SE, Shyu JY, Weaver MJ, Sodickson AD, Khurana B. Proximal femoral fractures: what the orthopedic surgeon wants to know. Radiographics. 2015;35:1563–84.

Case 4.6

Indication A 28-year-old basketball player with sudden onset of right gluteal pain and swelling during a game. MRI performed to rule out hamstring tendon tear.

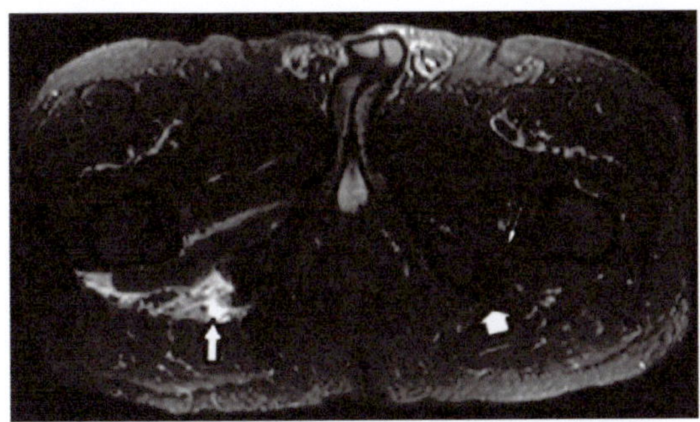

Axial T2 fat saturated

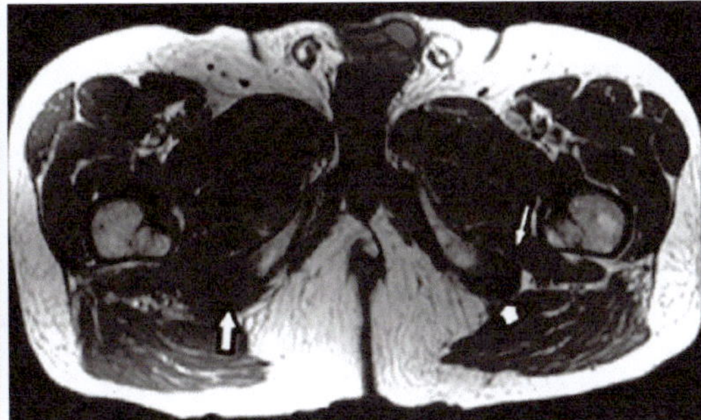

Axtial T1

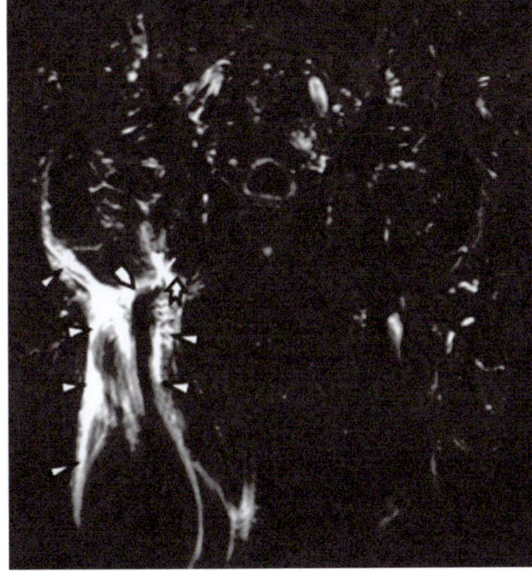

Coronal STIR

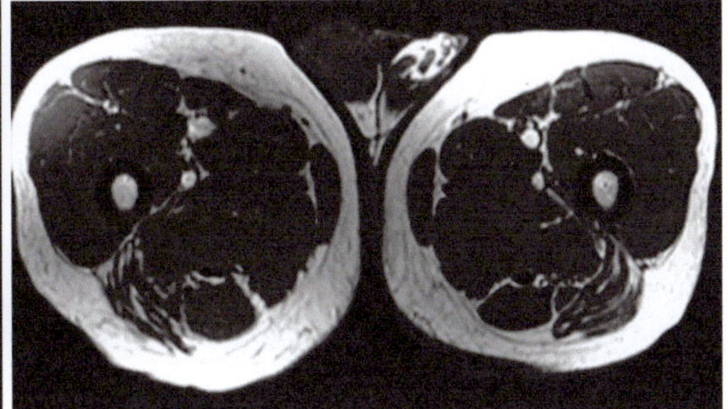

Axial T1

Findings

The left semimembranosus (thin arrow) and conjoined tendon (biceps femoris and semitendinosus (thick arrow)) are normal. There is complete rupture of the right hamstrings at the ischial tuberosity with nonvisualization of the tendon near the ischial tuberosity (arrows). There is tendon retraction measuring 2.2 cm (thin line) with a prominent amount of fluid/edema (arrowheads) at the myotendinous junction and surrounding the retracted tendon free edge (block arrow). There is a tiny 0.5 cm tendon stump (notched arrow) on the ischial tuberosity. No bony avulsion or marrow edema in the right ischial tuberosity is seen. There is no fatty atrophy of the hamstring muscle bellies on the T1-weighted images.

Impression/Recommendation

Proximal avulsion at the origin of the right hamstring tendons (grade 3 – complete rupture).

Discussion: Hamstring Tendon Injuries

The hamstring muscle complex is composed of three muscles: the biceps femoris, the semimembranosus, and the semitendinosus muscles which arise from the ischial tuberosity. The common origin (conjoined tendon) of the long head of biceps femoris and the semitendinosus tendons arises from the inferomedial aspect of the ischial tuberosity. The semimembranosus tendon originates from the superolateral aspect of the ischial tuberosity. The hamstring tendons span the entire length of the thigh and cross both the hip and knee joints to insert on the tibia and fibula. Muscles that cross two joints, like the hamstrings, gastrocnemius, and biceps, are more susceptible to injury. Hamstring injuries tend to heal slowly and are a significant cause of prolonged absence from sports.

Injury to the hamstring tendons includes tendinosis, partial and complete tears, as well as avulsions at the bone-tendon interface. The diagnosis of hamstring injury is usually made clinically where patients present with gluteal pain and point tenderness at the ischial tuberosity. MRI, however, is being increasingly utilized to evaluate these injuries and can help determine the size, extent, and location of the injury.

On MRI, tendinosis is suggested when there is thickening at the hamstring tendon origin with increased signal intensity in the tendon on both the T1- and T2-weighted images. However, interpretation of these images is somewhat inconclusive as it is also common to visualize these same findings in asymptomatic patients, and hence if you are to describe them in your report, it is important to have the clinician correlate with patient's presenting symptoms as well as point tenderness at the ischial tuberosity. The presence of surrounding soft tissue edema and bone marrow edema at the ischial tuberosity is more frequently seen in symptomatic patients and should be noted in the report.

Acute injuries to the hamstring tendons frequently occur at the proximal myotendinous junction. The most important sequence is the fluid-sensitive sequence where there will be hyperintense fluid signal suggesting the site of the tear. Grade 1 strains are considered a mild injury with small disruptions at the myotendinous junction. On MRI, this is seen as feathery-like edema within the muscle belly on the fat-suppressed fluid-sensitive sequences. A grade 2 strain represents a partial tear at the myotendinous junction with surrounding hyperintense hematoma at the site of tear. If possible, in your report, it is helpful to the surgeon if you can calculate an approximate involvement of the cross-sectional area of the muscle belly involved. Grade 3 strain represents a complete tear at the myotendinous junction with hyperintense fluid gap and retraction of the torn tendon stump. Avulsion injuries at the bone-tendon interface can occur with or without an avulsion fracture from the ischial tuberosity. It is sometimes difficult to visualize tiny cortical avulsions, and hence correlation with plain radiographs is essential. The amount of tendon retraction in the craniocaudal length should be measured. Complete chronic tears are characterized by muscle atrophy and fatty replacement of the muscle.

Hamstring tendon injuries are usually treated conservatively with rest, ice, compression, and elevation. The recovery may take up to 6 months. Surgery is usually reserved for complete tears with significant retraction greater than 2 cm.

Report checklist

1. Is there tendinosis at the hamstring origin? Is it associated with surrounding soft tissue edema and bone marrow edema at the ischial tuberosity? If yes, then this should be correlated with point tenderness at the ischial tuberosity.
2. Is there a tendon tear? Which tendon is involved? Where is the precise location of the tear (tendon/bone interface, tendon, proximal myotendinous junction, or muscle belly)?
3. What is the extent of the tear (grade 1, 2, or 3 strain)?
4. How much of the cross-sectional area of the muscle belly is involved?
5. Is there tendon retraction? If yes, what is the tendon gap?
6. Is there an associated cortical avulsion from the ischial tuberosity?
7. Is there muscle fatty atrophy to suggest a chronic injury?

Suggested Reading

Greenky M, Cohen SB. Magnetic resonance imaging for assessing hamstring injuries: clinical benefits and pitfalls – a review of the current literature. Open Access J Sports Med. 2017;8:167–70.

Rubin DA. Imaging diagnosis and prognostication of hamstring injuries. AJR Am J Roentgenol. 2012;199(3):525–33.

Case 4.7

Indication A 49-year-old female with severe lateral right hip pain and significant soft tissue swelling. MRI to rule out greater trochanteric bursitis.

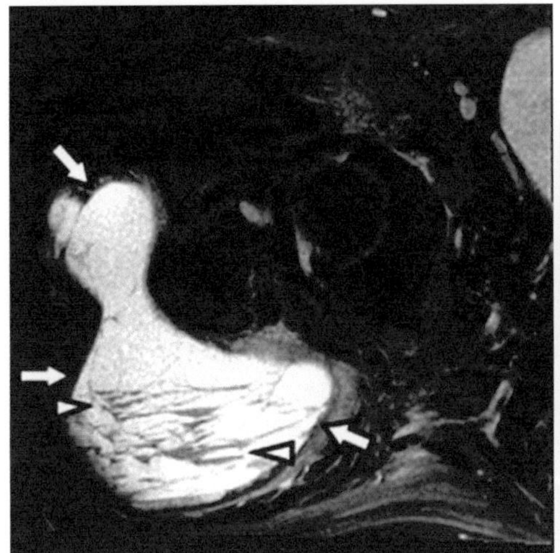

Axial STIR

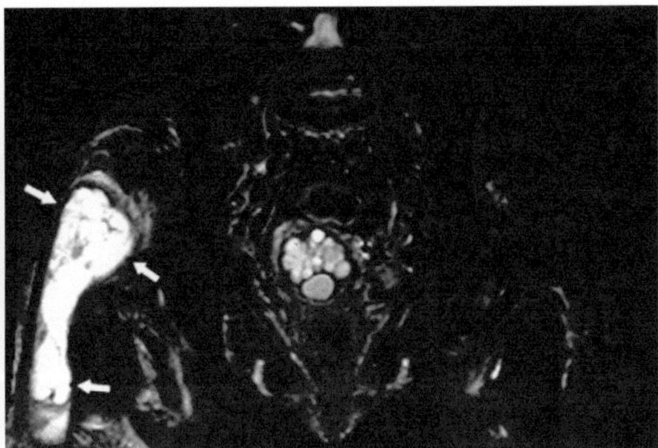

Coronal STIR

Findings

There is a large T2 hyperintense fluid collection within the right greater trochanteric bursa compatible with bursitis (arrows). The collection measures 8 × 6 cm and contains multiple fluid-fluid levels (arrowheads) along the dependent potion suggestive of debris and/or hemorrhage. There is mild tendinosis of the right gluteus medius tendon but without focal tear. The gluteus minimus tendon is intact. There is no strain or atrophy of the gluteal muscles.

Impression/Recommendation

Severe greater trochanteric bursitis.

Discussion: Greater Trochanteric Pain Syndrome

The greater trochanter has four facets (anterior, lateral, posterior, and superoposterior) and serves as the site of attachment of the gluteal abductors. The anterior facet serves as the insertion site for the gluteus minimus tendon. The gluteus medius tendon has two attachments: the anterior aspect of the tendon attaches on the lateral facet, while the posterior aspect of

the tendon attaches on the superoposterior facet. The posterior facet has no tendon attachments and is covered by the larger trochanteric (subgluteus maximus) bursa. There are two other smaller bursae: the subgluteus medius bursa, underneath the gluteus medius tendon, and the subgluteus minimus bursa, underneath the gluteus minimus tendon. The anterior facet and gluteus minimus tendon are best visualized on axial and sagittal planes, while the lateral facet and gluteus medius tendon are best evaluated on axial and coronal planes.

Greater trochanteric pain syndrome (GTPS) refers to pain in the lateral hip which is most commonly related to pathology of the gluteal tendons and inflammation of their bursae. Clinically, it presents as pain that is exacerbated by abduction of the hip joint or point tenderness at the greater trochanter. This condition generally arises in women aged 40–60 years but is increasingly seen in young athletic individuals.

On MRI, it is common to see minimal edema around the insertion of the gluteal tendons and trace (<3 mm) inflammation of the greater trochanteric bursa in older asymptomatic individuals and should not be interpreted as bursitis when it is minimal and symmetric bilaterally. Gluteal tendinosis appears as hyperintense signal on the T2-weighted images within an intact tendon. Thickening of the tendon and calcification at the insertion site may also be noted. The gluteus medius tendon is most often affected. Partial-thickness tears appear as focal discontinuity of tendon fibers, while in complete tears, there is complete loss of tendon fibers with or without tendon retraction. This can lead to fatty atrophy of the muscle bulk in chronic cases. Greater trochanteric bursitis is related to distention of the bursa with fluid and is commonly seen in patients with gluteal pathology. It appears as a focal area of T2 hyperintense fluid collection within the region of the trochanteric bursa and ranges from small to massive collections which can be complicated with internal hemorrhage or debris.

Most cases of GTPS respond to conservative treatment involving weight loss, nonsteroidal anti-inflammatory medication, and physiotherapy. More chronic conditions may require corticosteroid injections into the area.

Report checklist

1. Is there tendinosis of the gluteus medius or minimus tendons?
2. Are there focal tears of the gluteal tendons? Is it partial or complete?
3. Is there a muscle strain or fatty atrophy of the gluteal muscles?
4. Is there distention of the greater trochanteric bursa? Is it mild, moderate, or severe? If moderate to large, then give approximate size of the collection.
5. Is there internal hemorrhage or debris within the greater trochanteric bursitis?

Suggested Reading

Chowdhury R, Naaseri S, Lee J, Rajeswaran G. Imaging and management of greater trochanteric pain syndrome. Postgrad Med J. 2014;90:576–81.

Pfirrmann CW, Chung CB, Theumann NH, Trudell DJ, Resnick D. Greater trochanter of the hip: attachment of the abductor mechanism and a complex of three bursae--MR imaging and MR bursography in cadavers and MR imaging in asymptomatic volunteers. Radiology. 2001;221(2):469–77.

Case 4.8

Indication A 22-year-old male cyclist with anterior left hip pain and snapping sensation. MRI to assess the iliopsoas tendon.

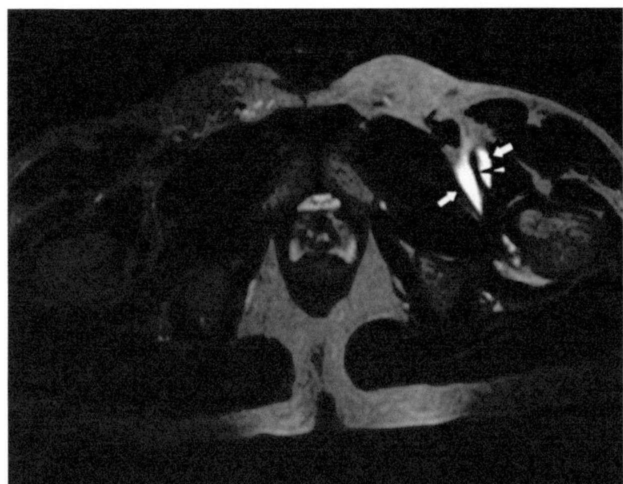

Axial T2

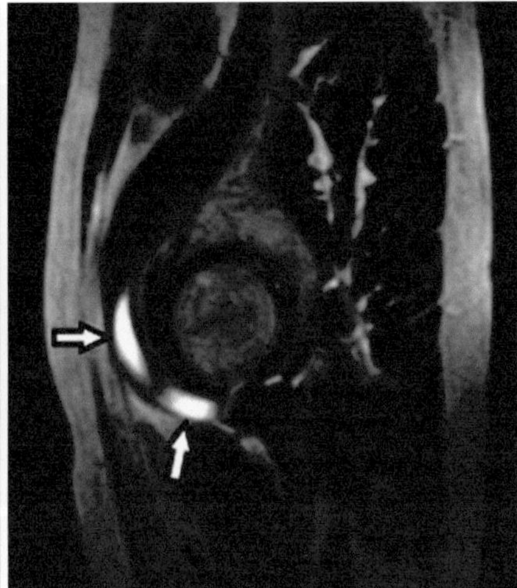

Sagittal T2

Findings
There is distention of the left iliopsoas bursa with a small amount of fluid measuring 5 cm in the craniocaudal dimension compatible with mild iliopsoas bursitis (arrows). The underlying iliopsoas tendon is intact without focal tear (arrowhead). The left hip joint is normal without significant degenerative changes or hip joint effusion.

Impression/Recommendation
Mild left iliopsoas bursitis.

Discussion: Iliopsoas Bursitis
The iliopsoas, or iliopectineal, bursa is located between the iliopsoas tendon and the anterior acetabular rim of the hip joint. It is the largest bursa in the human body and extends from the anterior aspect of the iliacus muscle superiorly to the lesser trochanter inferiorly and is in close relation with the femoral neurovascular bundle. In approximately 15% of patients, the bursa normally communicates with the hip joint.

Inflammation of the iliopsoas bursa is known as iliopsoas bursitis. Although it is more commonly seen in patients with advanced degenera-tive changes of the hip, it can also be seen in young athletic individuals due to repetitive overuse from mechanical friction of the iliopsoas tendon as it moves over the iliopectineal eminence. Other less likely causes include acute trauma, inflammatory arthropathies, or patients with total hip arthroplasty. Clinically, patients present with groin pain or a focal mass that can be exacerbated with hip extension.

MRI demonstrates a localized fluid collection deep to the iliopsoas tendon and anterior to the hip capsule that is homogeneously hyperintense on T2-weighted images and hypointense on T1-weighted images. Presence of internal hemorrhage or proteinaceous material may cause the fluid signal to appear slightly heterogeneous. The axial T2-weighted sequences are the most helpful in assessing the iliopsoas bursitis and documenting communication with the hip joint. The severity and craniocaudal extent of the inflamed bursa should be documented. Associated hip joint effusion or degenerative changes may be visualized. MRI is also helpful in differentiating iliopsoas bursitis from a paralabral cyst. Paralabral cysts are usually more localized and multiloculated in appearance and rarely extend inferior to the hip joint capsule.

The close intimate relation of the iliopsoas bursa to the adjacent iliopsoas tendon also helps in differentiating these two conditions.

The initial treatment involves conservative therapy such as rest and nonsteroidal anti-inflammatory agents. If these fail, then ultrasound-guided aspiration with injection of corticosteroids can be performed.

Report checklist

1. What is the severity (mild, moderate, or severe) of the iliopsoas bursitis and craniocaudal extent in centimeters?
2. Is the underlying iliopsoas tendon intact? Does it have tendinosis or tear?
3. Are there degenerative or inflammatory changes in the adjacent hip joint?
4. Is there a hip joint effusion?
5. Is the condition unilateral or bilateral?

Suggested Reading

Kozlov DB, Sonin AH: Iliopsoas bursitis: diagnosis by MRI. J Comput Assist Tomogr. 1998;22:625–8.

Wunderbaldinger P, Bremer C, Schellenberger E, Cejna M, Turetschek K, Kainberger F. Imaging features of iliopsoas bursitis. Eur Radiol. 2002;12(2):409–15.

Case 4.9

Indication: A 14-year-old gymnast with sudden left hip pain while competing with point tenderness at the left lesser trochanter. Plain radiographs suggest lesser trochanter fracture. MRI for further evaluation.

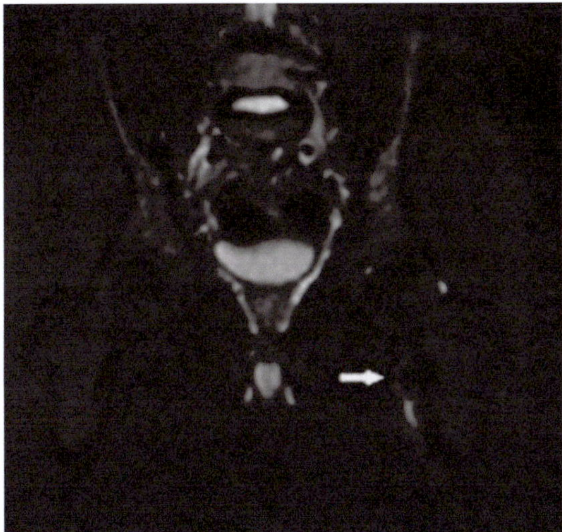

Coronal T2 fat saturated

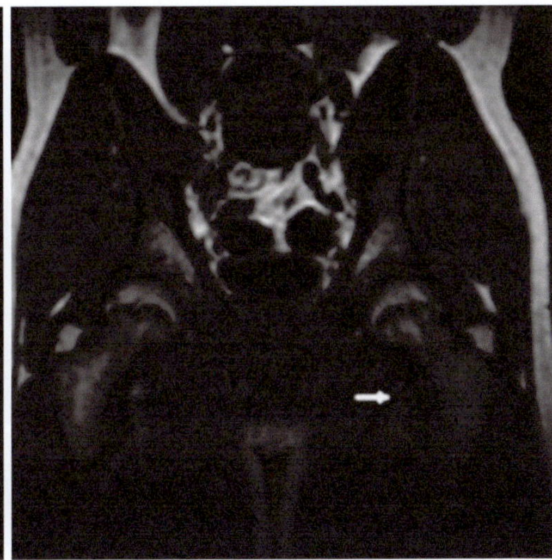

Coronal T1

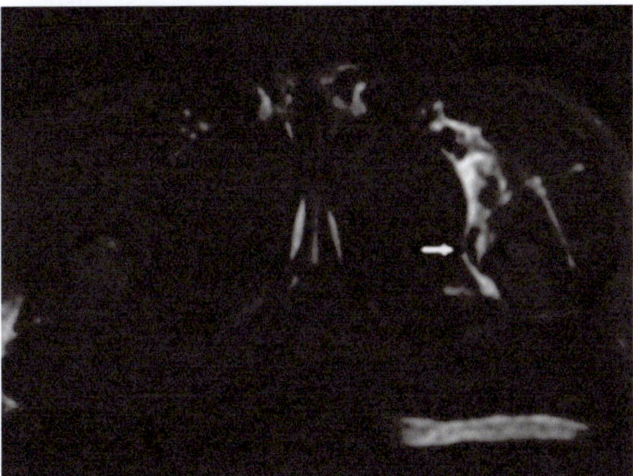

Axial T2 fat saturated

Findings

There is bony avulsion at the left lesser trochanteric apophysis at the insertion of the iliopsoas tendon without significant retraction (arrows). There is mild surrounding soft tissue edema and hemorrhage. There is no underlying bony lesion. There is no fatty atrophy of the iliopsoas muscle belly.

Impression/Recommendation

Bony avulsion at the left lesser trochanteric apophysis without significant retraction.

Discussion: Avulsion Fractures at the Pelvis

Avulsion fractures usually result from a sudden tensile force. Children and adolescents are particularly prone to such injuries as their apophyses have not yet ossified. The hip and pelvis are the most commonly affected regions, possibly because the apophyses in these regions tend to fuse relatively late and many of the muscles cross two joints. Patients typically experience a popping sensation at the site of the injury, followed by pain and local tenderness in the area.

Although clinical examination and plain radiographs are usually sufficient to diagnose avulsion fractures, findings may sometimes be equivocal. In such cases, MRI is useful; for example, an MRI can help detect a non-displaced apophyseal avulsion or avulsion of a non-ossified apophysis. MRI can also quantitatively assess the degree of tendon retraction. The amount of retraction directly influences prognosis; retraction greater than 2 cm is often associated with impaired healing and prolonged disability.

On MRI, the involved tendon can have a lax configuration due to retraction. The avulsed fragment of bone can often be seen attached to the tendon. However, if only the cortical bone is avulsed, it may be missed on MRI, as it does not contain marrow and appears hypointense and therefore indistinguishable from adjacent tendons. Hence, correlation with plain radiographs is important. On fluid-sensitive sequences, variable degrees of edema may be noted in the bone and adjacent soft tissues.

In the follow-up of acute lesions, MRI can help assess the presence and extent of muscle atrophy and fatty infiltration. During the healing phase of avulsion fractures, MRI may show extensive callus formation with deformity of the adherent cortex at the fracture sites. This can easily be mistaken for osteosarcoma or exostosis if clear patient history is not present.

Depending on the type of activity and age of the individual, a pelvic avulsion fracture may occur in any of the following locations:

1. *Ischial tuberosity:* The ischial tuberosity is the most common site for avulsion injuries of the pelvis. Ossification of the ischial apophysis begins at approximately 14 years of age and completes by age 24. The conjoined tendon (biceps femoris and semitendinosus) and semimembranosus of the hamstrings originate at this location.

2. *Anterior inferior iliac spine (AIIS):* The AIIS is the site of origin of the direct head of the rectus femoris. Ossification of the apophysis begins at approximately 13 years of age and completes by 18 years.

3. *Anterior superior iliac spine (ASIS):* The sartorius muscle originates from the ASIS. Ossification of the apophysis at this site begins at 13 years and completes in the early 20s.

4. *Other locations:* The following are locations where avulsion fractures may occur on rare occasions: the symphysis pubis (at the origin of rectus abdominis, gracilis, adductor brevis, or adductor longus), the iliac crest (at the insertion of abdominal musculature), the greater trochanter (at the insertion of gluteus minimus, obturators, and gemelli), and the lesser trochanter (at the insertion of the iliopsoas muscle).

Acute avulsion injuries are treated conservatively with bed rest, restriction of activity, and physical therapy. Avulsion fractures take, on average, 4–8 weeks to heal. If, however, the fractured bone fragment is displaced more than 2 cm, surgery may be required.

Report checklist
1. Which tendon is injured?
2. Where is the tendon injured (bony avulsion, tendon substance, myotendinous junction, muscle belly)?
3. If there is a complete tear, how much tendon retraction or tendon gap is present?
4. Is there an associated hematoma or fluid collection?
5. Is there muscle belly edema or fatty atrophy?

Suggested Reading

Nachtrab O, Cassar-Pullicino VN, Lalam R et al. Role of MRI in hip fractures, including stress fractures, occult fractures, avulsion fractures. Eur J Radiol. 2012;81(12):3813–23.

Vandervliet EJ, Vanhoenacker FM, Snoeckx A, Gielen JL, Van Dyck P, Parizel PM. Sports-related acute and chronic avulsion injuries in children and adolescents with special emphasis on tennis. Br J Sports Med. 2007;41(11):827–31.

Case 4.10

Indication A 58-year-old male status post bilateral total hip replacement (metal on metal) 5 years ago. Now presenting with left hip pain. Radiographs show lucency surrounding the femoral stem. MRI performed for further assessment.

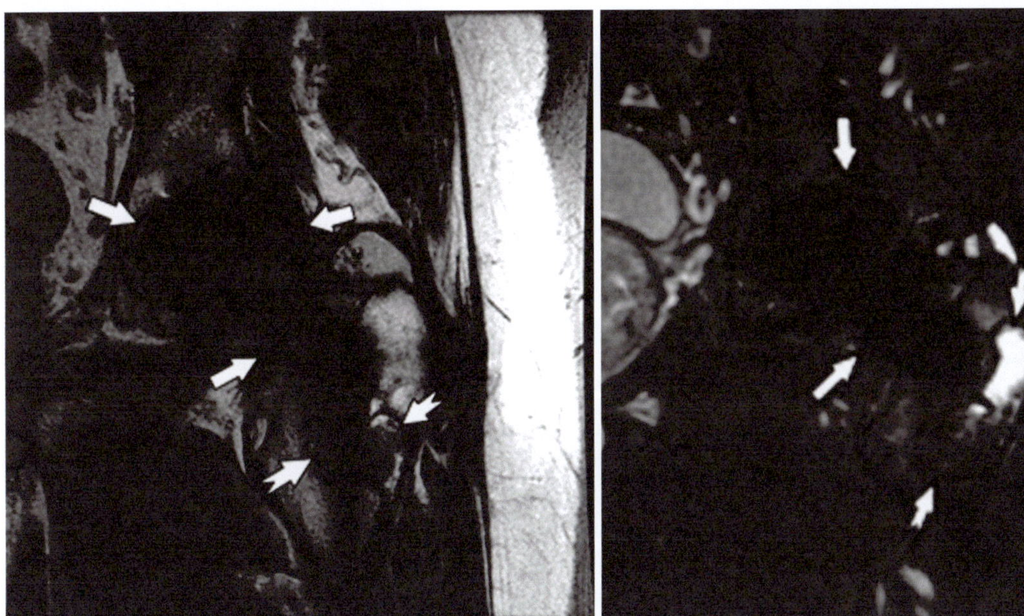

Coronal T2

Coronal STIR

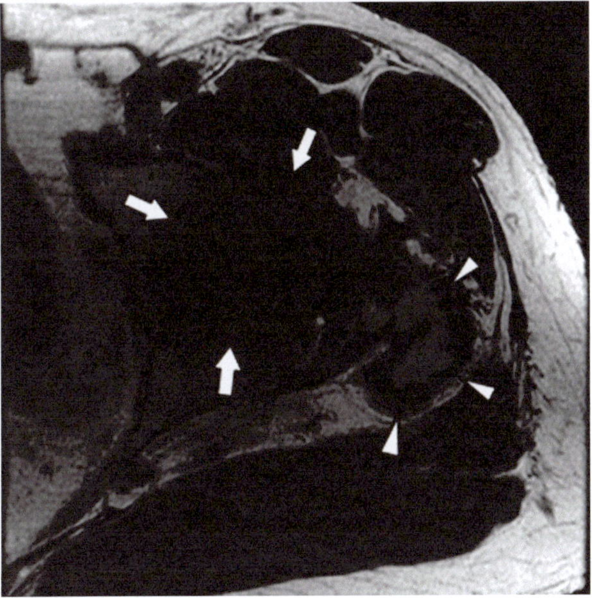

Axial T2

Findings

There is a left total hip prosthesis which causes some susceptibility artifact (arrows). There are well-defined cystic lesions in the proximal femoral shaft surrounding the femoral prosthesis containing internal hypointense foci as well as a well-defined hypointense rim (notched arrows). The collection extends beyond the bone into the left greater trochanteric bursa (arrowheads). There is no significant hip joint effusion.

Impression/Recommendation

Multiloculated cystic collection around the left hip prosthesis, most compatible with small particle disease/ALVAL.

Discussion: Small Particle Disease/ Pseudotumors/ALVAL/Metallosis

The number of hip arthroplasty procedures is increasing annually and is being performed in younger patients. Eventually, with time, many arthroplasties will fail. Plain radiography is the primary imaging modality used to evaluate patients after hip arthroplasty, and MRI typically has a limited role given the extensive susceptibility artifact caused by the metal components. Although this remains true, it is now known that plain films underestimate the extent of osteolysis associated with hip arthroplasty and provides poor assessment of the periarticular soft tissues. The most common complications associated with hip arthroplasty include aseptic loosening, infection, osteolysis, adverse reaction to metal debris, tendon avulsions, and periprosthetic fractures.

The metal components of the hip prosthesis distort the regional magnetic field and hence degrade the image quality. Several special considerations must be made to minimize metal artifact for accurate imaging of the hip prosthesis. These include (1) orienting the prosthesis longitudinally within the main magnetic field to reduce misregistration artifact, (2) using STIR sequences rather than spectral fat saturation and avoiding use of GRE sequences, (3) using a wide receiver bandwidth, (4) increasing the frequency encoding gradient strength, (5) reducing voxel size, and (6) reducing slice thickness. There are also new metal artifact reduction sequences available which include MAVRIC (multi-acquisition variable resonance image combination) and SEMAC (slice encoding for metal artifact correction).

Adverse local tissue reaction is an umbrella term describing reactions and histological changes to arthroplasty-related metal products and include small particle disease, pseudotumor of the hip, and aseptic lymphocyte-dominant vasculitis-associated lesion (ALVAL). They are thought to be related to hypersensitivity reaction that occurs in response to the release of small particles of debris due to wear of various components of the implant, either due to particles of metal, polyethylene or cement. ALVAL is a hypersensitivity reaction to metal ions seen in patients who have metal-on-metal arthroplasties. Adverse local tissue reaction can result in aggressive soft tissue destruction, and therefore early diagnosis and assessment of disease severity are essential for appropriate timing of revision surgery.

On MRI, the earliest findings of adverse local soft tissue reaction are a joint effusion and synovitis. There can be low signal intensity debris within the joint effusion. As the disease progresses, osteolysis ensues. This can be either focal or diffuse and can involve any portion of the implant from the acetabulum to the tip of the femoral stem. This is seen as an intermediate signal around the prosthesis on both the T1- and T2-weighted images. A typical finding is the presence of low signal intensity rim which outlines the osteolysis. In more aggressive reactions, the osteolysis can expand the bone cortex with extra-osseous extension, termed pseudotumors. Pseudotumor appears as complex cystic/solid masses in the periprosthetic soft tissues with a well-defined low signal intensity wall. They tend to occur more commonly at the posterolateral aspect of the joint which can then disrupt the joint capsule and extend to the greater trochanteric bursa. Alternatively, they may arise in the anterior aspect of the joint and extend into the iliopsoas bursa.

The primary differential diagnosis of pseudotumors is malignancy and infection. The presence of a low signal intensity rim around the cystic collection as well as the presence of low signal intensity foci within the collection should suggest pseudo-tumor/ALVAL rather than malignancy. Infectious collections are usually less well defined with surrounding inflammatory changes and fluid as well as lack of a low signal intensity rim.

Management of these lesions typically requires a revision arthroplasty.

Report checklist

1. Is the patient status post hip arthroplasty?
2. Are there any complex cystic/solid collections surrounding the prosthesis to suggest osteolysis?
3. Does the collection extend beyond the bone to the periarticular soft tissues?
4. Are there internal hypointense foci and/or is there a well-defined hypointense rim?
5. Is there a hip joint effusion or synovitis?
6. Does the patient have a history of malignancy or have symptoms of infection?

Suggested Reading

Hart AJ, Satchithananda K, Liddle AD, et al. Pseudotumors in association with well-functioning metal-on-metal hip prostheses: a case-control study using three-dimensional computed tomography and magnetic resonance imaging. J Bone Joint Surg Am. 2012;94(4):317–25.

Yanny S, Cahir JG, Barker T, Wimhurst J, Nolan JF, Goodwin RW, Marshall T, Toms AP. MRI of aseptic lymphocytic vasculitis-associated lesions in metal-on-metal hip replacements. AJR Am J Roentgenol. 2012;198(6):1394–402.

Case 4.11

Indication A 27-year-old rugby player with worsening subacute left-sided pubic pain.

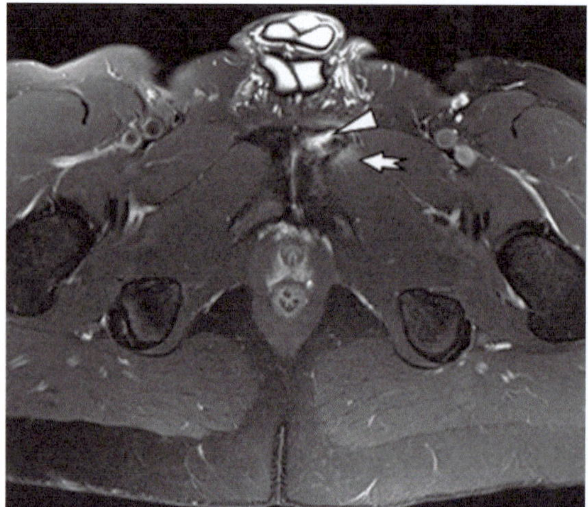

Axial T2 fat saturated

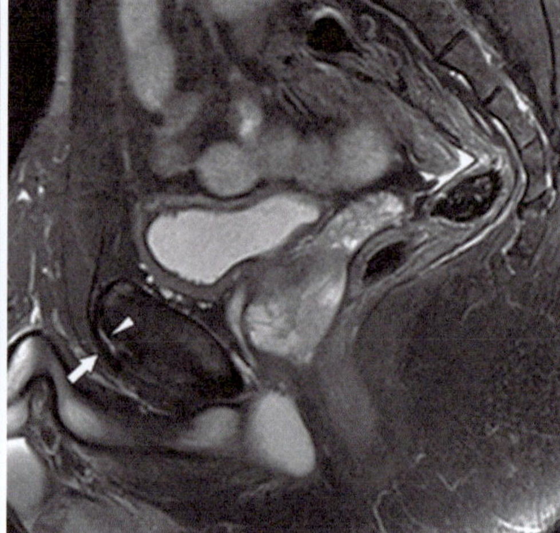

Sagittal T2 fat saturated

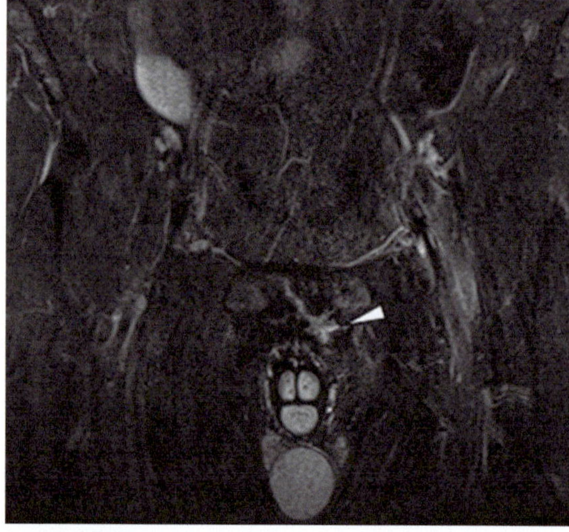

Coronal STIR

Findings

There is abnormal fluid/edema (arrowhead) at the attachment of the left rectus abdominis/adductor longus aponeurosis (arrow) to the pubic symphysis. Mild edema is seen near the bony attachment of the adductor longus muscle (notched arrow). There is no marrow edema or fluid at the pubic symphysis. The visualized hip joints are within normal limits.

Impression/Recommendation

Detachment (tear) of the left rectus abdominis/adductor longus aponeurosis.

Discussion: Athletic Pubalgia/sportsman's Hernia

The term "athletic pubalgia" is used to describe exertional pubic or groin pain observed in athletes, more commonly seen in athletes who play in sports that involve twisting at the waist, sudden directional change, and sideways movements. These disorders have been described by a myriad of names in the literature, including sport's hernia and sportsman's hernia, to name a few. It represents a constellation of injuries to the core muscles at the pubic symphysis. Patients usually present with insidious onset of groin pain that worsens with physical activity. Patients may also present acutely after a severe injury. On physical examination, there is pain to palpation at the external inguinal ring without a palpable hernia.

The normal anatomy at the pubic symphysis is complex with multiple musculotendinous, aponeurotic, and ligamentous attachments that act to stabilize the anterior pelvis. At the symphysis pubis, there is a fibrocartilaginous articular disc between the pubic bones which is supported by multiple small pubic ligaments. There are also various tendinous and muscle attachments at the symphysis pubis; however, the most important are the rectus abdominis and the adductor longus. The distal rectus abdominis muscle, and the proximal adductor longus fibers, blend together at the symphysis pubis to form a common rectus abdominis-adductor aponeurosis that broadly attaches to the periosteum at the anterior aspect of the pubic bones.

Clinically, it is often difficult to accurately evaluate these patients given that many different conditions may lead to groin pain including musculotendinous, osseous, or visceral pathology. Hence, MRI is usually the imaging modality of choice in these clinical situations. If an injury at the pubic symphysis is suspected, then MR imaging with a dedicated pubalgia protocol is recommended. In addition to the standard large field of view sequences to image the entire pelvis to evaluate for other pathologies that may cause referred groin pain such as internal derangement at the hip, osseous injury, sacroiliac pathology, and soft tissue masses, obtaining supplementary small field of view images centered at the pubic symphysis and the rectus abdominis-adductor aponeurosis is recommended. Small field of view axial oblique images are prescribed from a sagittal localizer paralleling the arcuate line of the pelvis to evaluate the aponeurosis better. Also, a true sagittal T2 fat-suppressed sequence center at the pubic symphysis is obtained to better evaluate the aponeurosis with its periosteal attachments on the anterior pubic bones.

On MRI, a linear cleft of fluid signal intensity is seen undermining the rectus abdominis-adductor aponeurosis which signifies detachment. These lesions can be unilateral; however, in other cases, it can be centered at the midline and extend to both aponeuroses on either side. Osteitis pubis is a common coexistent entity seen with detachment of the aponeurosis, whereby instability at the symphysis pubis results in shearing forces and secondary osseous stress response. This is seen on MRI as subchondral bone marrow edema at the pubic bones bilaterally, often asymmetric to one side. In more severe cases, there may be complete avulsion of the common adductor tendon from its proximal attachment with distal retraction and surrounding edema and hemorrhage. Other findings that can also be seen include tendinosis at the proximal adductor tendons. There may also be myotendinous strains of either the proximal adductors or distal rectus abdominis.

Treatment of these injuries depends on many factors, including the degree of injury, level of athletic participation, and patient's symptoms. Conservative management with rest and physiotherapy is usually recommended initially. Patients may be offered imaging-guided corticosteroid injections in the symphysis pubis or adductor tendons. Surgery is generally reserved for patients who do not improve with conservative management.

Report checklist

1. Is there detachment of the rectus abdominis-adductor aponeurosis?
2. Is it unilateral or bilateral?
3. Is there complete avulsion of the adductor longus tendon origin?
4. Is there bone marrow edema at the pubic bones to suggest osteitis pubis?
5. Is there muscle strains at the rectus abdominis and/or adductor longus?
6. Is there adductor longus tendinosis?
7. Is there an inguinal hernia?
8. How are the hip joints?

Suggested Reading

Khan W, Zoga AC, Meyers WC. Magnetic resonance imaging of athletic pubalgia and the sports hernia: current understanding and practice. Magn Reson Imaging Clin N Am. 2013;21:97–110.

Omar IM, Zoga AC, Kavanagh EC, Koulouris G, Bergin D, Gopez AG, Morrison WB, Meyers WC. Athletic pubalgia and "sports hernia": optimal MR imaging technique and findings. Radiographics. 2008;28:1415–38.

Case 5.1

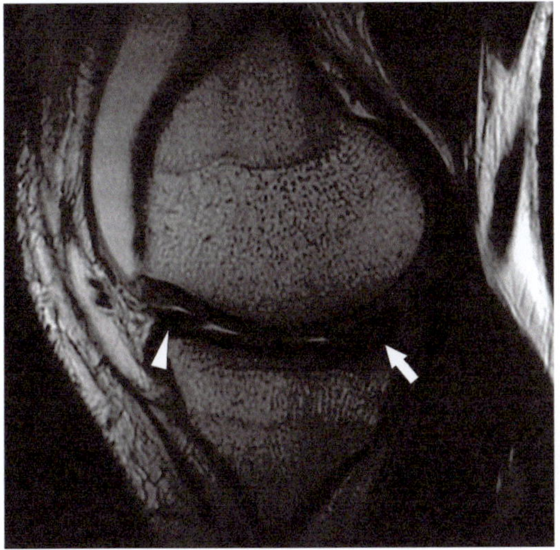

Sagittal PD

Normal appearance of the medial meniscus with the posterior horn (arrow) larger in size than the anterior horn (arrowhead)

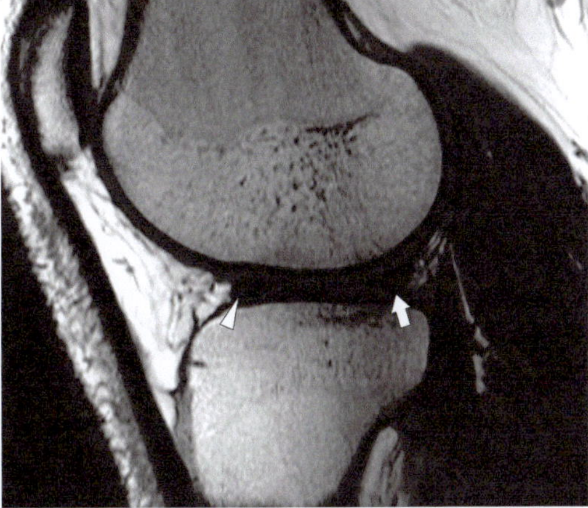

Sagittal PD

Normal appearance of the lateral meniscus with both the anterior (arrowhead) and posterior (arrow) horns similar in size

© Springer Nature Switzerland AG 2020
T. M. Hegazi, J. S. Wu, *Musculoskeletal MRI*, https://doi.org/10.1007/978-3-030-26777-3_5

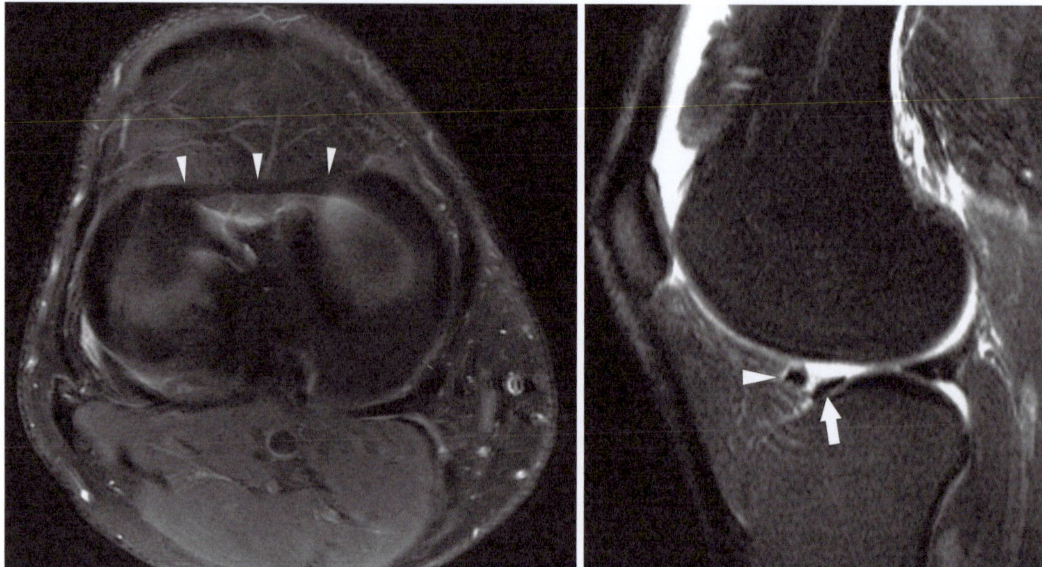

Axial PD fat saturated   Sagittal T2 fat saturated

Normal transverse meniscal ligament (arrowheads) which can sometimes mimic a meniscal tear of the anterior horn. Fluid is seen between the transverse ligament and the anterior horn (arrow) of the lateral meniscus

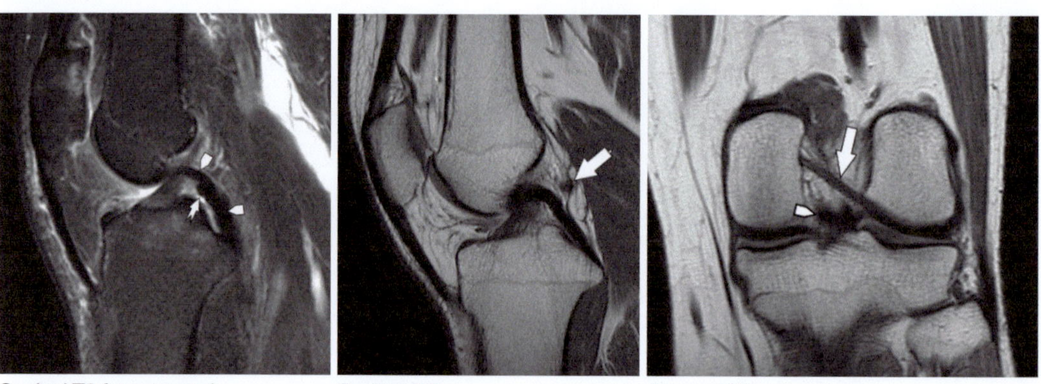

Sagittal T2 fat saturated   Sagittal PD   Coronal PD

Normal meniscofemoral ligaments of Humphrey (notched arrow) and Wrisberg (arrows) are anterior and posterior to the PCL (arrowheads), respectively

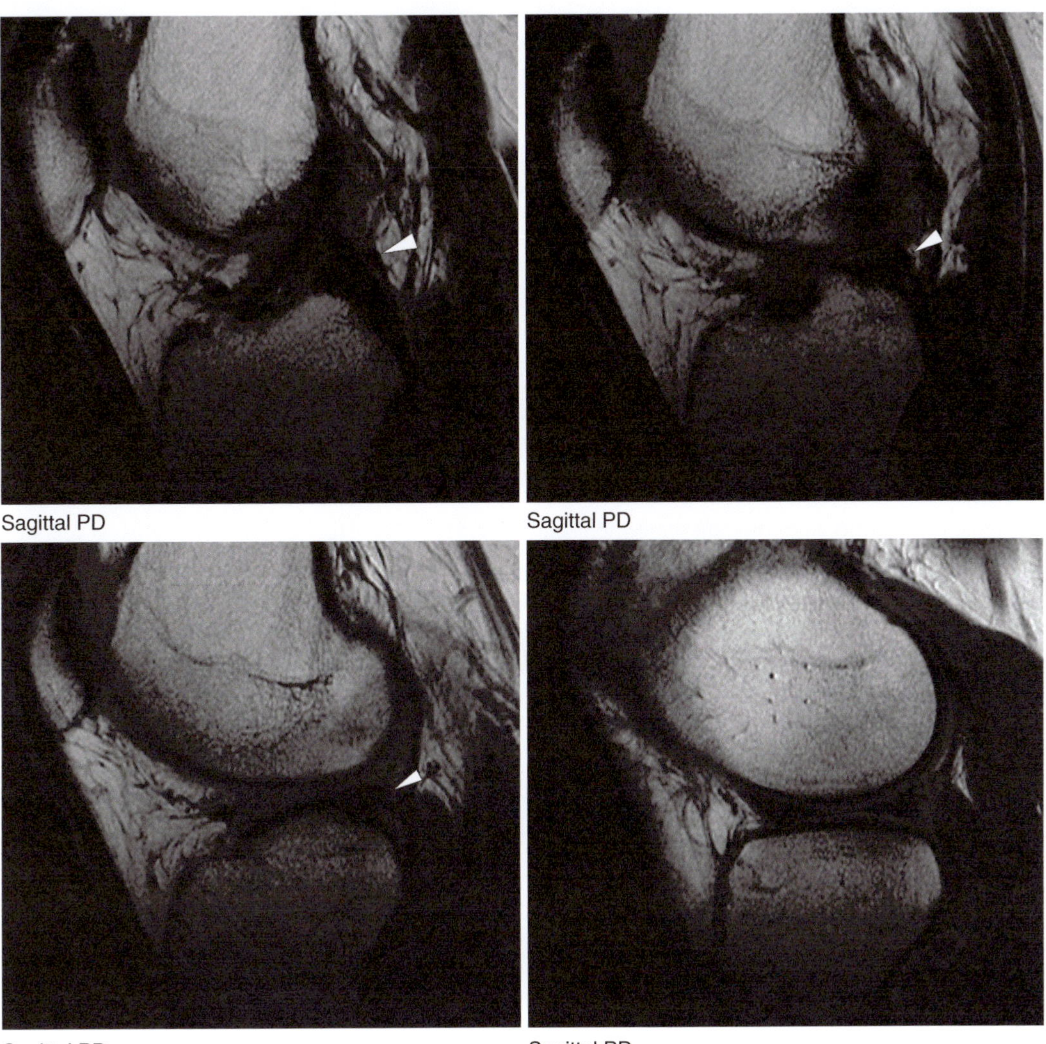

Sagittal PD

Sagittal PD

Sagittal PD

Sagittal PD

Normal meniscofemoral ligament of Wrisberg. Consecutive images mimicking a vertical tear of the lateral posterior horn by the meniscofemoral ligament of Wrisberg (arrowheads)

Discussion: Normal Meniscus and Normal Variants Mimicking Tears

The menisci are C-shaped fibrocartilaginous structures which lie between the articular surfaces of the femoral condyles and tibial plateaus. In cross-section, they are wedge shaped with a thick peripheral portion that tapers centrally to a thin free edge. The menisci are made of two types of collagen fibers. The first is circumferential collagen fibers that sweep along the long axis of the meniscus and help absorb axial load. The second are radially oriented fibers extending from the meniscal periphery to the free margin which help resist meniscal extrusion.

Each meniscus is divided into three segments, the anterior horn, the body, and the posterior horn, and each meniscus is attached to the tibia via anterior and posterior root attachments. Only the peripheral 15–20% of the meniscus is vascularized (red zone) from branches of the genicular arteries, while the majority of the meniscus is avascular (white zone).

The medial meniscus is larger and semilunar in shape. The posterior horn is wider than the anterior horn and is less mobile given its firm attachment to the joint capsule and deep fibers of the medial collateral ligament. The lateral meniscus is smaller in size than the medial meniscus, with uniform width of the anterior and posterior horns and is more mobile given its loose attachments to the joint capsule. The posterior horn of the lateral meniscus may also have attachments to the medial femoral condyle via the anterior and posterior meniscofemoral ligaments of Humphry and Wrisberg, respectively.

Anteriorly, the anterior horns of both menisci are attached via the anterior transverse meniscal ligament which can mimic a meniscal tear. The key is identifying the transverse ligament extending from one meniscus through Hoffa's fat pad and inserting to the other. Sometimes, the anterior horn of the lateral meniscus may appear speckled or striated near its anterior root attachment which can simulate a tear and hence should be reviewed cautiously. An important note is that isolated tears of the anterior horn of the lateral meniscus are uncommon.

On MRI, the sagittal plane is the primary plane for evaluating the anterior and posterior horns of the menisci, while the coronal plane is used for evaluating the body. Rarely, the axial plane may help visualize some tears (mainly radial tears). The normal meniscus appears dark on all pulse sequences with even contours and a triangular shape.

Suggested Reading

De Smet AA. How I diagnose meniscal tears on knee MRI. AJR Am J Roentgenol. 2012;199(3):48199.

Nguyen JC, De Smet AA, Graf BK, Rosas HG. MR imaging-based diagnosis and classification of meniscal tears. Radiographics. 2014;34(4):98199.

Case 5.2

Indication A 39-year-old male with medial knee pain and with positive McMurray test with external rotation and valgus stress.

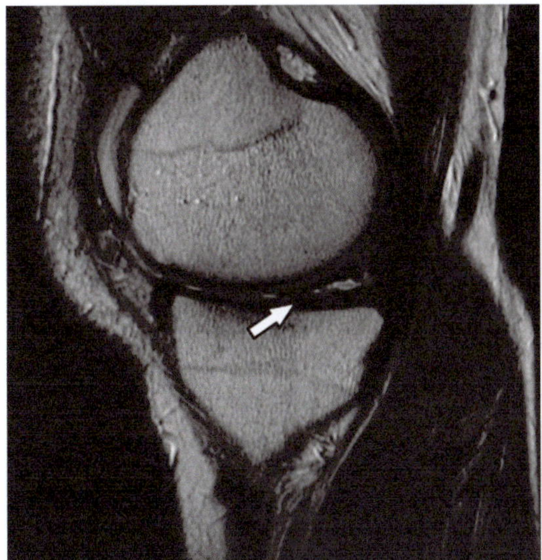

Sagittal PD

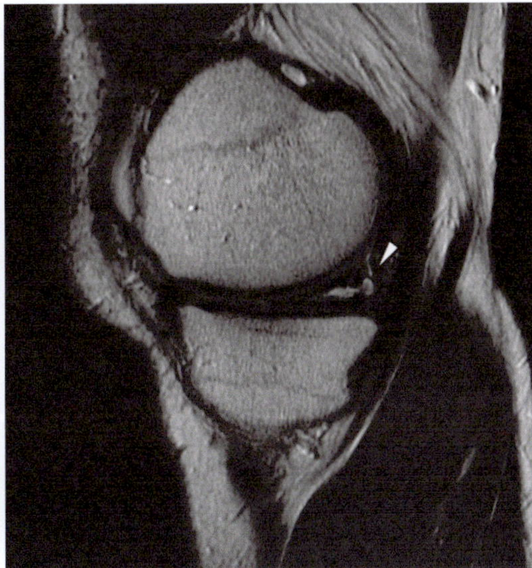

Sagittal PD

Findings

There is a horizontal tear involving the posterior horn of the medial meniscus (arrow) touching the inferior articular surface. There is an associated small 5 mm parameniscal cyst (arrowhead) located just posterior to the posterior horn of the medial meniscus. There is no displaced meniscal fragment. There are no focal chondral defects or subchondral marrow edema in the medial tibio-femoral compartment.

Impression/Recommendation

Horizontal tear at the posterior horn of the medial meniscus with a 5 mm parameniscal cyst.

Discussion: Menisci – Horizontal Tear

Roughly 12–14% of people have a meniscal tear in the United States, and having a meniscal tear increases the risk of developing osteoarthritis twofold compared to people without a tear. Patients with meniscal tears typically complain of pain at the joint line and can have a locking sensation. The McMurray test is a commonly performed clinical test and has sensitivity and specificity values of 55–80% for the diagnosis of a meniscal tear. In this test, the patient lies supine and has the hip and knee both flexed at 90 degrees. The examiner supports the ankle and grabs the knee with the thumb and side finger at the joint line. To test the medial meniscus, the lower leg is externally rotated and valgus stress is applied to the outside of the knee as the knee and hip are extended. To test the lateral meniscus, the lower leg is internally rotated and varus stress is applied to the inside of the knee as the hip and knee are extended. Pain, palpable snapping, or audible clicking indicates a positive test.

MRI has a high sensitivity and specificity for diagnosing a meniscal tear, and in today's clinical practice, it is uncommon for a surgeon to perform knee arthroscopy without a prior MRI. With advancing age, the meniscus undergoes myxoid degeneration which appears as intermediate signal intensity in the meniscus but should not reach an articular surface. These signal abnormalities have not been associated with tears at arthroscopy and do not increase the risk of developing a tear in the future.

MRI criteria for diagnosing meniscal tears can be divided into primary and secondary signs. There are two primary signs: (1) abnormal morphology or distortion (seen as blunting or truncation at the free edge of the meniscus) in the absence of prior surgery and (2) increased intrasubstance signal intensity that unequivocally contacts an articular surface on two or more images. This "two-slice-touch" rule has a positive predictive value (PPV) of 94% for medial meniscus and 96% for the lateral meniscus and hence should be reported as a meniscal tear. However, if the abnormal signal touches the articular surface on only one image, then the sensitivity of detecting a tear decreases to about 30–50% and should be reported as a "possible" tear. Secondary criteria for meniscal tears include meniscal extrusion, subchondral bone marrow edema, and presence of parameniscal cyst.

In general, meniscal tears are most common in the posterior horns, most frequently in the medial meniscus due to its strong attachments to the joint capsule. Isolated tears of the anterior horns are uncommon. There is no standard classification system for meniscal tears. However, the most common tear types described in the literature include horizontal, longitudinal, radial, root, complex, and bucket handle tears.

Horizontal tears are one of the most common tear patterns. These tears are often seen in patients older than 40 years of age without a known initiating traumatic event. They are also commonly seen in the setting of underlying degenerative joint disease and hence have also been classified as "degenerative" meniscal tears. Horizontal tears run parallel to the tibial plateau extending from the free edge toward the periphery splitting the meniscus into superior and inferior portions.

Think of viewing an ocean sunset where the horizon is the tear separating the sky from the water. On MRI, they appear as abnormally increased signal intensity that is horizontally oriented extending to the superior or inferior articular surface near the free edge.

Parameniscal cysts are most commonly seen with horizontal tears which can range from a few millimeters to several centimeters in size. On MRI, parameniscal cysts appear as fluid signal intensity lesions that have direct contact with an adjacent meniscal tear. These parameniscal cysts can dissect into the subcutaneous soft tissues of the knee or rarely have intraosseous extension which can make interpretation confusing. The presence of a parameniscal cyst should always alert you to look for an underlying meniscal tear. The only exception to this association is at the anterior horn of the lateral meniscus where it is also common to have ganglion cysts without a meniscal tear.

Occasionally, horizontal tears can become unstable and have a displaced meniscal fragment commonly called a flap tear or flipped fragment. Patients usually present with knee locking in these situations, and detection of these types of tears is important as they can be easily missed at arthroscopy. The majority of the displaced fragments are found at the posterior joint recess near or posterior to the posterior cruciate ligament. They can also be seen displaced in the superior or inferior knee recess/gutter above or below the body of the meniscus, respectively *(see supplementary images)*.

Surgical treatment of horizontal meniscal tears involves either meniscal debridement or partial meniscectomy, ideally with decompression of any associated parameniscal cysts.

Supplementary Images

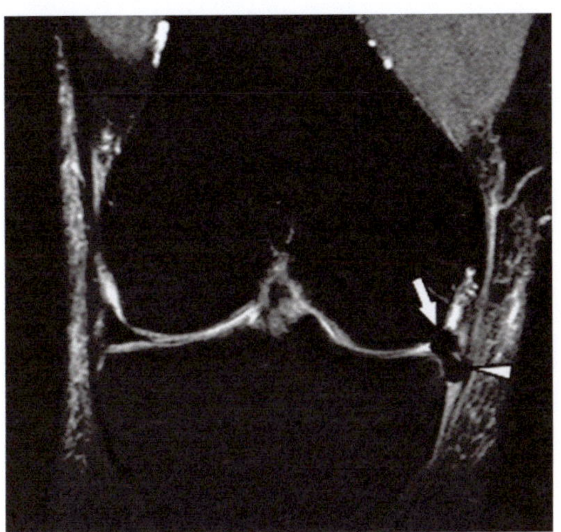

Coronal PD fat saturated

Displaced meniscal body tear. There is a tear at the body of the medial meniscus (arrow) with a small inferiorly displaced meniscal fragment into the meniscotibial recess/gutter (arrowhead)

Report checklist

1. Where is the meniscal tear located? medial or lateral meniscus? anterior horn, body, or posterior horn? inner two thirds or outer third of the meniscus?

2. Plane of the meniscal tear (horizontal, longitudinal, radial, root, bucket handle, complex)

3. Completeness of the tear (partial-thickness or complete width of the meniscus) as well as length of the tear

4. Is there a displaced or flipped meniscal fragment? If yes, its exact location

5. Is there an associated parameniscal cyst? If yes, its precise location and size

6. Any associated cartilage loss or subchondral marrow edema?

Suggested Reading

De Smet AA. How I diagnose meniscal tears on knee MRI. AJR Am J Roentgenol. 2012; 199(3):481–99.

Nguyen JC, De Smet AA, Graf BK, Rosas HG. MR imaging-based diagnosis and classification of meniscal tears. Radiographics. 2014;34(4):981–99.

Case 5.3

Indication A 27-year-old male with trauma 3 weeks ago presenting now with knee locking and pain. Evaluate for meniscus tear.

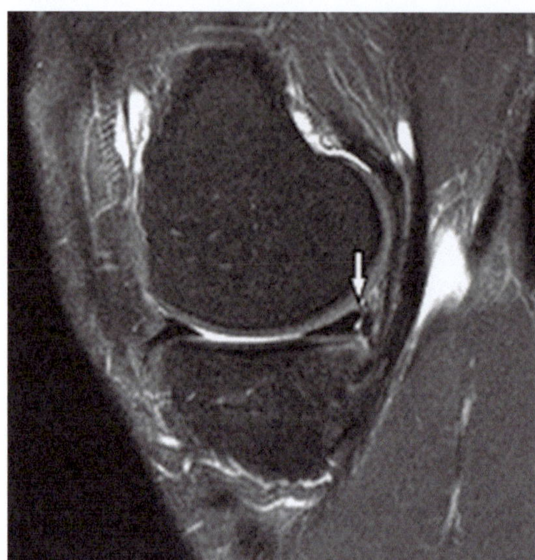

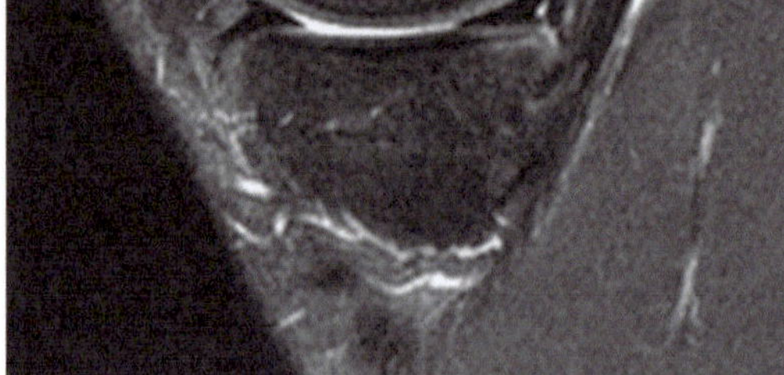

Sagittal T2 fat saturated

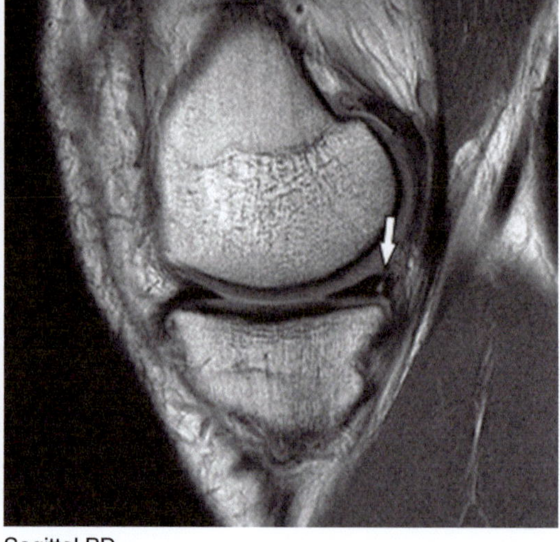

Sagittal PD

Findings

There is a longitudinal vertical tear at the posterior horn of the medial meniscus (arrows) involving the peripheral third of the meniscus (red zone) without a displaced meniscal fragment. There is no parameniscal cyst. There are no associated chondral defects or marrow edema.

Impression/Recommendation

Longitudinal vertical tear at the posterior horn of the medial meniscus.

Discussion: Menisci – Longitudinal Tear

Meniscal tears are the most common intra-articular knee injury and are the most common reason for knee arthroscopy performed by orthopedic surgeons. MRI is the preferred noninvasive imaging modality for evaluating internal derangement of the knee, especially meniscal tears. *Please refer to case 5.2 for further discussion on MRI criteria for diagnosing meniscal tears.*

Longitudinal tears typically occur in younger patients as compared to horizontal tears, and there is often a history of significant knee injury, especially an ACL tear. They also tend to involve the peripheral third (red zone) of the meniscus, particularly at the posterior horns of the medial and lateral menisci. Longitudinal tears typically have a vertical orientation running perpendicular to the tibial plateau and parallel to the circumference of the meniscus. They, therefore, divide the meniscus into peripheral and central halves.

On MRI, they are seen as a vertical line of increased signal intensity that contacts one or both articular surfaces. Longitudinal tears involving the peripheral third of the posterior horn of the lateral meniscus may be difficult to appreciate given the complex anatomy at that region. If the tear extends significantly through the long axis of the meniscus, the central (inner) fragment of the meniscus can become unstable and displaces centrally into the intercondylar notch creating a bucket handle tear. The "double PCL" sign can be seen in bucket handle tears involving the menisci. It is related to the flipped meniscus fragment sitting in the intercondylar notch just inferior and paralleling the PCL and hence gives the appearance of two PCLs on the sagittal plane *(see supplementary images)*. These bucket handle tears are much more common in the medial meniscus. When a bucket handle tear involves the lateral meniscus, it does not result in a double PCL sign as the ACL blocks the "handle" fragment from reaching the intercondylar notch. Alternatively, a bucket handle tear can displace into the anterior compartment of the knee rather than the intercondylar notch. The displaced meniscal fragment usually lies adjacent to the anterior horn of the meniscus giving the appearance of a "double anterior horn" sign with a diminutive posterior horn *(see supplementary images)*. This occurs most commonly with the lateral meniscus due to its looser posterior menisocapsular attach-

ments when compared to the more rigid attachments on the medial side.

It is important to be familiar with the normal anatomical structures that can mimic longitudinal tears. These structures include the insertion of the transverse meniscal ligament to the anterior horns of both menisci and the popliteal tendon sheath and meniscofemoral ligaments posteriorly for the lateral meniscus. No normal anatomic mimics exist for the posterior horn of the medial meniscus.

Peripheral longitudinal tears are usually treated with primary meniscal repair.

Supplementary Images

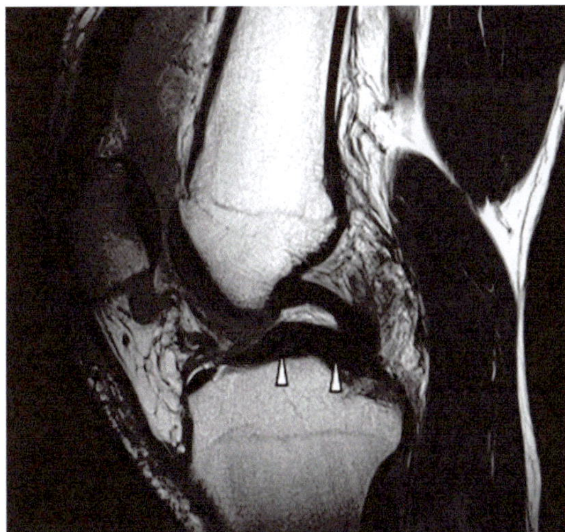

Sagittal PD

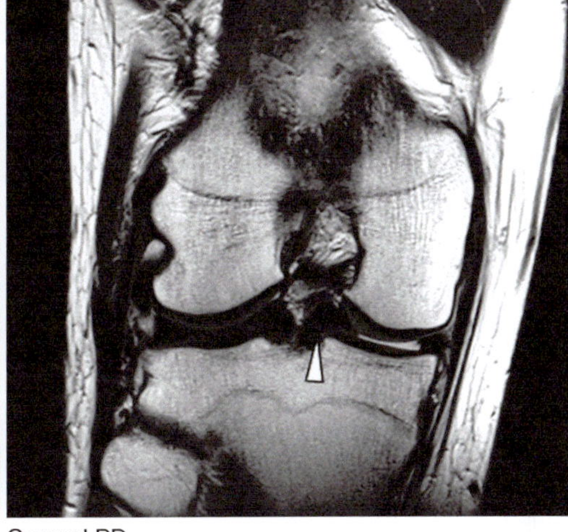

Coronal PD

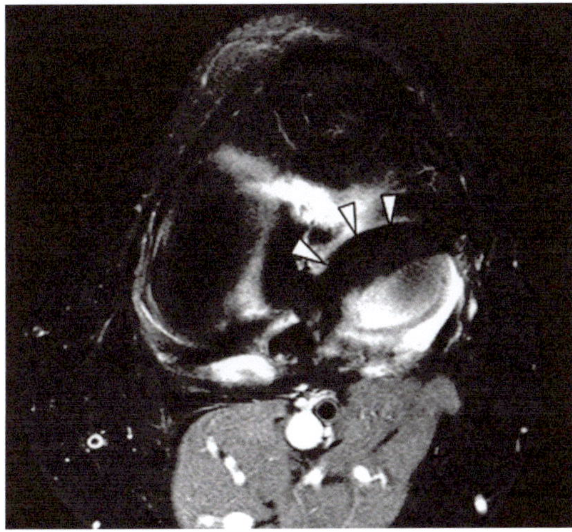

Axial PD fat saturated

"Double PCL" sign. There is a bucket handle tear involving the posterior horn and body of the medial meniscus with a displaced meniscal fragment (arrowheads) in the intercondylar notch, giving the "double PCL" sign on the sagittal plane

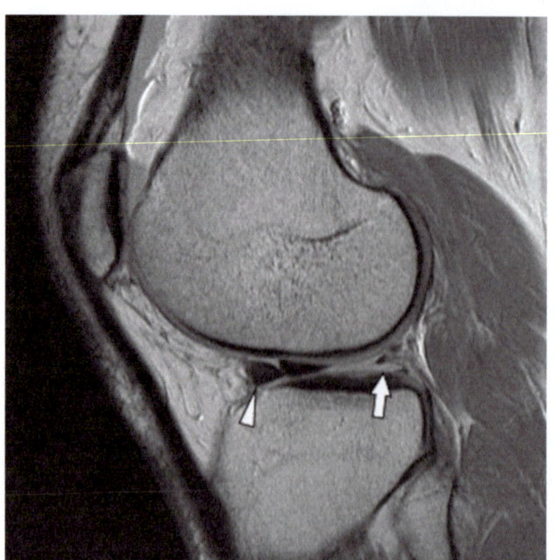

Sagittal PD

"Double anterior horn" sign. There is absence of the posterior horn of the lateral meniscus in its expected anatomic location (arrow). The posterior horn of the lateral meniscus is displaced anterior to the normal anterior horn giving the "double anterior horn" sign

Report checklist

1. Where is the meniscal tear located (medial or lateral meniscus? anterior horn, body or posterior horn? inner two thirds or outer third of the meniscus?
2. Plane of the meniscal tear (horizontal, longitudinal, radial, root, bucket handle, complex)
3. Completeness of the tear (partial-thickness or complete width of the meniscus) as well as length of the tear
4. Is there a displaced or flipped meniscal fragment? If yes, its exact location
5. Is there an associated parameniscal cyst? If yes, its precise location and size
6. Any associated cartilage loss or subchondral marrow edema?

Suggested Reading

De Smet AA. How I diagnose meniscal tears on knee MRI. AJR Am J Roentgenol. 2012; 199(3): 481–99.

Nguyen JC, De Smet AA, Graf BK, Rosas HG. MR imaging-based diagnosis and classification of meniscal tears. Radiographics. 2014;34(4):981–99.

Case 5.4

Indication A 41-year-old male with twisting injury 2 months ago. Now presenting with medial joint line pain and tenderness. Evaluate for medial meniscus tear or MCL injury.

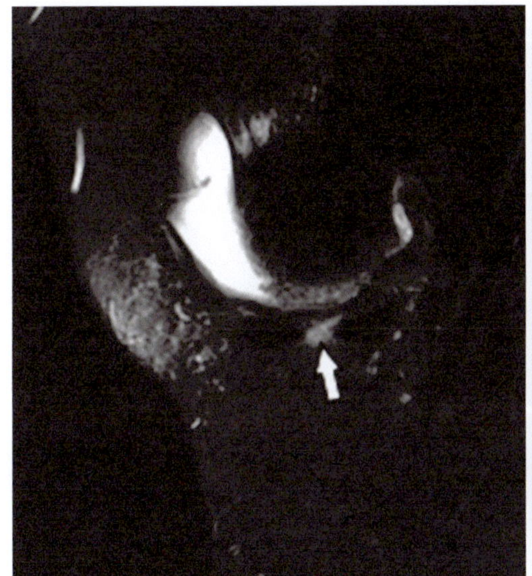

Sagittal T2 fat saturated

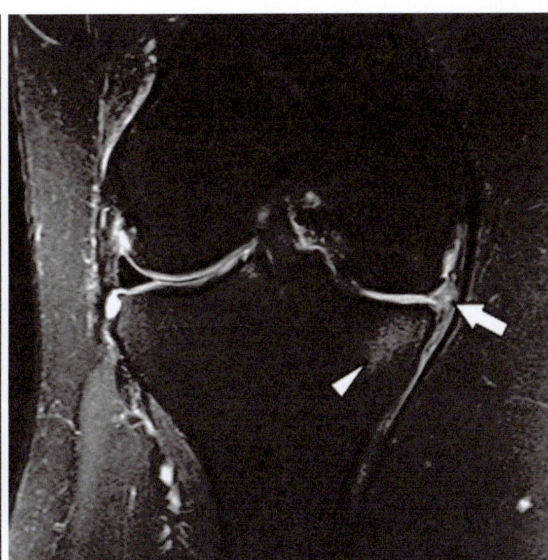

Coronal PD fat saturated

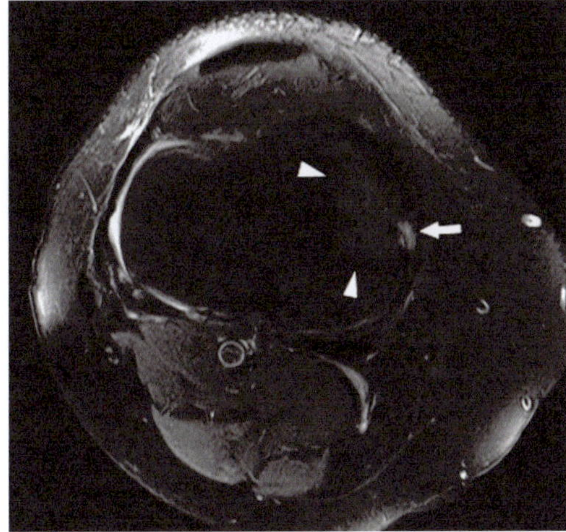

Axial PD fat saturated

Findings

There is a complete radial tear at the body of the medial meniscus (arrows). *[this is seen as a cleft sign on the sagittal plane and a "ghost meniscus" sign on the coronal plane].* There is no displaced meniscal fragment or parameniscal cyst. There are areas of high-grade partial-thickness chondral loss at the medial tibiofemoral compartment with underlying bone marrow edema (arrowheads).

Impression/Recommendation

Complete radial tear at the body of the medial meniscus.

Discussion: Menisci – Radial Tear

Meniscal tears are the most common intra-articular knee injury and are the most common reason for knee arthroscopy performed by orthopedic surgeons. MRI is the preferred noninvasive imaging modality for evaluating internal derangement of the knee, in particular, for evaluating meniscal tears. *Please refer to case 5.2 for further discussion on MRI criteria for diagnosing meniscal tears.*

Radial tears are vertically oriented tears that run perpendicular to both the tibial plateau and the long axis of the meniscus. They often begin at the free edge of the meniscus and extend toward the periphery. They can be either partial or complete, depending on the degree of involvement of the width of the meniscus. Since radial tears transect the longitudinal collagen fibers of the meniscus, they compromise the normal hoop strength of the meniscus resulting in severe loss of function and meniscal extrusion.

Various signs have been used to describe radial tears on MRI. These signs depend on the location of the tear relative to the imaging plane:

1. Cleft sign: this represents a vertical high signal intensity line passing through the meniscus. This sign is seen on sagittal images of a radial tear through the meniscal body, or on coronal images of a radial tear through the horns.
2. Truncated meniscus sign: represents abrupt truncation of the normal triangular meniscal contour at the free margin with preservation of the peripheral portion. This is usually related to a partial-thickness tear.
3. Ghost meniscus sign: is related to a complete radial tear. It represents a hyperintense area with no meniscal tissue seen due to the image slice passing through the meniscal tear. There is normal appearance of the meniscus seen on the adjacent slices. A truncated or ghost meniscus sign is seen on sagittal images of radial tears through the horns and on coronal images of radial tears through the body.

Symptomatic radial tears are usually treated by meniscal debridement at the tear site.

> **Report checklist**
> 1. Where is the meniscal tear located? medial or lateral meniscus? anterior horn, body or posterior horn? inner two thirds or outer third of the meniscus?
> 2. Plane of the meniscal tear (horizontal, longitudinal, radial, root, bucket handle, complex)
> 3. Completeness of the tear (partial-thickness or complete width of the meniscus) as well as length of the tear
> 4. Is there a displaced or flipped meniscal fragment? If yes, its exact location
> 5. Is there an associated parameniscal cyst? If yes, its precise location and size
> 6. Any associated cartilage loss or subchondral marrow edema?

Suggested Reading

Harper K, Helms CA, Lambert HS 3rd, Higgins LD. Radial meniscal tears: significance, incidence, and MR appearance. AJR Am J Roentgenol. 2005;185:1429–34.

Magee T, Shapiro M, Williams D. MR accuracy and arthroscopic incidence of meniscal radial tears. Skeletal Radiol. 2002;31(12): 686–9.

Nguyen JC, De Smet AA, Graf BK, Rosas HG. MR imaging-based diagnosis and classification of meniscal tears. Radiographics. 2014;34(4):981–99.

Case 5.5

Indication A 54-year-old female with chronic medial knee pain. Not responding to conservative management. Evaluate for meniscus tear or other intra-articular cause.

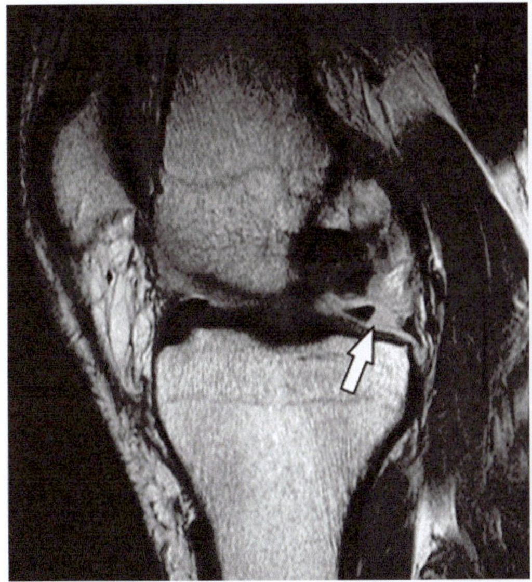

Sagittal PD

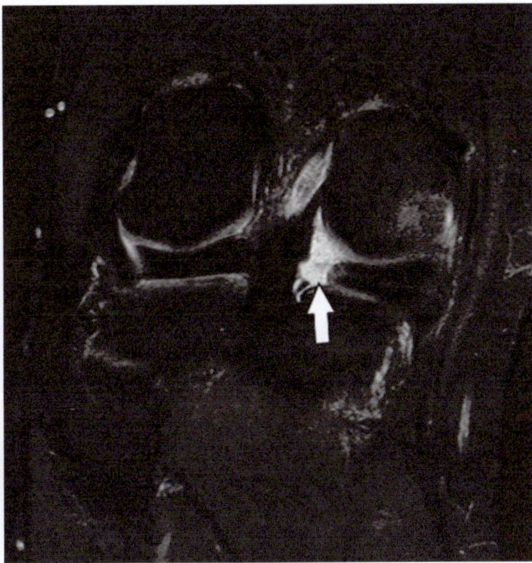

Coronal T2 fat saturated

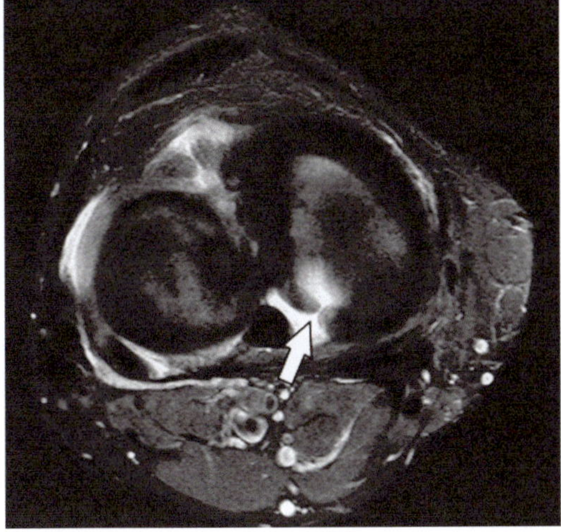

Axial PD fat saturated

Findings

There is a large complete radial tear at the posterior root of the medial meniscus (arrows) about 5 mm from its tibial attachment without extension of the tear into the posterior horn. There is a small amount of root meniscus still attached to the tibia. There is minimal extrusion of the meniscus body beyond the medial joint line. There is no parameniscal cyst and no focal chondral defects.

Impression/Recommendation

Complete radial tear near the posterior root of the medial meniscus.

Discussion: Menisci – Root Tear

MRI has high sensitivity and specificity for the identification of meniscal tears. MRI criteria for meniscal tears include abnormal morphology or abnormal fluid signal intensity extending to an articular surface. *Please refer to case 5.2 for further discussion on MRI criteria for diagnosing meniscal tears.*

Root tears have been receiving high attention in the radiology and orthopedic literature due to the recognition of the importance of this structure. The meniscal roots prevent meniscal extrusion which is vital in transmitting axial load into hoop stress. Each meniscus has anterior and posterior root attachments. Injuries to the meniscal root range from degeneration with thickening to a frank tear. Root tears are most commonly a radial-type tear and often occur in elderly patients.

MRI findings of a root tear include a linear defect on axial MR images perpendicular to the long axis of the meniscus. On the coronal plane, a vertical fluid cleft of high signal intensity can be seen (cleft sign). On the sagittal plane, a truncated meniscus or ghost meniscus sign will be visualized. *Please refer to case 5.4 for further discussion on radial tear signs.* When describing a root tear, it is important to describe whether there is root degeneration, a partial radial tear or complete radial tear. Also the distance of the tear from the root attachment and whether the tear extends into the respective anterior or posterior horn should be described in the report.

Complete root tears have a high association with meniscal extrusion beyond the margin of the tibia. Meniscal extrusion is considered present when there is >3 mm extrusion of the body of the meniscus at the level of the mid-joint line on a coronal image *(see supplementary images).* However, meniscal extrusion can also be seen with large radial tears, complex tears, and degenerative changes at the tibiofemoral knee compartments. When the meniscus extrudes peripherally, the axial load on the knee is not distributed appropriately, and this is a predisposing factor for developing osteoarthritis of the knee as well as a precursor for subchondral insufficiency fracture of the femoral condyles. Radial tears near the meniscal root attachment can function similar to a root tear.

Given the importance of meniscal root injury, novel surgical techniques have been developed to repair meniscal root injuries to prevent long-term complications. These include transtibial pullout repair and suture anchor repair techniques.

Supplementary Images

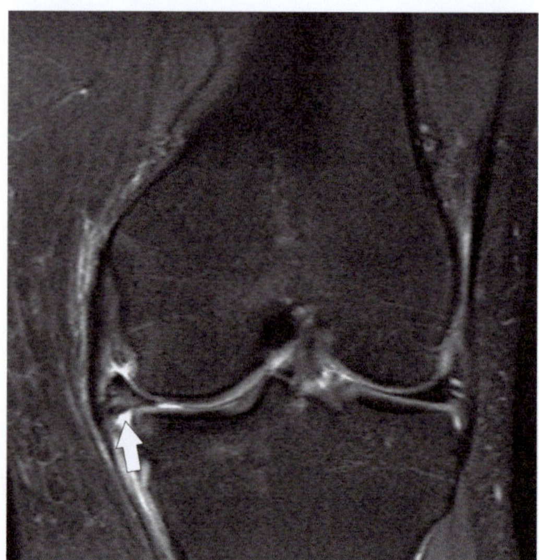

Coronal PD fat saturated

Meniscal extrusion. There is 5 mm of extrusion of the body of the medial meniscus (arrow) beyond the medial joint line

Report checklist

1. Where is the meniscal tear located? medial or lateral meniscus? anterior horn, body or posterior horn? inner two thirds or outer third of the meniscus?
2. Plane of the meniscal tear (horizontal, longitudinal, radial, root, bucket handle, complex)
3. Completeness of the tear (partial-thickness or complete width of the meniscus) as well as length of the tear
4. Is there a displaced or flipped meniscal fragment? If yes, its exact location
5. Is there an associated parameniscal cyst? If yes, its precise location and size
6. Any associated cartilage loss or subchondral marrow edema?

Suggested Reading

Choi CJ, Choi YJ, Lee JJ, Choi CH. Magnetic resonance imaging evidence of meniscal extrusion in medial meniscus posterior root tear. Arthroscopy. 2010;26:1602–1606.

Lee SY, Jee WH, Kim JM. Radial tear of the medial meniscal root: reliability and accuracy of MRI for diagnosis. AJR Am J Roentgenol. 2008;191:81–85.

Case 5.6

Indication   A 28-year-old male with recent twisting knee injury and medial joint line pain. Rule out internal derangement.

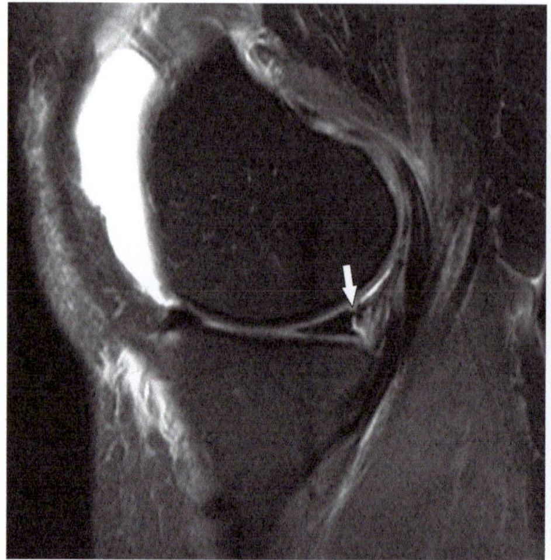

Sagittal PD fat saturated

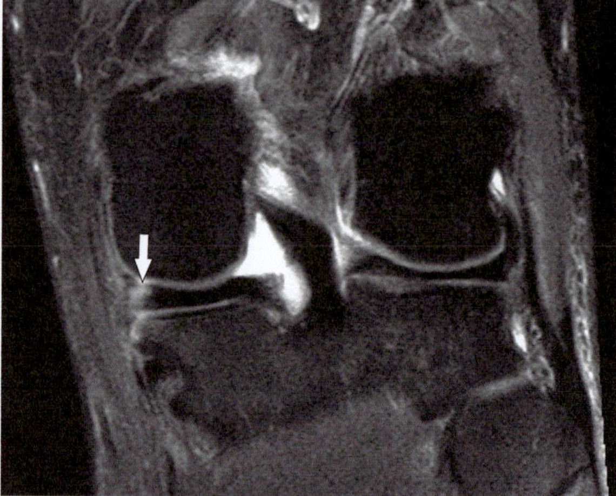

Coronal PD fat saturated

Findings

There is a vertically oriented fluid-filled cleft (arrows) at the junction of the posterior horn of the medial meniscus and the adjacent capsule. On the coronal image, there is irregularity and fraying of the peripheral aspect of the meniscus.

Impression/Recommendation

Meniscocapsular separation.

Discussion: Menisci – Meniscocapsular Separation

Meniscocapsular separation is defined as the detachment of the peripheral portion of the meniscus from its capsular attachment. The meniscus itself is normal in morphology and hence results in a floating meniscus. This type of injury is relatively uncommon and is usually missed clinically and on MRI. Meniscocapsular separation usually involves the less mobile medial meniscus and is often associated with other ligamentous injuries, especially anterior cruciate ligament (ACL) and medical collateral ligament (MCL) tears. Therefore, patients usually present with tenderness and persistent pain over the medial joint line. This injury should be suspected in individuals with an ACL tear who complain of medial knee pain without any obvious abnormality of the medial meniscus or the MCL.

Meniscocapsular separations are hard to diagnose based on clinical findings as the symptoms are nonspecific. MRI can potentially aid in diagnosis; however, it is essential to be familiar with the normal anatomy and MR appearance of the medial meniscocapsular area to appreciate this lesion and avoid pitfalls. The medial meniscus has strong peripheral attachments to the joint line and the deep fibers of the MCL, and there is usually no fluid present between the periphery of the meniscus and the joint capsule. Sometimes small recesses can be seen posterior to the posterior horn of the medial meniscus; however, these are usually small and do not extend along the entire craniocaudal length of the meniscus.

Meniscocapsular separation should be suspected on MRI if there is irregularity at the peripheral margin of the medial meniscus with fluid signal intensity extending in a vertical orientation between the periphery of the meniscus and the adjacent joint capsule from the superior to inferior surface.

Meniscocapsular separation can be repaired surgically by using all-inside nonabsorbable sutures.

> **Report checklist**
> 1. Is there excess fluid between the posterior horn of the medial meniscus and joint capsule with a normal appearing meniscus?
> 2. Is there an associated ACL tear?
> 3. Are there any associated articular cartilage loss or subchondral marrow edema?

Suggested Reading

De Maeseneer M, Shahabpour M, Vanderdood K, Van Roy F, Osteaux M. Medial meniscocapsular separation: MR imaging criteria and diagnostic pitfalls. Eur J Radiol. 2002;41(3): 242–52.

Nguyen JC, De Smet AA, Graf BK, Rosas HG. MR imaging-based diagnosis and classification of meniscal tears. Radiographics. 2014;34(4):981–99.

Case 5.7

Indication A 29-year-old female with severe knee pain after an injury while playing soccer. Rule out ACL tear.

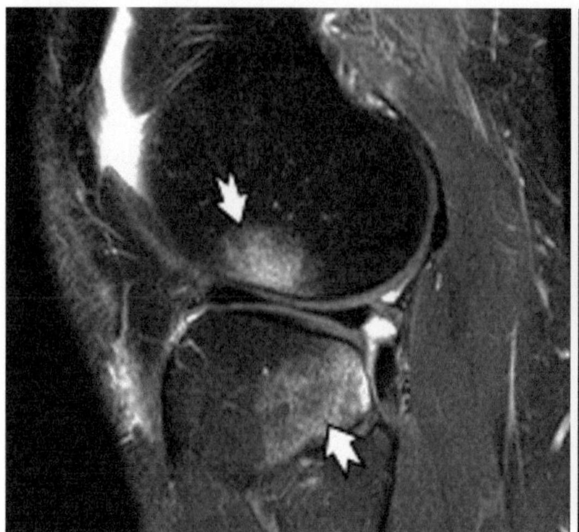

Sagittal T2 fat saturated

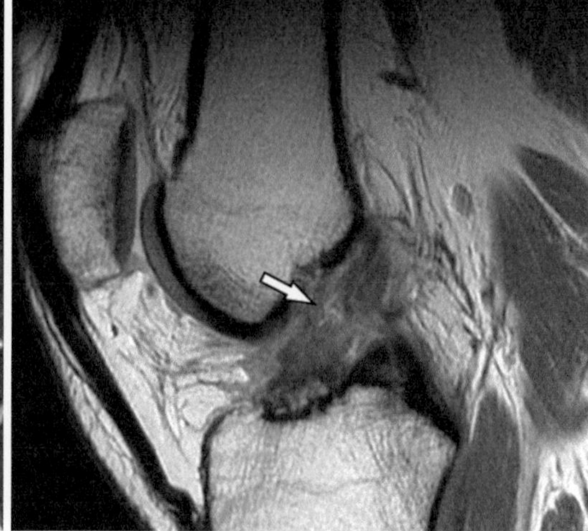

Sagittal PD

Findings

There are bone contusions (notched arrows) at the lateral femoral condyle and posterior aspect of the lateral tibial plateau consistent with a pivot-shift type mechanism of injury. There is a complete tear at the mid-substance of the anterior cruciate ligament (arrow) with surrounding soft tissue edema compatible with an acute tear. There is no meniscus tear or focal chondral defects. There is a small joint effusion.

Impression/Recommendation

Complete tear of the anterior cruciate ligament at its mid-substance.

Discussion: Anterior Cruciate Ligament Injury

The normal anterior cruciate ligament (ACL) has an oblique course in the intercondylar notch of the knee originating from the posteromedial aspect of the lateral femoral condyle extending anteriorly and medially parallel to the roof of the intercondylar notch (Blumensaat's line) to insert onto the tibia, anterolateral to the medial tibial spine. The ACL is an intra-articular, extra-synovial structure and is composed of two discrete bundles – the larger and stronger anteromedial bundle and smaller posterolateral bundle.

On MRI, the normal ACL appears hypointense on both T1- and T2-weighted images; however distally, the ligament fans out at its tibial insertion with a striated appearance of high signal intensity due to the presence of normal interspersed fat and should not be mistaken for a tear. When assessing the ACL, if both bundles are visualized from their origin to insertion, then this indicates an intact ligament. Assessing the ACL on only the sagittal plane can be problematic as many ACL tears occur at the femoral origin, and there can be partial volume averaging artifact at this region between the ACL and the lateral femoral condyle. Therefore, it is essential to evaluate the ACL on all (axial, coronal, and sagittal) planes to thoroughly evaluate the ACL in order to avoid this pitfall.

Tears of the ACL are one of the most frequently encountered knee ligament injuries. Several mechanisms of injury can result in ACL tears including "dashboard" and hyperextension injuries; however, the most common mechanism is related to a valgus force on the knee with flexion and external rotation of the tibia or internal rotation of the femur, the so-called "pivot-shift" mechanism of injury. ACL tears most commonly occur at its mid-substance followed by its femoral origin. Tibial avulsions are rare and usually occur in the pediatric population. The majority of ACL injuries can be diagnosed from history and physical examination in the hands of an experienced clinician. The role of MRI is to define the extent of the injury (partial-thickness or complete tear) and location of the tear (mid-substance, femoral avulsion or tibial avulsion). MRI can also assess associated abnormalities such as meniscal tears, other ligamentous injuries, and assess for cartilaginous and osseous abnormalities.

The major finding of an acute ACL tear on MRI is an enlarged and edematous ligament with ill-definition and fiber discontinuity either at its mid-substance or femoral origin. In the case of a femoral avulsion, there can be fluid signal intensity at the normal attachment of the ACL seen on the axial and coronal images referred to as the "empty notch" sign. The ACL may have posterior bowing and a horizontal orientation, no longer parallel Blumensaat's line. Tibial avulsions of the ACL are rare (5%) with the osseous avulsed fragment either non-displaced or minimally displaced. Bone marrow edema at the fracture site is usually minimal and hence can be easily missed; therefore, correlation with plain radiographs is important *(see supplementary images)*.

Many secondary signs of ACL tears have been described. They, however, do not significantly improve the accuracy of diagnosing an ACL tear. To name a few, there can be bone marrow contusions at the lateral femoral condyle and the posterior aspect of the lateral tibial plateau related to the pivot-shift mechanism of injury. There may also be an osteochondral impaction fracture at the lateral femoral condyle with irregularity of the articular surface and underlying bone marrow edema referred to as the "deep femoral sulcus" sign. There is also the "anterior drawer" sign which is anterior subluxation of the lateral tibial plateau relative to the femur by >5 mm measured on a sagittal slice through the middle of the lateral femoral condyle and posterior margin of the lateral tibial plateau *(see supplementary images)*. The "vertical fibular collateral" sign is when the entire length of the fibular collateral ligament is seen on one coronal slice *(see supplementary images)*. A Segond fracture is an avulsion injury of the lateral rim of the tibia at the attachment site of the anterolateral ligament and is suggestive of an ACL tear in 90–100% of cases *(see supplementary images)*.

A partial ACL tear is more difficult to appreciate on MRI and can sometimes mimic a complete rupture. This is seen as edema and ill-definition of the ligament with some areas of fiber discontinuity; however, some fibers remain intact throughout the normal course of the ligament. This is best evaluated on the coronal and axial images. The anteromedial bundle is most commonly injured in partial tears. In addition, ganglia in the ACL can also mimic a partial tear *(please refer to case 5.17 for further discussion on ACL ganglia)*. The ligament will be enlarged; however, there should be normal fibers coursing through the ligament which will be absent in an ACL tear. A chronic tear (>8 weeks) may have a variable appearance on MRI. It can be completely absent or have a severely attenuated appearance *(see supplementary image)*. The ligament may also become fibrosed and fused to the intercondylar roof or the posterior cruciate ligament.

When an ACL tear is suspected, special attention should be made to the posterior horn of the lateral and medial menisci due to the increased association with peripheral longitudinal vertical tears. Also, assessment of other ligamentous injuries should be sought.

Treatment of ACL injuries depends on many factors such as the degree of the ACL injury, presence of other ligamentous or meniscal injuries, patient's age, and level of activity. However, ACL deficient knees are at increased risk for secondary meniscal tears, articular damage, and early osteoarthritis, and thus in young individuals, the ACL is usually repaired or reconstructed.

Supplementary Images

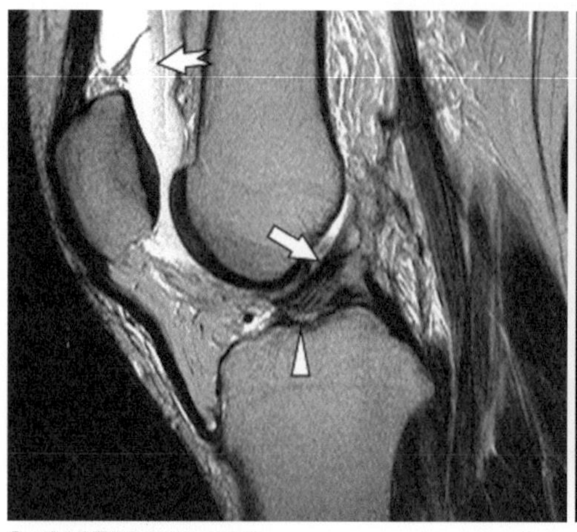

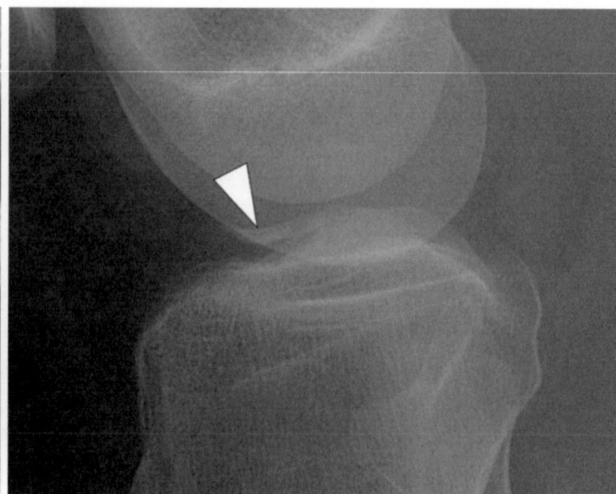

Sagittal T2 fat saturated

Tibial avulsion of the ACL (arrow) with a small osseous fracture fragment (arrowheads). This is better seen on the plain radiograph. There is an associated knee joint effu-sion (notched arrow). These avulsion injuries are more common in young patients

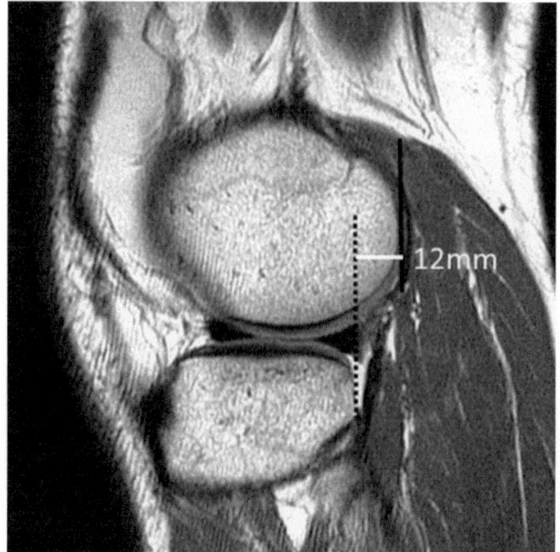

Sagittal PD

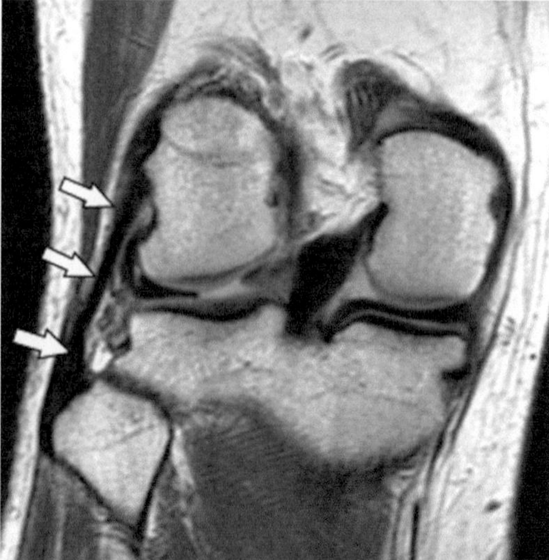

Coronal PD

There is anterior translation of the posterior margin of the lateral tibia (dotted black line) relative to the posterior margin of the lateral femoral condyle (solid black line), measuring 12 mm (white line). This is a secondary sign of ACL rupture. Normal distance should be <5 mm

The fibular collateral ligament is seen in its entirety on a single coronal slice (arrows), a secondary sign of ACL rupture

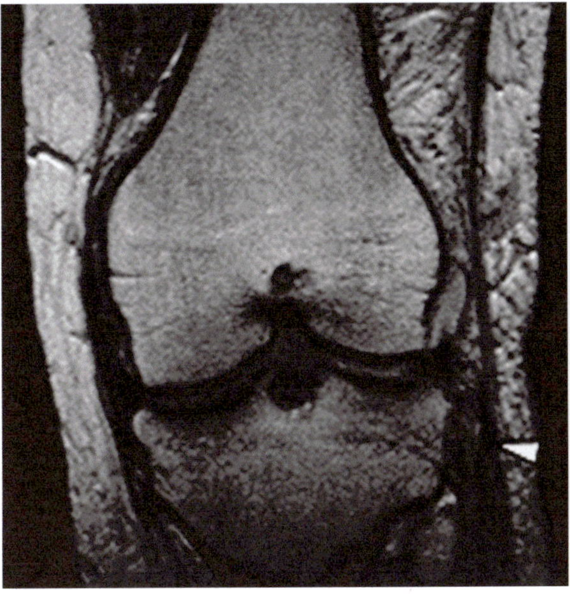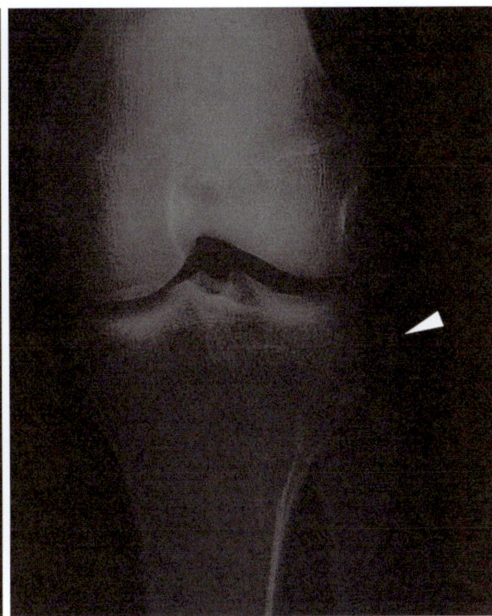

Coronal PD

Small cortical avulsion from the lateral rim of the tibia (arrowheads) compatible with a Segond fracture. This is confirmed on the plain radiographs

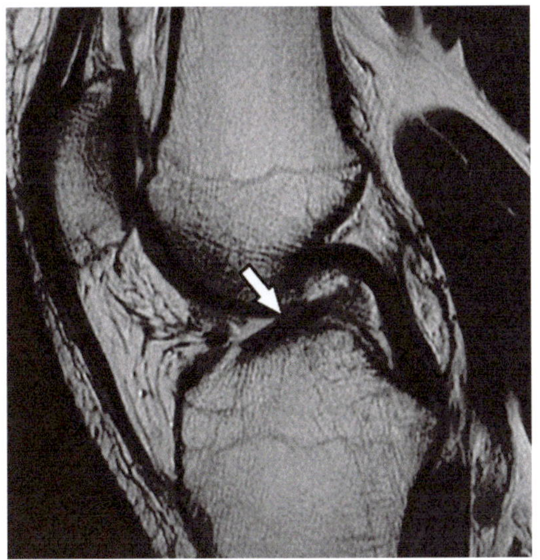

Sagittal PD

There is a chronic tear of the ACL (arrow). The ligament is attenuated and the distal fibers have a flatten orientation

Report checklist

1. Where is the location of the ACL injury (femoral, mid-substance, tibial)?
2. Is the ACL sprained, partially torn or completely disrupted? Could this be an ACL ganglion mimicking a tear?
3. Is there an associated avulsion fracture (often tibial avulsion)?
4. Is there intraligamentous and surrounding soft tissue edema to suggest an acute tear?
5. Are there bony contusions at the lateral femoral condyle and posterior aspect of lateral tibial plateau suggesting a pivot-shift mechanism of injury?
6. Is there an osteochondral impaction at the sulcus terminalis of the lateral femoral condyle?
7. Are there meniscal tears? Especially at the posterior horn of either menisci? Any chondral defects?
8. Any other ligamentous injury?
9. Presence of joint effusion/hemarthrosis?
10. Could this be a chronic ACL tear?

Suggested Reading

Lee K, Siegel MJ, Lau DM et-al. Anterior cruciate ligament tears: MR imaging-based diagnosis in a pediatric population. Radiology. 1999;213(3):697–704.

Volokhina YV, Syed HM, Pham PH, Blackburn AK. Two helpful MRI signs for evaluation of posterolateral bundle tears of the anterior cruciate ligament: a pilot study. Orthop J Sports Med. 2015;3(8).

Case 5.8

Indication A 28-year-old male with medial knee pain and tenderness after a fall. Assess medial collateral ligament and medial meniscus.

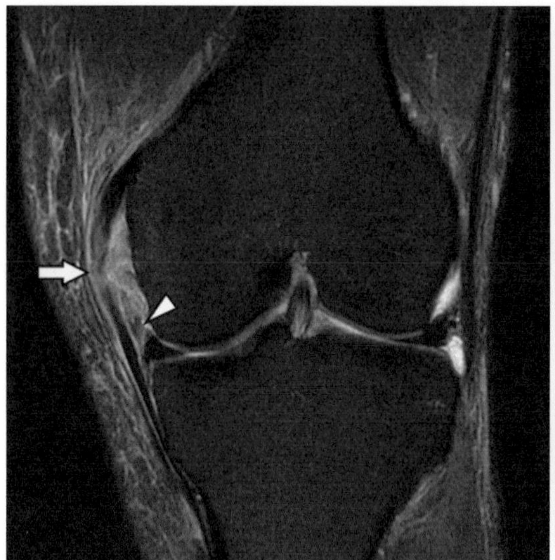

Coronal T2 fat saturated

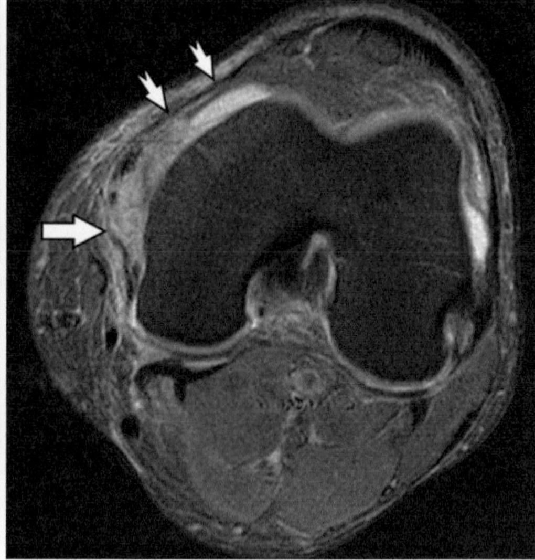

Axial PD fat saturated

Findings

There is partial disruption of the proximal fibers of the superficial medial collateral ligament (arrows) with irregularity and periligamentous edema compatible with an acute grade 2 sprain. There is also a tear of the deep meniscofemoral ligament (arrowhead). The meniscotibial ligament, medial patellofemoral retinaculum (notched arrows), and the posteromedial corner structures are intact. The ACL and menisci are normal. No focal bony contusion or fractures are seen.

Impression/Recommendation

Acute grade 2 sprain of the medial collateral ligament and tear of the deep meniscofemoral ligament.

Discussion: Medial Collateral Ligament Injury

The superficial medial collateral ligament (MCL) runs vertically along the middle third of the knee medially originating from the adductor tubercle of the medial femoral condyle and inserting dis-

tally on the tibia approximately 6–7 cm distal to the joint line and deep to the pes anserine tendons. The ligament measures approximately 1.5 cm in anterior to posterior width. There are smaller but functionally important deep fibers of the MCL which are thickening of the medial joint capsule and lie deep to the superficial MCL referred to as the meniscofemoral and meniscotibial ligaments. The superior meniscofemoral ligament attaches the superior aspect of the medial meniscus to the femur while the inferior meniscotibial ligament (also referred to as the coronary ligament) extends from the inferior aspect of the medial meniscus attaching to the tibia. The MCL functions as the primary restraint for valgus and external rotation stress. Between the superficial and deep layers of the MCL lies a small potential space known as the MCL bursa which can sometimes be inflamed resulting in bursitis and should not be mistaken for MCL injury or meniscocapsular separation. These structures are best evaluated on coronal and axial fat-suppressed fluid-sensitive sequences *(see supplementary images)*.

Injuries to the MCL are usually the result of a valgus stress, however, sometimes injured in more complex twisting injuries which may result in multiple ligamentous injuries as ACL tear as well as meniscal tears.

On MRI, the normal MCL is denoted as a low signal intensity band that extends from its femoral epicondylar attachment to the medial tibia. After a traumatic event, a grade 1 injury is demonstrated as thickening and edema within the ligament as well as periligamentous edema more commonly involving the proximal femoral attachment, however no focal ligament tear. It is important to understand that edema superficial to the MCL is a nonspecific finding, and although it can be seen with MCL injuries, it can also be present with meniscal tears, osteoarthritis, and Baker's cyst rupture. Therefore care should be taken in diagnosing MCL sprain in the absence of knee trauma. Grade 2 injuries represent a partial-thickness tear which appears as high fluid signal intensity signal within the ligament with irregularity and attenuation of the fibers of the MCL. This is also more commonly seen at its proximal femoral origin or the mid-substance. Complete tears (grade 3 injury) are diagnosed when there is complete disruption of the fibers with fluid signal gap and retraction of the torn ligament. It is also important to look for and comment on the integrity of the deep meniscotibial, and meniscofemoral ligaments as these may also need to be surgically fixed.

Characteristic bony contusions or osteochondral impaction fractures can be seen at the lateral femoral condyle and lateral tibial plateau related to the valgus injury. Injuries of the MCL can propagate both anterior or posteriorly to involve the anterior medial patellofemoral ligament (MPFL) or the posteromedial supporting structures as the posterior oblique ligament (POL) and posterior capsule. A chronic injury may be accompanied with thickening of the ligament and intraligamentous or periligamentous ossification or calcification which is known as Pellegrini-Stieda disease.

In general, grade 1 and 2 injuries are treated conservatively; however, grade 3 injuries are usually treated surgically especially if it is associated with other ligamentous injuries as an ACL tear.

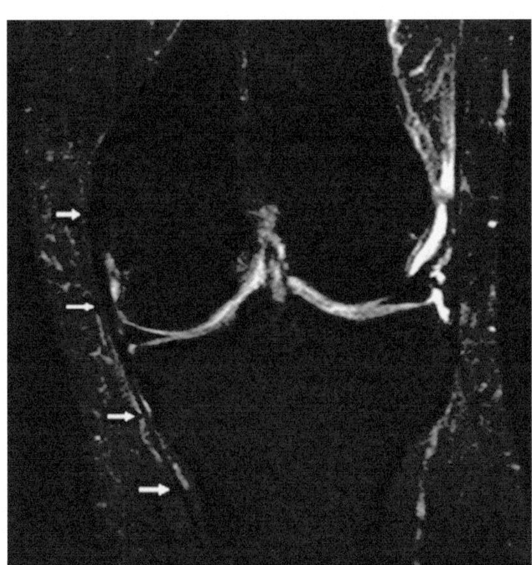
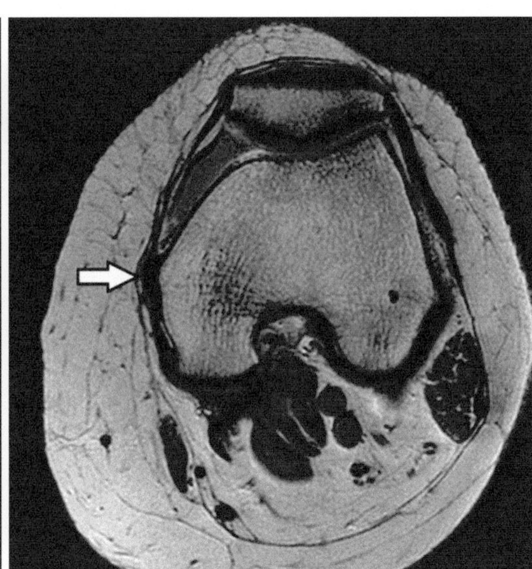

Coronal PD fat saturated   Axial PD

Normal appearance of the superficial MCL (arrows)

Report checklist

1. Where is the location of the MCL injury (proximal, mid-substance, distal)? Superficial and/or deep components?
2. Is the MCL sprained, partially torn or completely disrupted? Is there an associated avulsion fracture?
3. How are the deep meniscotibial and meniscofemoral ligaments?
4. Does the injury extend anteriorly to the MPFL or posteriorly to involve the posteromedial structures (POL, posterior capsule)?
5. Are there other ligamentous injuries (ACL tear, meniscal tears)?
6. Are there focal bone contusions or osteochondral impaction fractures at the lateral tibiofemoral compartment?

Suggested Reading

Ikuma H, Abe N, Uchida Y, Furumatsu T, Fujiwara K, Nishida K, et al. Novel magnetic resonance imaging evaluation for valgus instability of the knee caused by medial collateral ligament injury. Acta Med Okayama. 2008. 62(3):185–91.

Miller TT. Imaging of the medial and lateral ligaments of the knee. Semin Musculoskelet Radiol. 2009;13:340–52.

Case 5.9

Indication A 27-year-old male with sports injury while playing football. Patient has severe pain and tenderness at the lateral aspect of the knee. Evaluate for ligamentous injury.

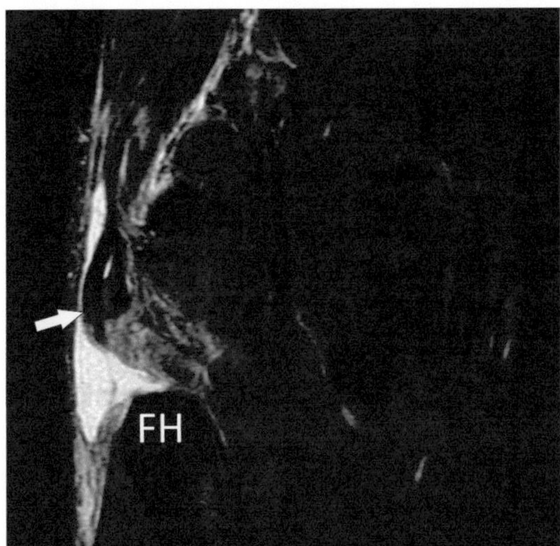

Coronal T2 fat saturated

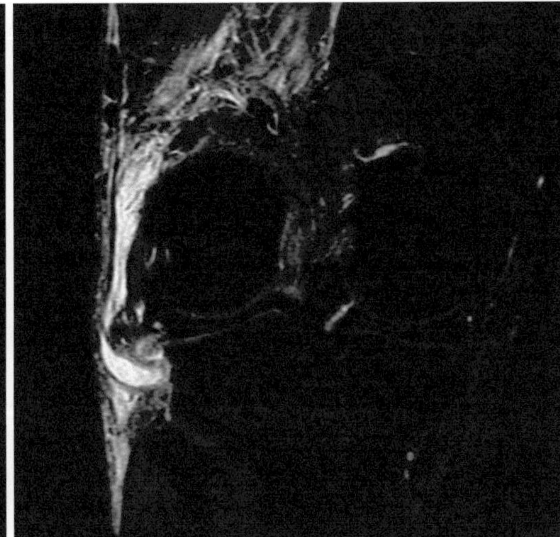

Coronal T2 fat saturated

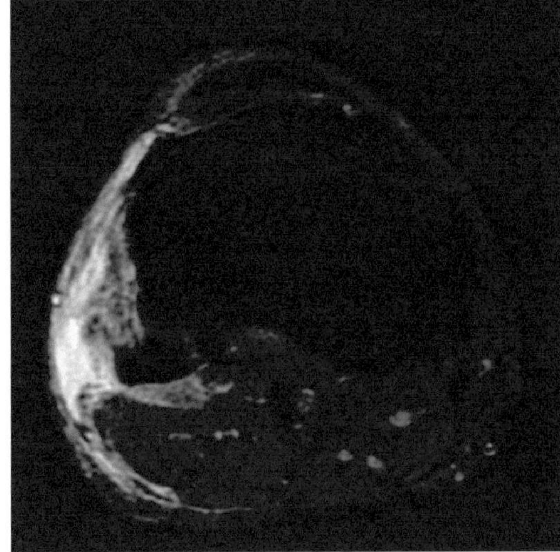

Axial T2 fat saturated

Findings

There is complete avulsion of the conjoined tendon of the biceps femoris and lateral collateral ligament (arrow) from its distal attachment on the fibular head (FH). There is 2 cm of proximal retraction of the torn tendon stump. There is surrounding soft tissue edema and hemorrhage. No associated avulsion fracture is seen on the radiographs (not shown). The iliotibial band is intact.

Impression/Recommendation

Complete avulsion of the conjoined tendon from its fibular attachment.

Discussion: Lateral Collateral Ligament Complex Injury

At the lateral compartment of the knee, there are many ligamentous and tendinous structures collectively known as the lateral collateral ligament (LCL) complex. These are the primary restraint against varus angulation. The LCL complex consists of three layers:

- Superficial layer: consists of the iliotibial band anteriorly and the biceps femoris tendon posteriorly.
- Middle layer: consists of the patellar retinaculum anteriorly and the lateral collateral ligament (also called the fibular collateral ligament) posteriorly.
- Deep layer: consists of the joint capsule with its insertion on the femur and tibia.

The fibular collateral ligament originates from the external tuberosity of the lateral femoral condyle and descends obliquely while the biceps femoris descends posterior to the fibular collateral ligament. Both of which insert as the conjoined tendon onto the fibular head. The iliotibial band descends to insert on the anterolateral aspect of the tibia at Gerdy's tubercle. MRI has an accuracy of 90% in determining the extent of LCL injury. The LCL complex is best visualized on axial and coronal images; however, it can also be assessed on the most peripheral sagittal images.

Injuries to the LCL complex are uncommon; however, they may occur in a varus-type mechanism of injury while in knee extension. LCL complex injuries may be either isolated or more commonly occur in combination with other ligamentous injuries including the cruciate ligaments and injuries to the posterolateral corner ligamentous structures.

Fibular collateral ligament injuries range from a low-grade sprain which is seen as mild periligamentous edema in an otherwise normal appearing ligament. Grade 2 sprains are seen as thickening or attenuation of the ligament with high signal intensity within its mid-substance. Grade 3 sprains are seen as a complete disruption of the ligament which can occur either at its origin, mid-substance or at its distal attachment. The most common type of injury of the LCL complex is avulsion of the conjoined tendon from its attachment on the fibular head which may or may not have an associated osseous avulsion fracture. This will be better seen on plain radiographs. In chronic cases, the tendon may appear diffusely thickened without surrounding edema.

Injuries to the iliotibial band also range from minor sprains (grade 1), to complete disruption (grade 3) which also most commonly occurs at its distal attachment on the tibia. An avulsion fracture of Gerdy's tubercle may also occur.

Treatment options depend on the extent of the injury. Conservative approaches include rest and rehabilitation. Surgery includes either repair or reconstruction of the components of the LCL complex.

Report checklist
1. Which of the LCL complex structures are injured?
2. Is the ligament sprained, partially torn or completely disrupted?
3. Where is the level of ligamentous injury (origin, mid-substance, or distal attachment)?
4. If there is complete avulsion of the ligamentous structures, is there an associated bony avulsion fracture?

Suggested Reading

Miller TT. Imaging of the medial and lateral ligaments of the knee. Semin Musculoskelet Radiol. 2009;13:340–52.

Recondo JA, Salvador E, Villanúa JA, Barrera MC, Gervás C, Alústiza JM. Lateral stabilizing structures of the knee: functional anatomy and injuries assessed with MR imaging. Radiographics. 2000;20:S91–102.

Case 5.10

Indication   A 27-year-old female cyclist with chronic lateral knee pain.

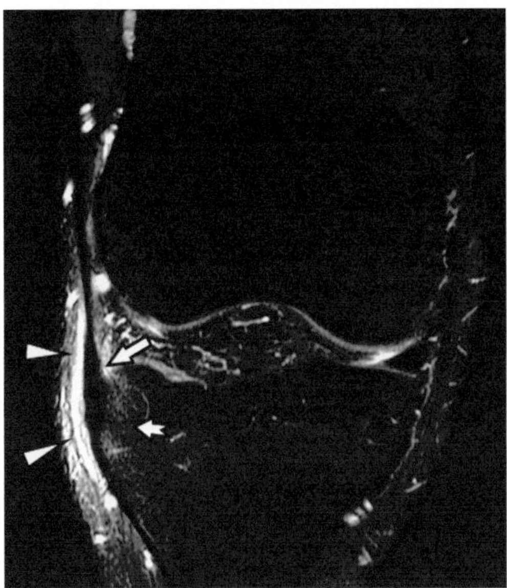

Coronal T2 fat saturated

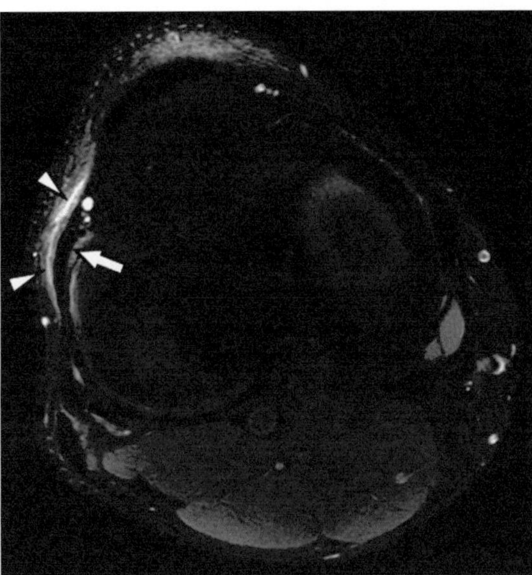

Axial PD fat saturated

Findings

There is thickening and abnormal increased signal intensity of the distal iliotibial band (ITB) at its tibial insertion (arrow). This is associated with soft tissue edema deep to the ITB at the level of the lateral femoral epicondyle as well as overlying subcutaneous soft tissue edema (arrowheads). There is minimal reactive bone marrow edema at the anterolateral aspect of the tibia (notched arrow).

Impression/Recommendation

Thickening of the iliotibial band with surrounding soft tissue edema, most compatible with iliotibial band friction syndrome.

Discussion: Iliotibial Band Friction Syndrome

The iliotibial band (ITB) represents the distal tendon of the tensor fascia lata that descends to the knee and attaches onto Gerdy's tubercle on the anterolateral aspect of the proximal tibia. Iliotibial band friction syndrome represents an inflammatory overuse injury, often occurring in long-distance runners and cyclists caused by repetitively rubbing of the ITB with the adjacent lateral femoral epicondyle during flexion and extension at the knee. Patients present with anterolateral knee pain, and there is usually point tenderness at the lateral femoral epicondyle just proximal to the joint line.

On MRI, the most characteristic finding is ill-defined edema in the soft tissues located deep to the distal ITB at the level of the lateral femoral epicondyle. This is best seen on the coronal and axial fluid-sensitive sequences. Usually, the ITB itself is normal in thickness and signal; however, in more severe or chronic cases, the ITB may become thickened with heterogeneous signal. Also, there can be reactive bone marrow edema at the anterolateral aspect of the tibia.

It is important to not confuse the normal joint recess that extends deep to the iliotibial band as ITB friction syndrome. To avoid this pitfall, do not rely merely on the coronal plane. Cross-reference should be made to the axial sequences to determine whether the fluid is located within the joint space or the adjacent soft tissues. Any soft tissue edema deep to the ITB and located outside of the joint should raise the suspicion of ITB friction syndrome.

Patients with ITB friction syndrome usually respond to conservative therapy which includes cessation of the inciting event and NSAIDs. Rarely orthotics or steroid injections are needed in refractory cases.

> **Report checklist**
> 1. Is there soft tissue edema deep to the ITB at the level of the lateral femoral condyle? Did you correlate with the axial plane to make sure it is not a normal joint recess?
> 2. Is there thickening and abnormal signal in the distal ITB? Is there a tear of the distal ITB?
> 3. Is there reactive bone marrow edema at the anterolateral aspect of the tibia?
> 4. Is there a lateral meniscus tear?

Suggested Reading

Haims AH, Medvecky MJ, Pavlovich R et-al. MR imaging of the anatomy of and injuries to the lateral and posterolateral aspects of the knee. AJR Am J Roentgenol. 2003;180(3): 647–53.

Muhle C, Ahn JM, Yeh L, Bergman GA, Boutin RD, Schweitzer M, Jacobson JA, Haghighi P, Trudell DJ, Resnick D. Iliotibial band friction syndrome: MR imaging findings in 16 patients and MR arthrographic study of six cadaveric knees. Radiology. 1999;212:103–10.

Case 5.11

Indication A 31-year-old female with recent lateral patellar dislocation. Has joint effusion and knee pain. Assess medial retinaculum and medial patellofemoral ligament.

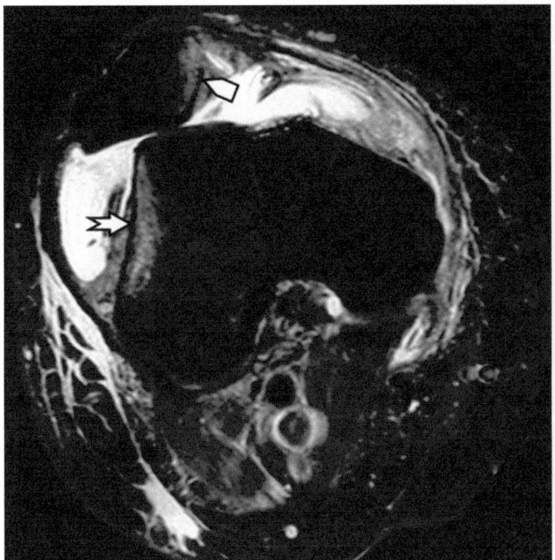
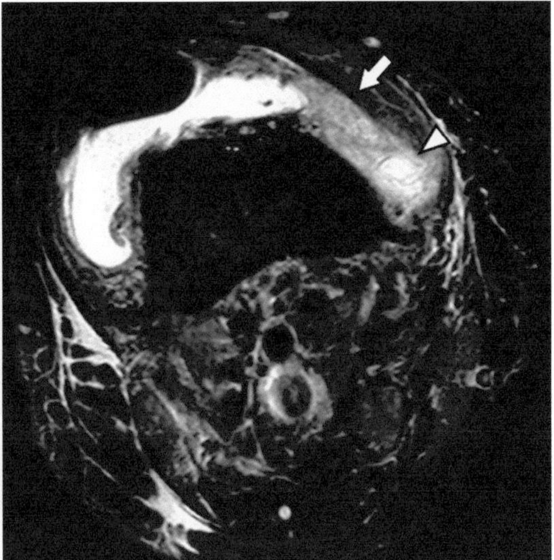

Axial T2 fat saturated   Axial T2 fat saturated

Findings
There are kissing bone contusions at the antero-lateral aspect of the lateral femoral condyle (notched arrow) and the medial aspect of the patella (block arrow), compatible with a recent transient lateral patellar dislocation. There is extensive soft tissue edema at the femoral attach-ment (arrowhead) of the medial patellofemoral ligament (MPFL, arrow) with uplifting of the vastus medialis obliquus muscle and fluid track-ing beneath the muscle consistent with complete rupture of the MPFL.

Impression/Recommendation
Transient lateral patellar dislocation with com-plete disruption of the MPFL.

Discussion: Transient Lateral Patellar Dislocation
Lateral patellar dislocations usually result from a twisting injury or from a direct trauma. Certain anatomical anomalies predispose to such lesions such as trochlear dysplasia, patella alta, and lateralization of the tibial tuberosity. The diagnosis is usually not evident clinically

due to the transient and brief nature of the injury, as the patella will often relocate. Transient lateral patellar dislocations usually result in osseous injuries as well as soft tissue injuries to the medial stabilizers of the patella. Most patients are at increased risk of recurrent dislocations in the future which can result in chronic patellofemoral instability and arthritis if left untreated.

MRI plays a crucial role in identifying this injury pattern and in general the orthopedic sur-geon is evaluating for complications of the tran-sient dislocation as oppose to assessing whether the patella is dislocated, which should be quite evident on physical exam unless the patient is obese. Osseous findings of a recent lateral patel-lar dislocation include bone marrow contusions at the anterolateral aspect of the lateral femoral condyle and at the inferomedial aspect of the patella. The majority of cases have a chondral or osteochondral injury at the medial patellar facet inferiorly. These osteochondral injuries may be displaced and result in an intra-articular loose body *(see supplementary images)* which may require surgical treatment.

Soft tissue injuries to the medial soft tissue stabilizers of the patella are also commonly seen and include the medial patellofemoral ligament (MPFL), medial retinaculum, and the medial patellotibial ligament. The MPFL is the most important of these stabilizing structures and should be carefully scrutinized on MRI as injury to this structure has the highest risk of subsequent dislocations. The MPFL originates from the adductor tubercle just proximal to the origin of the superficial fibers of the medial collateral ligament. It then extends anteriorly beneath the fascia of the vastus medialis obliquus (VMO) muscle to insert on the superior pole of the patella. The medial retinaculum originates from the fascia at the undersurface of the VMO and inserts onto the middle third of the patella. Lastly, the patellotibial ligament arises from the medial aspect of the tibia and extends in a cephalad direction to insert on the lower pole of the patella. Given that most surgeons will repair a disrupted MPFL while rarely reconstruct a medial retinaculum or patellotibial ligament, it is crucial to differentiate between an injury to the medial retinaculum and the MPFL for appropriate presurgical planning.

To differentiate between these two structures, the axial plane is very helpful. The MPFL lies more proximal to the medial retinaculum. Identifying the relationship of these structures to the overlying VMO muscle is key. If the distal aspect of the VMO is visualized on the axial plane, then the underlying ligamentous structure represents the MPFL. However, if you scroll more inferiorly and the VMO is not seen, then the medial linear hypointense structure represents the medial retinaculum. Injuries to these structures can be classified as sprain, partial-thickness tear, or complete disruption. The majority of injuries to the MPFL occur at the femoral attachment. At this region the MPFL is not clearly identified as a separate structure as its blends with the underlying fascia of the VMO. A disruption is suspected when there is significant soft tissue edema with anterior and superior displacement and uplifting away from the adductor tubercle with fluid and hemorrhage tracking beneath the muscle. When there is only soft tissue edema at the adductor tubercle however no significant displacement of the muscle or fluid tracking beneath the muscle, then this should suggest a sprain or partial-thickness tear. Less commonly, injuries of the MPFL occur at the patellar insertion which is more easily identified as disruption of the linear hypointense band with surrounding soft tissue edema. On the other hand, injuries of the medial retinauculum occur more commonly at the patellar attachment which is also easily identified as thickening or attenuation of the retinaculum with surrounding soft tissue edema depending on the degree of injury.

Associated findings on MRI include a large joint effusion/hemarthrosis. There is an association between transient patellar dislocation with meniscal tears and MCL injuries. It is also important to comment on any underlying abnormal patellofemoral alignment such as patella alta, lateral patellar tilt, or femoral trochlear dysplasia.

Most cases of first time patellar dislocation are treated conservatively unless there is significant rupture of the medial stabilizers, a displaced intra-articular chondral or osteochondral loose body. Surgical repair is most commonly directed to MPFL reconstruction.

Supplementary Images

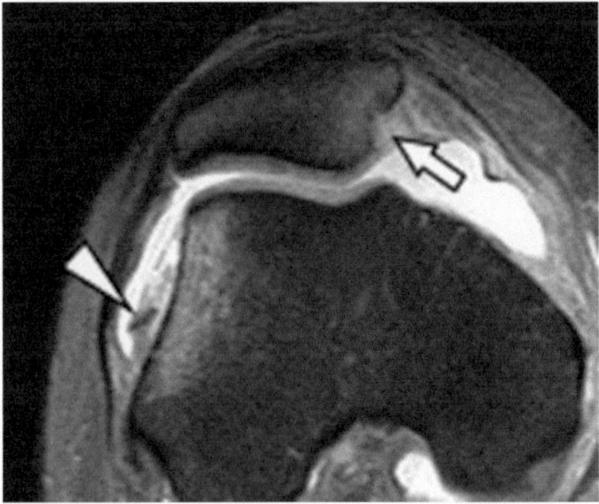

Axial PD fat saturated

Cartilage injury from transient patellar dislocation. There is osteochondral fragment (arrowhead) in the lateral joint space with the donor at the medial patella (arrow). Note the edema in the medial patella and the lateral femoral condyle indicating bone contusions from transient lateral patellar dislocation

Report checklist

1. Are there kissing bone contusions at the lateral femoral condyle and the medial patella to suggest a recent transient lateral patellar dislocation?
2. Is there a chondral or osteochondral defect from the medial patellar articular surface? If yes, what is the size and where is it located? Is there intra-articular displacement?
3. Is there uplifting of the VMO muscle with fluid tracking beneath it to suggest complete disruption of the MPFL? If not, is there just soft tissue edema at the adductor tubercle suggesting MPFL sprain or low-grade injury?
4. Is there a sprain or tear of the medial retinaculum (which lies more inferior to the MPFL)?
5. Is there a joint effusion or hemarthrosis?
6. How are the medial meniscus and the medial collateral ligament?
7. Are there any underlying anatomical anomalies at the patellofemoral compartment which could predispose the patient to recurrent dislocation (femoral trochlear dysplasia, patella alta, lateralization of the tibial tuberosity)?

Suggested Reading

Diederichs G, Issever AS, Scheffler S. MR imaging of patellar instability: injury patterns and assessment of risk factors. Radiographics. 2010;30 (4): 961–81.

Guerrero P, Li X, Patel K, Brown M, Busconi B. Medial patellofemoral ligament injury patterns and associated pathology in lateral patella dislocation: an MRI study. Sports Med Arthrosc Rehabil Ther Technol 2009;1(1):17.

Case 5.12

Indication A 32-year-old man presents with severe knee pain and swelling after feeling a popping sensation while playing basketball. Cannot extend his knee.

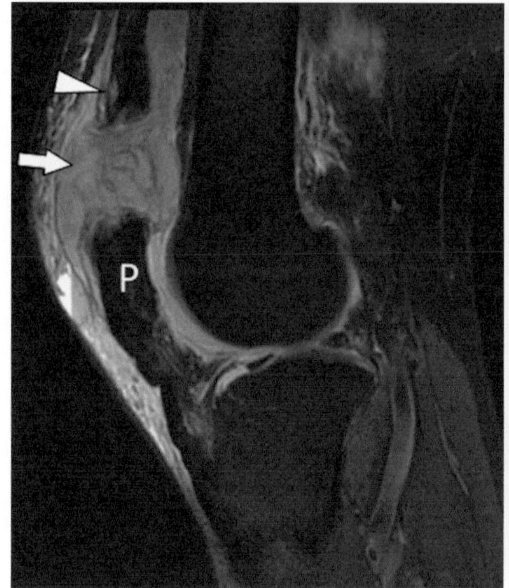

Sagittal T2 fat saturated

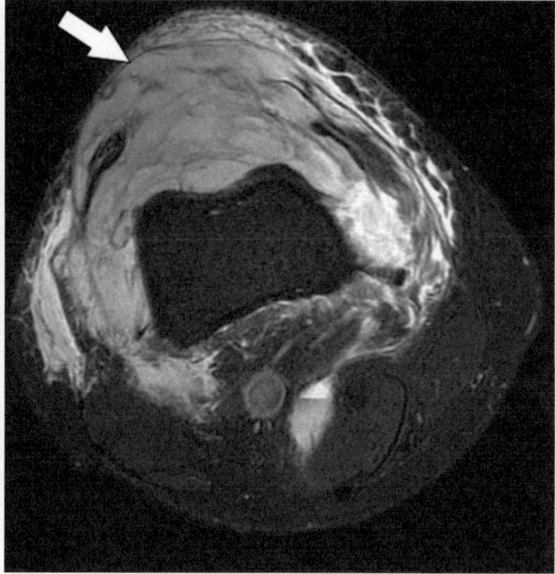

Axial T2 fat saturated

Findings

There is a complete rupture of the distal quadriceps tendon at its insertion onto the patella with retraction of the torn tendon fibers (arrowhead) by approximately 4 cm superiorly. This is associated with extensive surrounding soft tissue edema and hematoma (arrows). There is no bony avulsion fracture of the patella (P). There is mild patella baja. There is a large knee joint effusion.

Impression/Recommendation

Complete rupture of the quadriceps tendon. Orthopedic consultation for possible surgical repair is recommended.

Discussion: Quadriceps Tendon Tear

The quadriceps tendon is a multilayered structure formed by the coalescence of four separate muscles. On sagittal MRI images, the normal quadriceps tendon demonstrates a trilaminar striated appearance with intermediate signal intervening between the tendon layers (on T1- and T2-weighted images). The superficial anterior layer represents the rectus femoris tendon. The vastus medialis and lateralis tendons form the thick middle layer, while the vastus intermedius tendon forms the deep layer.

Quadriceps tendinopathy is most commonly the result of chronic overuse, but other predisposing factors such as diabetes, gout, and steroids have been identified which can result in tendon degeneration. Tears can be from a direct injury or from forceful muscle contraction. Spontaneous ruptures have been reported as well.

On MRI, tendinopathy is demonstrated by thickening of the distal tendon with high signal intensity both within the tendon substance and between the separate layers. There may be soft tissue edema within the suprapatellar fat pad just deep to the distal fibers of the quadriceps tendon.

Quadriceps tendon tears most commonly occur in the relatively hypovascular region

1–2 cm from its insertion on the superior patella. Partial tears most commonly involve the rectus femoris tendon insertion and appear as high signal intensity disruption of the tendon with some intact fibers. Complete tears, however, show no intact fibers and the torn tendon fibers may be retracted proximally due to muscular contraction. This is usually associated with extensive soft tissue edema and hemorrhage as well as patella baja. Both axial and sagittal fluid-sensitive sequences should be obtained to identify the precise muscle involved, the tear extent, and proximal retraction of the torn tendon stump. Chronic tears can have muscle atrophy and fatty infiltration which is best seen on the T1-weighted images as linear streaks of high signal intensity within the muscle belly.

Partial tears are usually treated conservatively with knee immobilization, while complete tears need urgent surgical intervention within 24–48 hours.

Report checklist

1. What is the degree of quadriceps tendinosis (mild, moderate, severe)?
2. Is there a tendon tear? Where is it located? Is it partial-thickness or complete rupture? Is it acute or chronic? Which muscles are involved?
3. Extent of retraction of the tendon stump
4. Any associated avulsion fracture from the superior pole of the patella?
5. Is there fatty atrophy of the quadriceps muscle?
6. How is the patellar tendon?

Suggested Reading

Bencardino JT, Rosenberg ZS, Brown RR, Hassankhani A, Lustrin ES, Beltran Traumatic musculotendinous injuries of the knee: diagnosis with MR imaging. Radiographics. 2000;20(suppl1):S103–20.

Ilan DI, Tejwani N, Keschner M, et al. Quadriceps tendon rupture. J Am Acad Orthop Surg. 2003;11:192–200.

Case 5.13

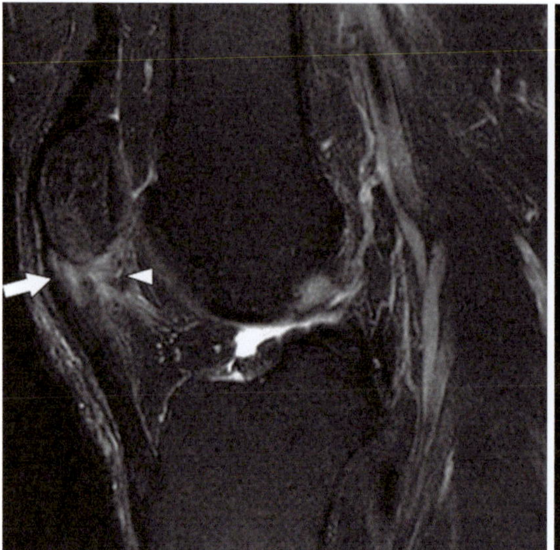

Sagittal T2 fat saturated

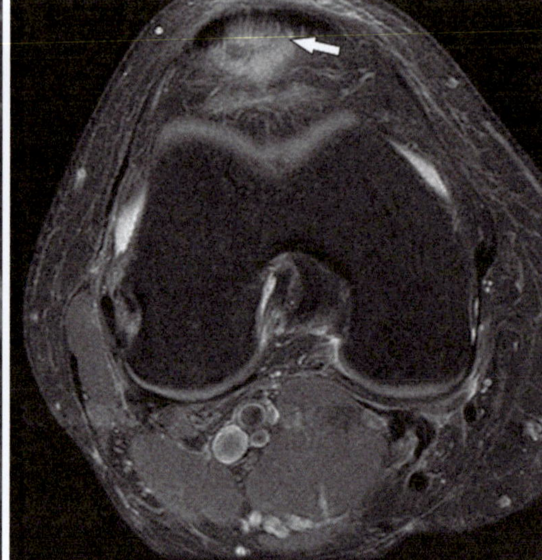

Axial PD fat saturated

Findings

There is moderate thickening at the proximal origin of the patellar tendon (arrows) with increased signal intensity within the tendon substance compatible with moderate tendinosis. This is minimal soft tissue edema in Hoffa's fat pad (arrowhead). There is no patellar tendon tear. The quadriceps tendon is normal.

Impression/Recommendation

Moderate proximal patellar tendinosis.

Discussion: Patellar Tendinopathy

The patellar tendon originates from the inferior aspect of the patella and inserts on the anterior tibial tuberosity. On MRI, the normal tendon appears as a uniformly hypointense band on all pulse sequences that is usually <7 mm in anteroposterior dimension. It is important to note that some variations on imaging may simulate pathology but are normal findings. First, there can be focal areas of hyperintense signal both at the proximal and distal ends of the tendon on the sagittal T1-weighted images due to magic angle effect; however, this should demonstrate normal low signal on the T2-weighted images. Also, there may be linear striations of intermediate signal within the mid portion of the tendon at its patellar origin which is a normal MRI finding seen in asymptomatic individuals and should not be misinterpreted as patellar tendinosis.

Patellar tendinosis (tendinopathy), also known as jumper's knee, is an overuse injury that typically occurs in athletes with repetitive jumping. Patellar tendon pathology usually occurs at its proximal attachment and ranges from mild tendinosis to partial-thickness tear and complete disruption of the tendon.

Tendinosis is usually seen as focal thickening of the patellar tendon with increased intrinsic signal at its proximal aspect and slight irregularity of the posterior border of the tendon. This is often associated with soft tissue edema in the underlying Hoffa's fat pad. With severe tendinosis, the tendon may be diffusely thickened and contain hyperintense signal on the T2-weighted images. The presence of fluid signal in the tendon substance represents a focal partial-thickness tear which usually begins at the posterior border of the tendon. Complete disruption of the tendon fibers will appear as discontinuity of the tendon with hemorrhage and edema at the tear site. This is usually associated with retraction and proximal migration of the patella (patella alta).

Conservative management with rest and later physical therapy is generally successful in treating patellar tendinosis. Recurrence is not uncommon. Severe and refractive cases may need to be surgically treated.

Report checklist

1. What is the degree of patellar tendinosis (mild, moderate, severe)?
2. Location of abnormality along the patellar tendon (proximal, mid-substance, distal)
3. Is there a focal tendon tear? Is it partial thickness or complete?
4. Any associated avulsion fracture from the inferior pole of the patella in cases of complete disruption?
5. How is the quadriceps tendon?
6. Is there edema in Hoffa's fat pad, patella alta, and/or lateral patellofemoral cartilage abnormality to suggest abnormal patellar tracking?

Suggested Reading

Dupuis Carolyn S., Sjirk J. Westra, Joseph Makris and E. Christine Wallace. Injuries and Conditions of the Extensor Mechanism of the Pediatric Knee. Radiographics. 2009;29(3):877–86.

Peers KH, Lysens RJ. Patellar tendinopathy in athletes: current diagnostic and therapeutic recommendations. Sports Med. 2005;35: 71–87.

Case 5.14

Indication A 19-year-old male with anterior knee pain at the proximal tibia. Radiographs show fragmentation at the tibial tuberosity. Assess the patellar tendon.

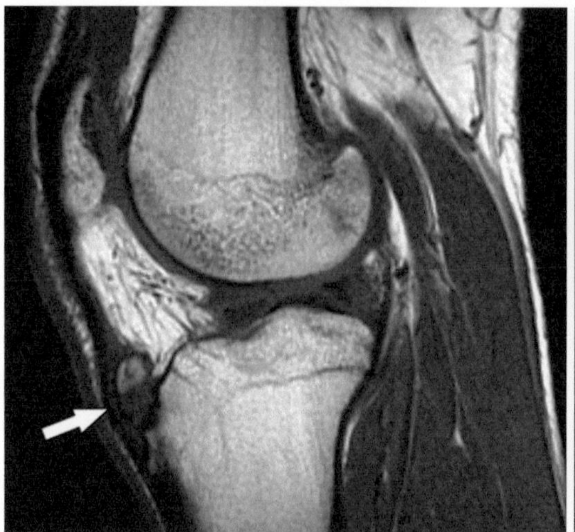

Sagittal T1

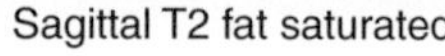

Sagittal T2 fat saturated

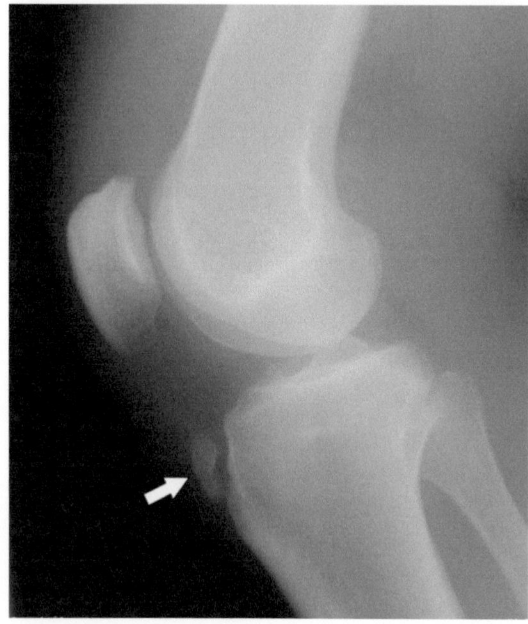

Findings

There is fragmentation at the anterior tibial tuberosity with bone marrow edema (arrows) compatible with Osgood-Schlatter disease. There is thickening of the distal patellar tendon compatible with tendinosis. There is no patellar tendon tear. There is no distention of the infra-patellar bursa with fluid.

Impression/Recommendation

Osgood-Schlatter disease with patellar tendinosis.

Discussion: Osgood-Schlatter Disease

The tibial tubercle develops as an anterior extension of the proximal tibial physis which is composed of fibrocartilage in young children and progressively ossifies into adolescence.

Osgood-Schlatter disease (OSD) represents a chronic avulsion injury "apophysitis" at the insertion of the patellar tendon-tibial tuberosity junction which leads to tendinosis of the distal patellar tendon with fragmentation and bone marrow edema of the tibial tuberosity. It typically develops during growth spurts of adolescence and is bilateral in 50% of patients. It is usually diagnosed clinically in active adolescence with tenderness and swelling over the tibial tuberosity.

Radiographs are helpful in confirming the diagnosis which shows sclerosis and fragmentation of the tibial tubercle with overlying soft tissue swelling; however, normal plain radiographs do not exclude the diagnosis. MRI demonstrates thickening and heterogeneous signal of the distal patellar tendon representing tendinosis with osseous fragmentation of the tibial tubercle. In active OSD, there may be edema at the tibial tubercle and in the fragmented ossicles as well as fluid in the deep infrapatellar bursa representing bursitis. Chronic OSD should only reveal bone fragmentation without significant osseous edema or bursitis.

OSD is usually treated conservatively by limiting physical activities and analgesia. Rarely, therapeutic casts and surgery are required.

Report checklist

1. Is there bone marrow edema in the fragmented ossicles or the anterior tibial tuberosity to suggest active OSD? Or is there just fragmentation without significant bone marrow edema suggesting chronic OSD?
2. Is there overlying soft tissue edema?
3. Is there distal patellar tendinosis? Is there a patellar tendon tear?
4. Is there deep infrapatellar bursitis?

Suggested Reading

Demirag B, Ozturk C, Yazici Z, Sarisozen B. The pathophysiology of Osgood-Schlatter disease: a magnetic resonance investigation. J Pediatr Orthop B. 2004;13:379–82.

Hirano A, Fukubayashi T, Ishii T et-al. Magnetic resonance imaging of Osgood-Schlatter disease: the course of the disease. Skeletal Radiol. 2002;31(6):334–42.

Case 5.15

Indication A 55-year-old female with sudden worsening knee pain medially and unable to weight-bear. Assess for internal derangement.

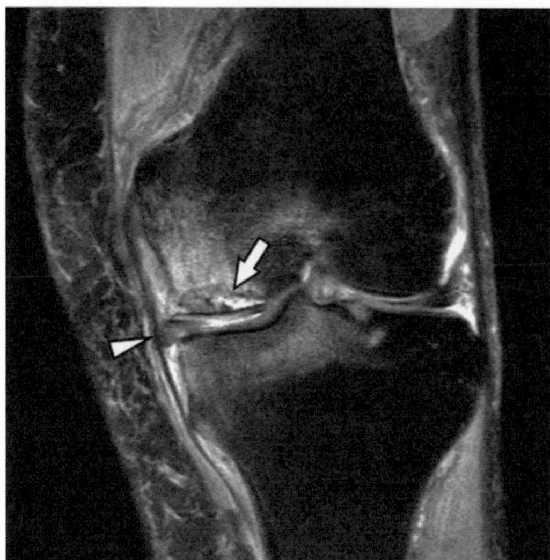

Coronal T2 fat saturated

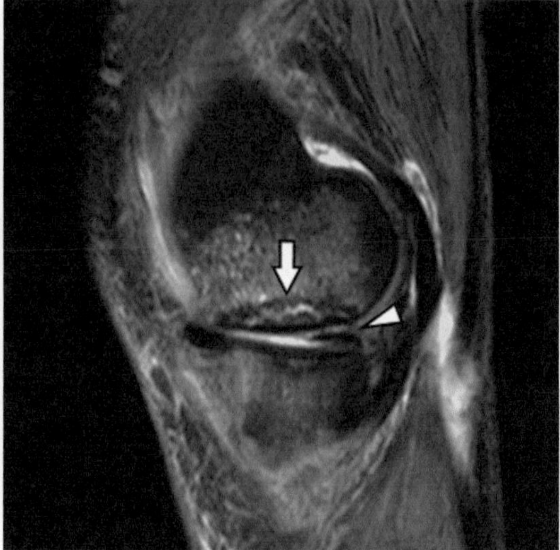

Sagittal T2 fat saturated

Findings

There is an irregular subchondral fracture line at the central weight-bearing portion of the medial femoral condyle (arrows) measuring 3.5 × 3 cm with marked surrounding reactive bone marrow edema compatible with a subchondral insufficiency fracture. There is high signal intensity fluid signal in the fracture line, but there is no collapse of the articular surface. There is a complex tear at the body of the medial meniscus (arrowheads). There are no full-thickness chondral defects.

Impression/Recommendation

Subchondral insufficiency fracture at the medial femoral condyle (previously called spontaneous osteonecrosis of the knee (SONK)).

Discussion: Subchondral Insufficiency Fracture of the Knee

Insufficiency fracture is a type of stress fracture resulting from normal stresses applied to abnormally weaken bone. In the knee, subchondral insufficiency fractures were previously termed spontaneous osteonecrosis of the knee (SONK); however, recent histopathological data demonstrates that the abnormality underlying this process is indeed a fracture without the presence of necrotic bone.

Subchondral insufficiency fractures typically occur in elderly women with osteoporosis and are most frequently encountered at the weight-bearing portion of the medial femoral condyle. They can also be seen in the lateral femoral condyle and tibial plateaus, although less common. No specific predisposing factors have been found; however, most patients have altered biomechanics of the joint related to underlying meniscal tears, prior meniscectomy, and osteoarthritis.

Initially, radiographs are normal or may have mild decrease bone density. However, MRI is the modality of choice in evaluating this injury which demonstrates irregular low signal intensity subchondral line representing a fracture line on all pulse sequences paralleling the subchondral bone often with marked surrounding bone marrow edema on edema-sensitive MR sequences. High signal intensity fluid may be seen in the fracture line which can suggest separation of the osteo-chondral fragment and hence increases the risk of articular collapse. As the disease progresses, there is usually collapse of the subchondral bone and secondary osteoarthritis. Note that many orthopedic surgeons may still use the term SONK to describe these lesions.

Patients are usually treated conservatively with limitation of weight-bearing activities which can lead to healing of the fracture line. However, if there is progressive subchondral collapse of the articular surface and secondary osteoarthritis, this may result in the need for knee arthroplasty.

Report checklist
1. Where is the location and size of the subchondral fracture line?
2. Is there surrounding bone marrow edema suggesting an acute fracture?
3. Is there collapse of the articular surface?
4. Are there any chondral defects or subchondral cystic changes to suggest secondary degenerative changes?
5. Are there signs of prior meniscal surgery or meniscal tears?
6. Is the patient elderly and at risk for low bone density?

Suggested Reading

An VV, Broek MVD, Oussedik S. Subchondral insufficiency fracture in the lateral compartment of the knee in a 64-year-old marathon runner. Knee Surg Relat Res. 2017;29(4): 325–8.

Gorbachova T, Melenevsky Y, Cohen M, Cerniglia BW. Osteochondral lesions of the knee: differentiating the most common entities at MRI. Radiographics. 2018;38(5): 1478–95.

Case 5.16

Indication A 39-year-old female with posterior knee pain and swelling. X-ray showed ossification posteriorly.

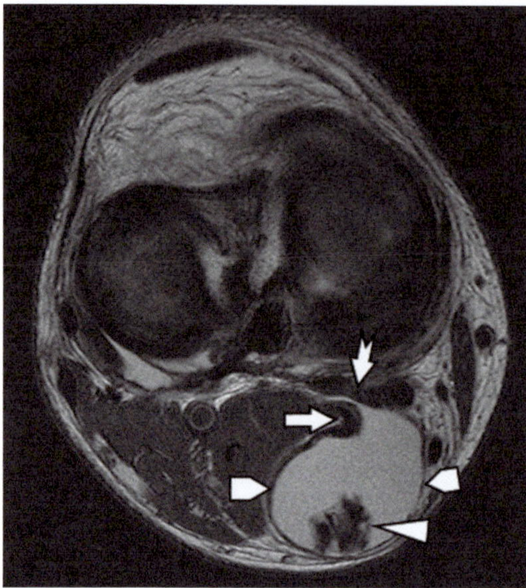
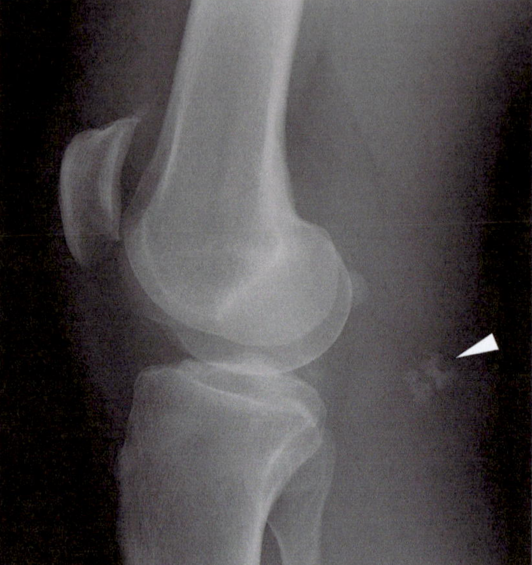

AxialT2

Findings

There is a moderate-sized 4 × 5 × 4 cm cystic mass (block arrows) within the popliteal fossa located between the tendons of the medial head of the gastrocnemius muscle (arrow) and the semimembranosus (notched arrow) compatible with a Baker's cyst. There is a 1 cm loose body (arrowheads) lying in the dependent portion of the cyst. There is no compression on the popliteal vessels, and there are no signs of cyst rupture.

Impression/Recommendation

Popliteal (Baker's cyst) with a 1 cm loose body corresponding to the ossification seen on X-ray.

Discussion: Baker's Cyst

The popliteal cyst (Baker's cyst) is a synovial cyst located in the popliteal fossa caused by extension of joint fluid into the normally occurring gastrocnemius-semimembranosus bursa. It is the most common cystic mass around the knee joint, seen in 30–40% of knee MRIs in daily clinical practice. They arise between the medial head of the gastrocnemius muscle and the semimembranosus tendons which is the key to making the diagnosis.

Baker's cysts have a normal communication with the posterior aspect of the knee joint which can have a ball valve-like mechanism, meaning that fluid can enter the cyst but have difficulty exiting. Any condition that causes an increase in synovial fluid within the joint can lead to secondary Baker's cysts.

On MRI, they are seen at the medial aspect of the popliteal fossa and usually demonstrate low signal intensity on T1-weighted images and high signal on T2-weighted images. They can have internal septations, be multiloculated, and can have heterogeneous signal intensity due to the presence of internal debris. Intra-articular loose bodies may also extend into the Baker's cyst and progressively increase in size. When they do become very large, they can fill the entire cyst and be confusing on MRI, mimicking a neoplasm.

The key again is to identify that it is located within the Baker's cyst. Plain radiographs can be helpful to show its ossified nature.

Most Baker's cysts are asymptomatic and only incidentally identified on MRI. However, when they are large, patients can present with a painful mass in the popliteal fossa with limitation of knee flexion. If the cysts rupture, they can mimic a DVT or thrombophlebitis clinically.

Baker's cyst may be complicated with internal hemorrhage which would demonstrate high signal intensity in the T1-weighted images and can have fluid-fluid levels. Also, Baker's cysts may rupture which will be seen as soft tissue edema extending inferiorly along the medial gastrocnemius muscle. If a Baker's cyst becomes very large, they can also compress the popliteal vessels resulting in DVTs. Since Baker's cysts are lined by synovium, they can be affected by synovial pathologies such as synovial chondromatosis or pigmented villonodular synovitis (PVNS).

It is crucial to differentiate a Baker's cyst from other cystic masses – particularly extra-articular ganglion cysts and parameniscal cysts. Extra-articular ganglion cysts appear as well-defined rounded or lobulated fluid collections with sharply defined internal septations (bunch of grapes appearance). As stated earlier, the key to diagnosing a Baker's cyst is the precise anatomic location at the site of the gastrocnemius-semimembranosus bursa. The characteristic feature of a meniscal cyst is a cystic mass accompanying a meniscal tear. Atypical popliteal cysts that are not located

within the gastrocnemius-semimembranosus bursa or have nonuniform signal intensity might need further evaluation with intravenous contrast to exclude a soft tissue sarcoma.

Most Baker's cysts are treated conservatively given that no vascular or neural compression is present. If the cyst is large and symptomatic, aspiration can be performed under ultrasound guidance. Surgery is rarely needed and is usually performed to correct the underlying intra-articular pathology rather than the Baker's cyst itself.

Report checklist
1. Is the cystic mass located between the medial head of gastrocnemius muscle and the semimembranosus tendon?
2. What is the size of the cystic mass?
3. Is there internal debris or hemorrhage? Any loose bodies?
4. Is there compression on the neurovascular structures?
5. Is there cyst rupture?
6. Could this be a solid mass? Consider IV contrast if unsure?

Suggested Reading

Marra MD, Crema MD, Chung M, Roemer FW, Hunter DJ, Zaim S, et al. MRI features of cystic lesions around the knee. Knee. 2008. 15(6):423–38.

Perdikakis E, Skiadas V. MRI characteristics of cysts and "cyst-like" lesions in and around the knee: what the radiologist needs to know. Insights Imaging. 2013;4(3):257–72.

Case 5.17a

Indication A 55-year-old male with chronic knee pain and swelling medially.

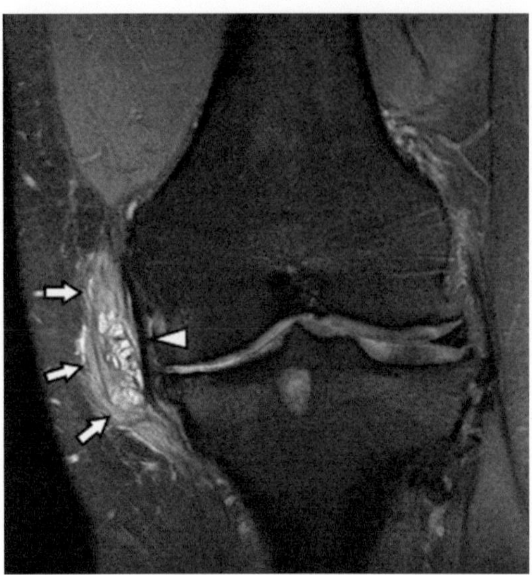

Coronal T2 fat saturated

Findings
There is a large cystic lesion (arrows) lateral to the medial collateral ligament (arrowhead) consistent with MCL bursitis.

Case 5.17b

Indication A 28-year-old female with medial knee pain and tenderness below the joint line not improving with conservative management.

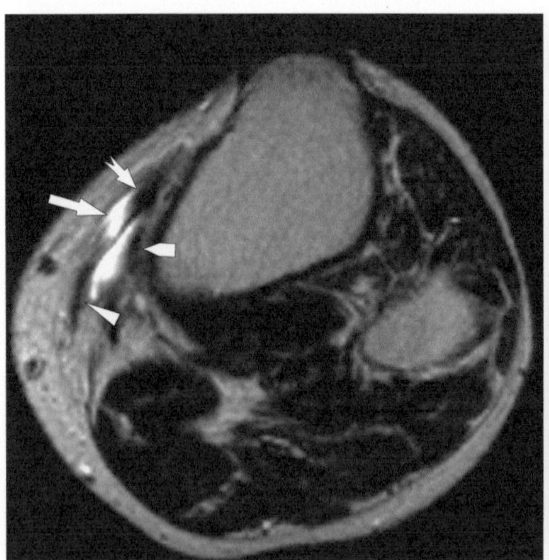

Axial T2

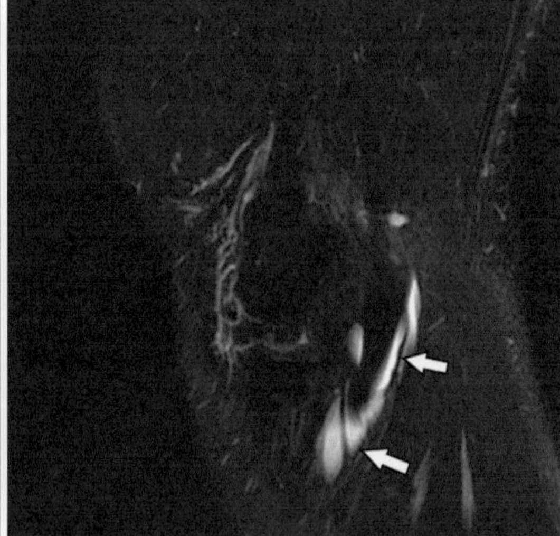

Sagittal T2 fat saturated

Findings
There is a lobular cystic fluid collection (arrow) deep to the pes anserine tendons: sartorius (notched arrow), gracilis (block arrow), semitendinosis (arrowhead) at the level of the proximal tibia medially consistent with pes anserinus bursitis.

Case 5.17c

Indication A 17-year-old male with severe anterior knee pain and swelling after a fall 6 weeks ago. On exam, there is skin thickening and cellulitis.

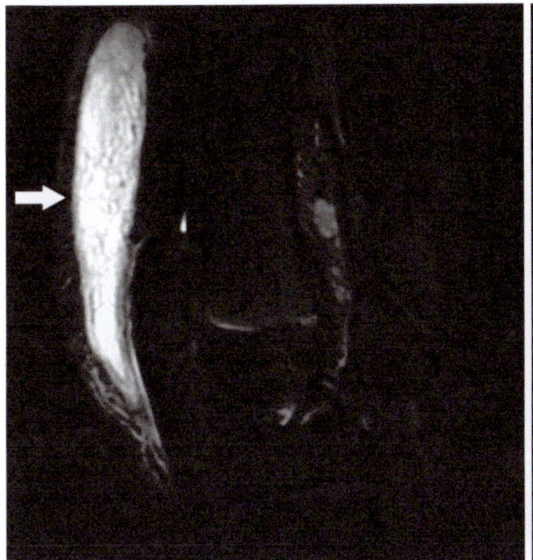

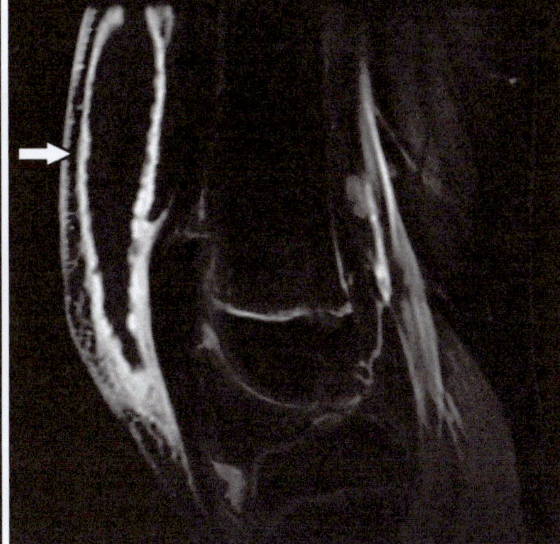

Sagittal T2 fat saturated   Sagittal T1 fat saturated post contrast

Findings
There is a large 9 × 4 cm localized cystic collection (arrows) within the soft tissues anterior to the patella and distal quadriceps tendon with peripheral rim enhancement (arrowheads) and surrounding soft tissue edema compatible with prepatellar bursitis.

Case 5.17d

Indication A 36-year-old female with anterior knee lump and swelling after fall 2 weeks ago. Assess for underlying soft tissue tumor.

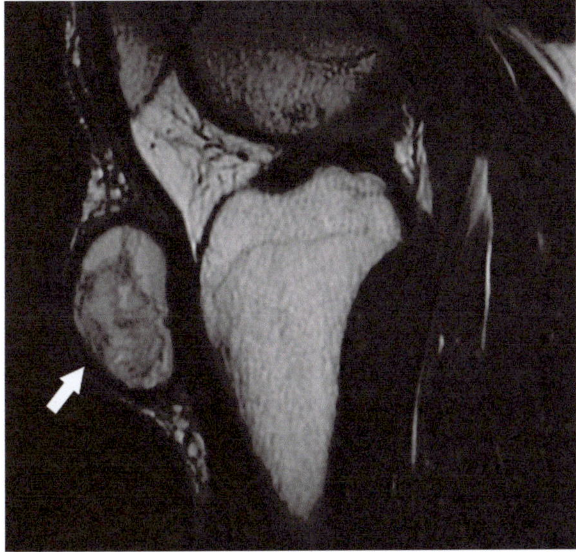

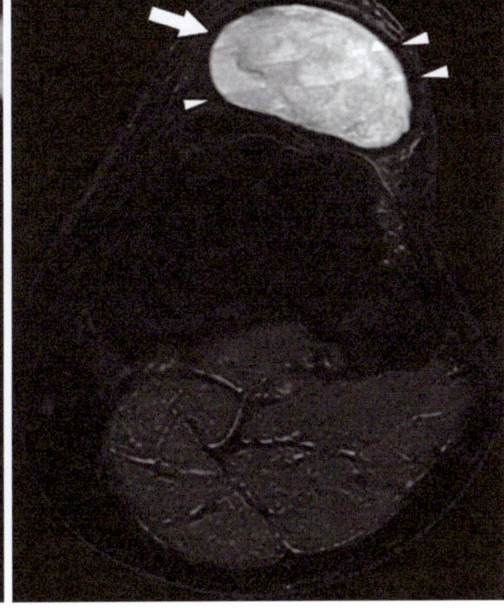

Sagittal T1   Axial T1 fat saturated

Findings
There is a 4 × 3 cm localized mass in the subcutaneous soft tissues anterior to the distal patellar tendon (arrows). On the T1 weighted fat suppressed images, there is internal hyperintense fluid with multiple fluid-fluid levels (arrowheads) suggestive of internal hemorrhagic products.

Case 5.17e

Indication A 32-year-old male with knee pain after fall. Rule out internal derangement.

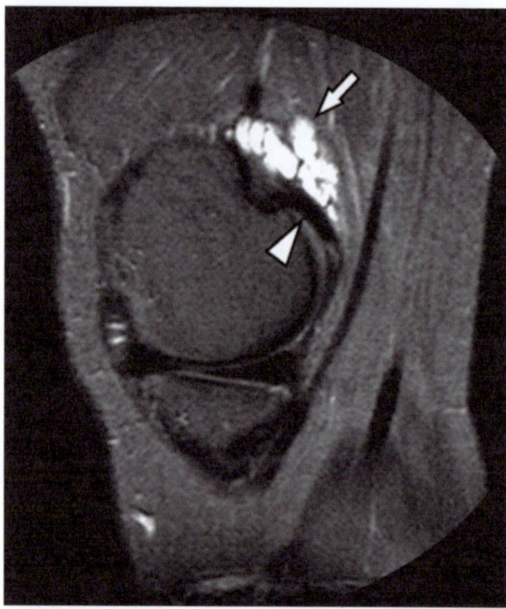

Sagittal T2 fat saturated

Findings
There is a small multiseptated cystic lesion (arrow) at the origin of the medial head of gas-

trocnemius (arrowhead) at the distal femur most compatible with a ganglion cyst. There is no intraosseous extension.

Case 5.17f

Indication A 34-year-old male with chronic knee pain and limited knee extension. Rule out ligament injury.

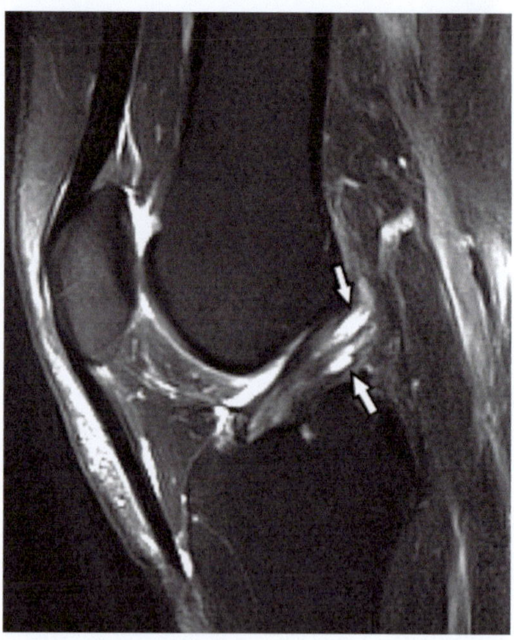

Sagittal T2 fat saturated

Findings
There is a small cystic lesion within the proximal fibers of anterior cruciate ligament (arrows), which expands the ligament fibers and produces a "drumstick" or "celery stalk" appearance. The ACL fibers are continuous without focal tear.

Case 5.17g

Indication A 38-year-old female with lump on the lateral aspect of the leg, increasing in size over last year. Is there a soft tissue mass?

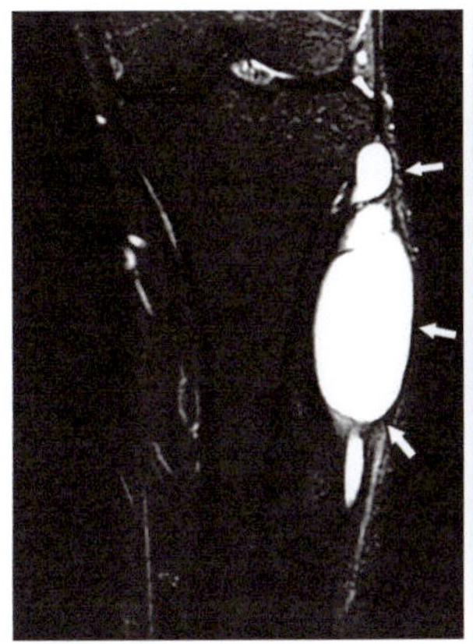
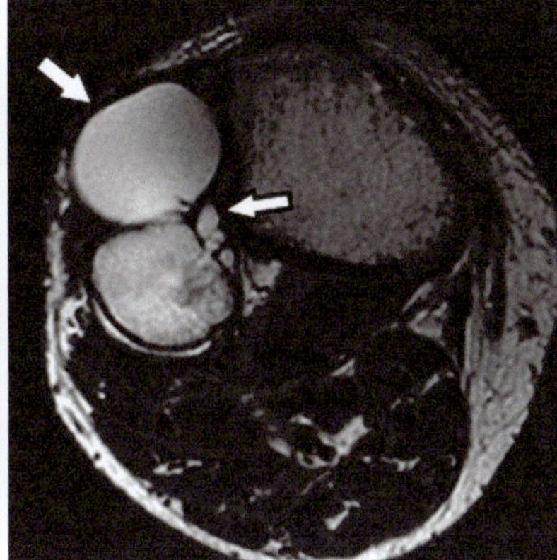
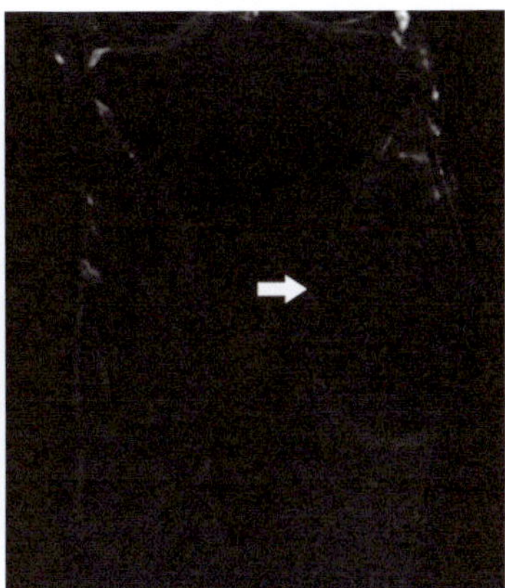

Coronal T2 fat saturated   Axial T2   Coronal T1 fat saturated post contrast

Findings

There is a large 10 × 4 cm cystic mass (arrows) with a small tail arising from the proximal tibiofibular joint extending into the anterior compartment of the leg most compatible with a synovial cyst. There is only faint peripheral rim enhancement on the contrast images. There is no visible compression of the common peroneal nerve.

Impression/Recommendation

Case 5.17a: Medial collateral ligament bursitis.

Case 5.17b: Pes anserinus bursitis.

Case 5.17c: Large rim enhancing prepatellar bursitis. Underlying infection cannot be ruled out. Aspiration of the collection is recommended for microbiology assessment.

Case 5.17d: Hemorrhagic superficial infrapatellar bursitis.

Case 5.17e: Ganglion cyst at the origin of the medial gastrocnemius muscle.

Case 5.17f: ACL ganglion cyst.

Case 5.17 g: Proximal tibiofibular joint ganglion cyst.

Discussion

Cysts and cystic lesions around the knee are common finding seen on routine MRIs of the knee. They can be confusing to the reader if one is not aware of the potential diagnosis and pitfalls. MRI helps delineate the precise anatomic location of the lesion and determines if the lesion is purely cystic or solid after the administration of intravenous contrast. Although the differential diagnosis of a cyst around the knee is wide, we will discuss the most common cysts in this section.

The most common cysts seen around the knee are related to distended bursas. A bursa is a fluid-filled sac or sac-like cavity that is lined by synovial membrane usually located around frictional surfaces such as tendons or muscles around a joint, but it does not have a direct connection to the joint. Its primary function is to facilitate smooth motion between such surfaces. Inflammation of these bursae as a result of trauma, overuse, infection, and hemorrhage is called bursitis. The most common bursa is the gastrocnemius-semimembranosus bursa which is commonly known as Baker's cyst *(please refer to case 5.16 for further details on Baker's cyst)*. The medial collateral ligament (MCL) bursa is typically located between the superficial and deep portions of the MCL. The bursa is best seen on a coronal T2-weighted fat-suppressed images as localized fluid collections between the superficial and deep fibers of the MCL. Pes anserinus bursitis appears as a lobular cystic lesion located deep to the pes anserine tendons (sartorius, gracilis, and semitendinosus) near their insertion on the medial aspect of the tibia about 4–6 cm distal to the joint line. The prepatellar bursa is located within the soft tissues superficial to the patella and the proximal patellar tendon usually occurring secondary to repeated trauma as kneeling (housemaid's knee). They can also occur secondary to a direct trauma which can be hemorrhagic with internal high signal on the T1-weighted images. There are two infrapatellar bursae; the superficial infrapatellar bursa is located within the subcutaneous soft tissues anterior to the tibial tuberosity, while the deep infrapatellar bursa is located posterior to the distal patellar tendon and the anterior tibial cortex inferior to Hoffa's fat pad and appears as a small triangular shaped fluid collection. Note should be made that a small amount of fluid in the deep infrapatellar bursa is usually a normal finding on MRI.

Other common cysts in and around the knee are ganglion cysts. Ganglia are myxoid lesions filled with gelatinous fluid of unknown etiology. They usually appear multiseptated and can occur at any tendon insertion. Long-standing ganglia can cause pressure erosions on the adjacent bone or have intraosseous extension. The most common location of ganglion cysts is at the tendon insertions of the medial and lateral gastrocnemius as well as the popliteus muscles. Ganglia can also be intra-articular with the most common location within the anterior cruciate ligament (ACL). The ACL usually appears thickened and striated with diffuse hyperintense signal on the T2-weighted images. These are commonly mistaken for partial ACL tears, but the key to diagnosis is that in ACL ganglia, the ACL fibers can still be traced from their origin to insertion without fiber discontinuity. Parameniscal cysts are easily diagnosed as they are usually located adjacent to a meniscal tear.

Another cystic lesion seen around the knee is proximal tibiofibular joint (PTFJ) cyst which is commonly mistaken for a tumor, and hence knowledge of this lesion is important to avoid this pitfall. It is a synovial cyst and thought to represent fluid accumulation from communication with the knee joint. They are relatively uncommon, and when seen are usually small and asymptomatic. However, they may become larger in size and compress on the adjacent common peroneal nerve causing a foot drop. On MRI, this is usually seen as denervation intramuscular edema within the muscle of the anterior leg compartment.

Other uncommon cystic lesion mimickers include hematoma, abscess, vascular malformations, and neoplastic lesions. Solid tumors around the knee that can appear cyst-like include synovial sarcomas, myxoid tumors, and peripheral nerve sheath tumors.

The exact anatomic location of the cystic lesions in the knee allows for its correct diagnosis. However, when a cystic lesion is in an atypical location or if there are internal solid enhancing nodular components, then this should raise suspicion for a neoplastic lesion and the need for further investigations and management.

> **Report checklist**
> 1. What is the size and anatomic location of the cystic mass?
> 2. Is the mass in a common location for cystic masses around the knee? If not, consider administering intravenous contrast to exclude a solid mass (synovial sarcoma, myxoma, nerve sheath tumor)
> 3. Is there injury of adjacent structures (ligaments, muscles, menisci, nerves)?

Suggested Reading

McCarthy CL, McNally EG. The MRI appearance of cystic lesions around the knee. Skeletal Radiol. 2004;33:187–209.

Telischak NA, Wu JS, Eisenberg RE. Cysts and cystic-appearing lesions of the knee: a pictorial essay. Indian J Radiol Imaging. 2014; 24(2):182–91.

Case 5.18

Indication A 45-year-old woman with medial knee pain.

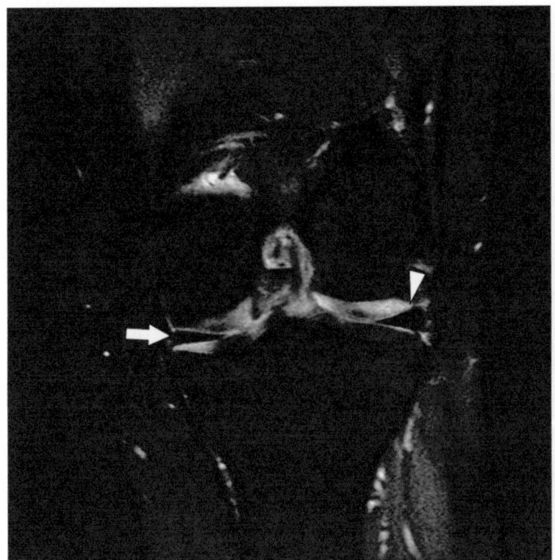

Coronal PD fat saturated

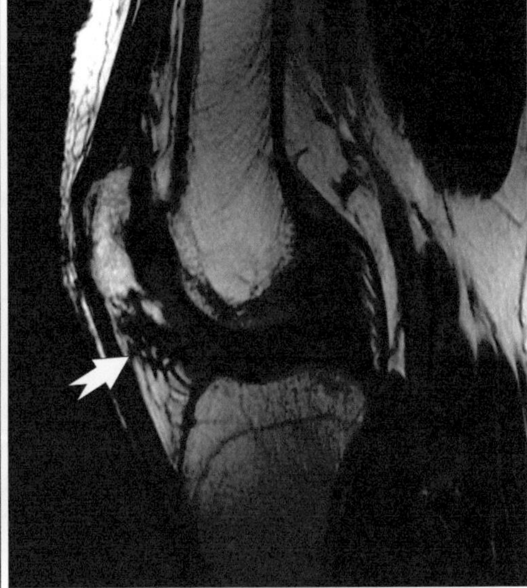

Sagittal PD

Findings
The body of the medial meniscus (arrow) is small in size when compared to the body of the lateral meniscus (arrowhead). However, there is no fluid signal in the medial meniscal remnant to suggest a meniscal re-tear. There is scarring in Hoffa's fat pad (notched arrow) consistent with prior arthroscopic surgery.

Impression/Recommendation
Partial meniscectomy changes in the medial meniscal body without meniscal re-tear.

Discussion: Postoperative meniscus.
Surgical procedures performed for meniscal tears are common and include partial meniscectomy or meniscal repair. Rarely meniscal transplants can also be performed. It is extremely important to be aware of prior meniscal surgery before interpreting a knee MRI. This can be obtained from the clinical information on the MRI requisition form or from the electronic medical records (EMR). This is to prevent the pitfall of overcalling the presence of a meniscal tear when the findings are due to postoperative changes. MRI can provide clues to prior arthroscopic surgery; however, knowledge of the patient's surgical history will greatly aid in interpretation of the MRI. Within Hoffa's fat pad, there may be linear hypointense areas on either side of the patellar tendon representing prior arthroscopy "scope scar". Another clue is a truncated or diminutive portion of the meniscus (absence of meniscal tissue) without visualizing a displaced meniscal fragment. These are all important information to be aware of while interpreting the study, as the MRI criteria normally used for diagnosing a meniscus tear cannot be applied in the setting of prior meniscal surgery. Also correlation with preoperative MRI, if available, is very useful in increasing the accuracy of differentiating a tear from normal healing granulation tissue.

Some patients who have had prior meniscal surgery may return to clinic with persistent or recurrent knee pain. The role of MRI in these situations is to identify whether the cause of knee symptoms is from the meniscus such as a persistent or recurrent meniscal tear or if the pain is related to non-meniscal causes such as chondral pathology, intra-articular loose bodies, or a subchondral insufficiency fracture.

What is considered a normal appearance of the postoperative meniscus depends on the type of surgery that was performed. In patients who have had a partial meniscectomy, then the free edge of the meniscus usually has a sharp, truncated, and blunted appearance *(see supplementary images);* however there should be no surfacing signal in the residual portion of the meniscus. Meniscal repairs are usually performed in tears within the peripheral vascularized third of the meniscus (red zone) using sutures or bioabsorbable arrows. In these cases, there can be intermediate signal intensity within the meniscus tissue touching an articular surface for up to 1-year post surgery representing granulation tissue. Although, following this period, MRI may demonstrate an almost normal appearing meniscus indicating complete healing.

Evaluating a postoperative meniscus for a meniscus re-tear is challenging as the majority of patients remain having signal alterations within the meniscus, mainly on the T1 and PD sequences which usually represent granulation tissue; however, this can be seen with re-tears as well. A re-tear can only be diagnosed on conventional MRI when (1) definite surfacing fluid signal is seen on the T2-weighted images, (2) a displaced meniscal fragment, and (3) a tear at a new site. If surfacing signal is seen on the T1 or PD sequences but not on the T2-weighted images, then this remains indeterminate for a tear as this could also represent granulation tissue. In these situations, MR arthrography can provide better accuracy in differentiating the two. A meniscal re-tear is diagnosed on MR arthrography when intra-articular gadolinium contrast is seen within the substance of the meniscus and reaching an articular surface *(see supplementary images).*

About 40% of patients with prior meniscal surgery have associated articular chondral abnormalities, and this should be routinely sought for. Also assessing for intra-articular loose bodies, synovitis, and bone marrow edema within the femoral condyles or tibial plateaus.

The value of repeated repair of the meniscus is debated, and clinical studies have demonstrated mixed results.

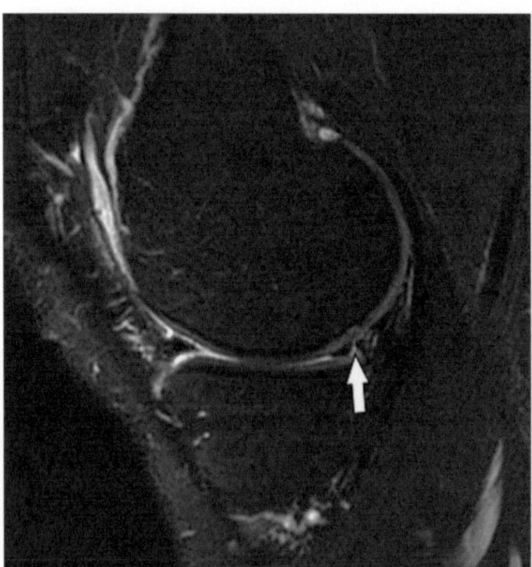

Sagittal T2 fat saturated

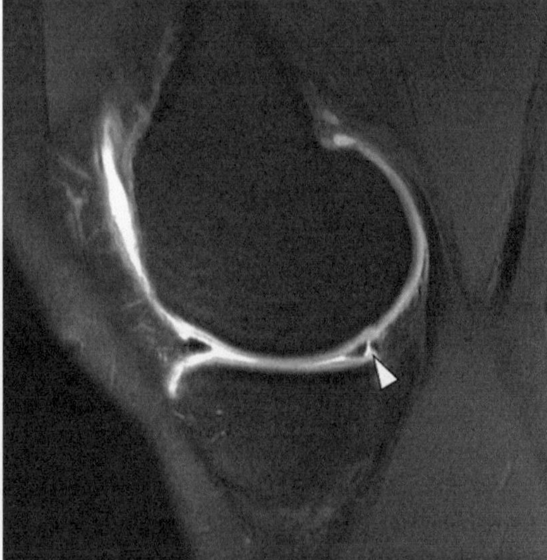

Sagittal T1 fat saturated (MR arthrogram)

Meniscal re-tear. There is high signal (arrow) in the diminutive posterior horn of the medial meniscus on the T2-weighted images which is equivocal for fluid signal. There is contrast *(arrowhead) extending into the meniscus on the arthrogram image confirming a re-tear*

Report checklist

1. Has the patient had prior meniscal surgery (look for scarring in Hoffa's fat pad)? Was it a partial meniscectomy, meniscal repair, or transplant? Location of the surgery?
2. Is there high signal intensity fluid on the T2-weighted images or intra-articular gadolinium contrast in the meniscus substance touching an articular surface to indicate a meniscal re-tear?
3. Is there a displaced meniscal fragment? Is there a tear at a new site?
4. Are there new focal chondral pathology?
5. Are there intra-articular loose bodies? synovitis? subchondral insufficiency fractures?

Suggested Reading

Davis KW, Tuite MJ. MR imaging of the postoperative meniscus of the knee. Semin Musculoskelet Radiol. 2002;6(1):35–45.

Nakayama H, Kanto R, Kambara S, et al. Clinical outcome of meniscus repair for isolated meniscus tear in athletes. Asia Pac J Sports Med Arthrosc Rehabil Technol. 2017;10:4–7.

Case 5.19

Indication A 39-year-old male with prior ACL reconstruction 5 years ago. Now presents with knee pain and giving way. Assess ACL graft.

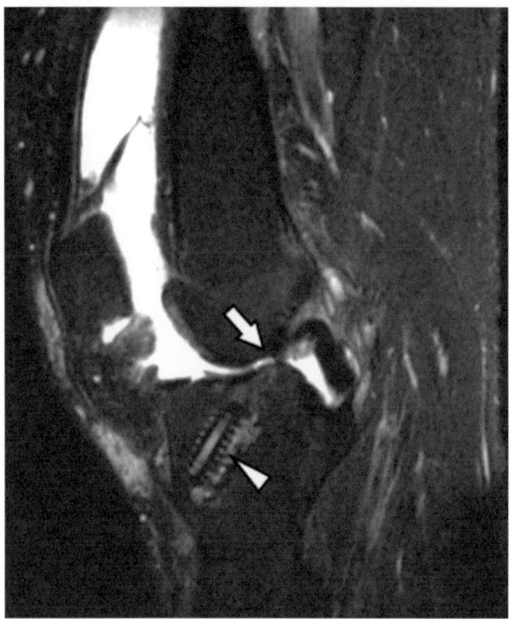

Sagittal T2 fat saturated

Findings
The patient is status post ACL reconstruction. The ACL graft is not visualized at its intra-articular portion (arrow). The tibial (arrowhead) and femoral interference screws are intact. There is a large knee joint effusion.

Impression/Recommendation
Complete ACL graft tear.

Discussion: Postoperative ACL Reconstruction
Orthopedic surgeons usually recommend ACL reconstruction in most patients with ACL tears since if left untreated, the patient can develop secondary meniscal tears and knee joint osteoarthritis. There are many graft options available for reconstruction; however, by far the two most common grafts used are (1) bone-patellar tendon-bone graft which is taken from the central third of the patellar tendon with proximal and distal bone plugs and (2) hamstring grafts, taken from the distal gracilis and semitendinosus tendons which do not include bone plugs and hence require fixation devices to secure the grafts inside the osseous tunnels. Both types of grafts have been shown to have similar long-term outcomes in regard to knee stability with graft selection usually based on surgeon preference. Currently, cadaveric ACL allografts are not routinely used.

Patients may return with persistent pain, knee instability, or acute re-injury after ACL reconstruction. MRI may be performed to assess the ACL graft as well as assess for other associated injuries in the knee. When evaluating these studies, one should always start with the position of the ACL graft and its appearance. The position can be optimally assessed on MRI and correct positioning of the graft is important for proper function of the graft. The optimal position of the tibial tunnel is located just posterior to Blumensaat's line seen on the sagittal plane. Placing the tibial tunnel too posterior may lead to instability while placing it too far anteriorly will cause abnormal contact of the graft with the intercondylar roof, "roof impingement." Roof impingement may cause knee pain and limitation of movement and places the graft at increased risk of degeneration and disruption. On MRI, roof impingement is present when the tibial tunnel is placed too far anteriorly with posterior bowing of the graft at the intercondylar notch *(see supplementary images)*. In chronic cases, increased signal intensity in the graft with partial-thickness tearing may also be visualized.

Next, the age of the graft should be taken into consideration. The ACL graft may demonstrate intermediate signal within the first 12–18 months post surgery due to the normal revascularization process of the graft; however, the graft should never be as bright as fluid in signal intensity. This is more commonly seen with a hamstring graft and should not be misinterpreted as graft disruption. After this period, the graft should demonstrate low signal intensity on both T1- and T2-weighted images. Any increased signal in the graft following this period should raise suspicion for graft impingement or graft disruption. Tears of the graft are seen as fluid signal intensity within the graft with either partial-thickness or complete disruption of the graft fibers and possible graft laxity.

Arthrofibrosis is intra-articular scarring that may occur following ACL reconstruction and can be either diffuse or focal. The most common focal form is termed a "cyclops" lesion which represents focal nodular fibrosis in the intercondylar notch anterior to the ACL graft. During arthroscopy, the arthrofibrosis can appear as a single "eye," hence its name. Patients usually present with anterior knee pain and loss of full extension. On MRI, this is seen as a well-defined soft tissue nodule abutting the anterior aspect of the ACL graft and demonstrates mixed heterogeneous signal intensities on T1- and T2-weighted images *(see supplementary images)*.

Lastly, tunnel cysts or ganglion cysts may form around the ACL graft within the osseous tunnels leading to knee laxity. Although a small amount of fluid is normal in the tunnels, large cysts or enlargement of the tunnels is abnormal. The exact etiology is unknown and is thought to be multifactorial but results in inadequate fixation of the graft within the tunnel. This has also been termed tunnel lysis or tunnel expansion and on MRI is seen as enlargement of the tunnel with fluid or ganglion cysts surrounding the intraosseous portions of the graft *(see supplementary images)*.

Supplementary Images

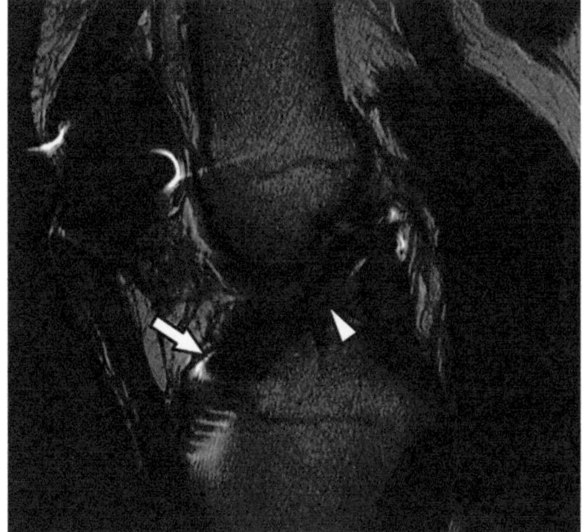

Sagittal PD

The tibial tunnel is placed too far anteriorly (arrow). This results in secondary graft roof impingement evident by posterior bowing of the graft and increased signal intensity within the graft substance (arrowheads). The graft is still intact

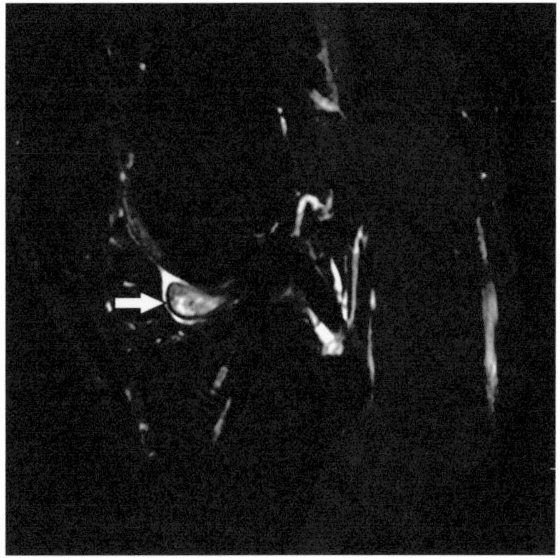

Sagittal T2 fat saturated

There is a well-defined soft tissue nodule with heterogenous signal anterior to the ACL graft in the intercondylar notch (arrow) compatible with focal arthrofibrosis (cyclops lesion)

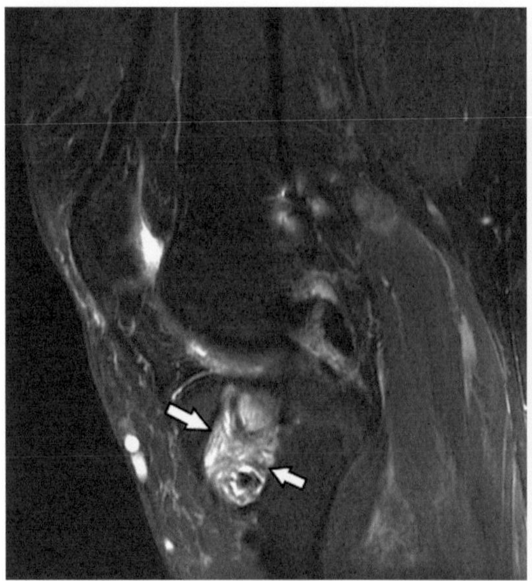

Sagittal T2 fat saturated

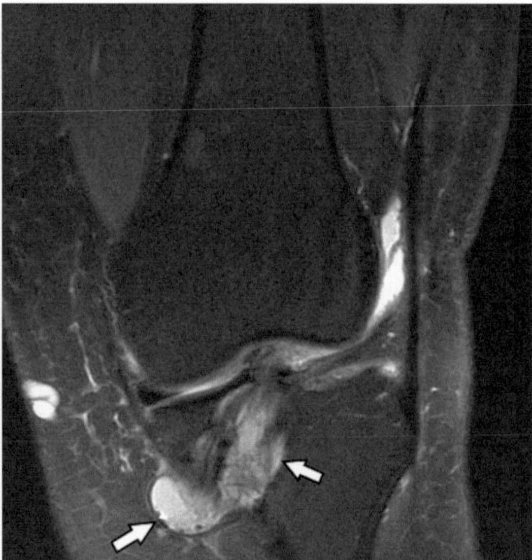

Coronal T2 fat saturated

There is significant widening of the tibial tunnel with multiple cysts surrounding the ACL graft (arrows) compatible with tunnel cysts/tunnel lysis

Suggested Reading

Bencardino JT, Beltran J, Feldman MI, Rose DJ. MR imaging of complications of anterior cruciate ligament graft reconstruction. Radiographics. 2009;29(7):2115–26.

Meyers AB, Haims AH, Menn K, Moukaddam H. Imaging of anterior cruciate ligament repair and its complications. AJR Am J Roentgenol. 2010;194(2):476–84.

© Springer Nature Switzerland AG 2020
T. M. Hegazi, J. S. Wu, *Musculoskeletal MRI*, https://doi.org/10.1007/978-3-030-26777-3_6

Case 6.1

Indication A 34-year-old female runner with foot pain for 2 weeks.

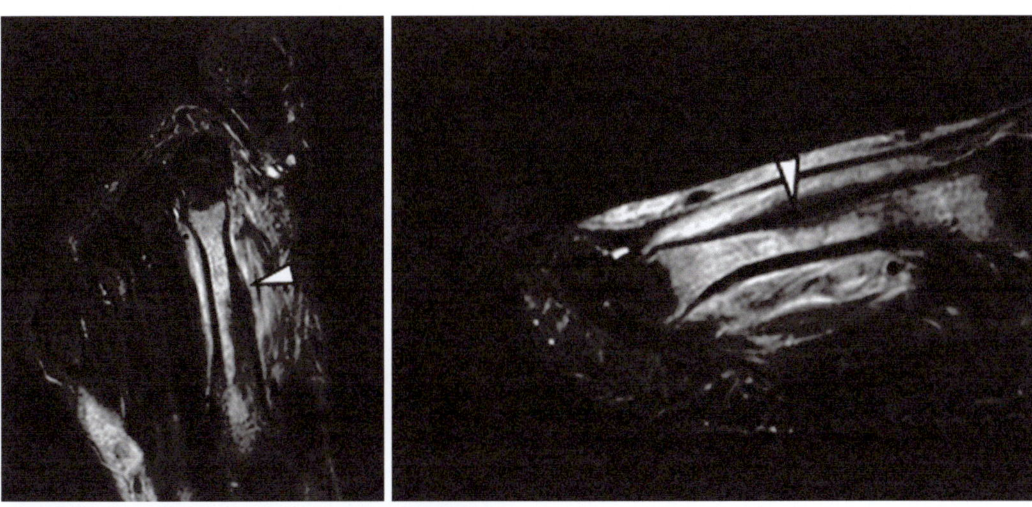

Axial T2 fat saturated   Sagittal T2 fat saturated

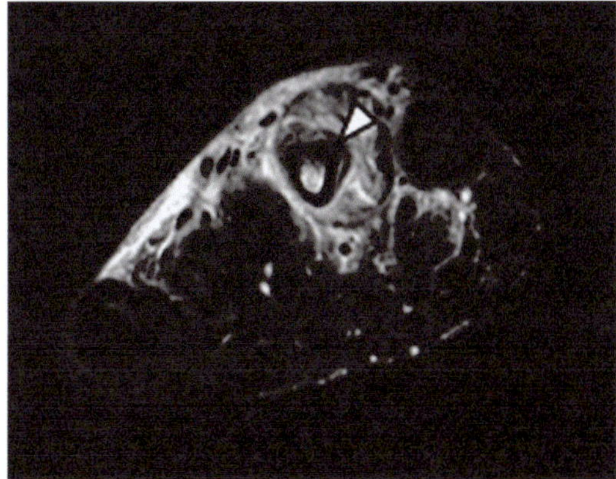

Coronal T2 fat saturated

Findings

There is marked reactive bone marrow edema at the 2nd metatarsal shaft with hypointense medial cortical thickening (arrowheads) compatible with a stress fracture. There is associated smooth periosteal reaction along the medial aspect of the metatarsal shaft and edema within the surrounding soft tissues.

Impression/Recommendation

Non-displaced 2nd metatarsal stress fracture. Limited weight-bearing is recommended.

Discussion: Metatarsal Stress Fractures

Stress fractures result from repetitive stress on bones and are classified as either fatigue or insufficiency fractures. Fatigue fractures occur from repetitive excessive stress onto normal bone and are commonly seen in athletes and military recruits. Insufficiency fractures are however related to normal stress on abnormally weaken bone, commonly seen in osteoporotic patients. Patients usually present with foot pain that worsens with weight-bearing and activity and typically improves with non-weight-bearing.

In the foot, stress fractures are most commonly seen at the mid-diaphysis or neck of the 2nd and 3rd metatarsals. MRI is a very sensitive modality in the detection of marrow changes related to repetitive osseous injury. Early on, osseous injury is usually seen as an area of poorly defined bone marrow edema within the shaft of the metatarsals on the fluid-sensitive sequences, without visualization of a hypointense fracture line. This is called stress response. As the stresses continue, a discrete fracture can occur and will typically appear as a hypointense line abutting the cortex usually perpendicular to the metatarsal shaft. This can be accompanied by smooth periosteal reaction seen as edema surrounding the bone cortex circumferentially. It is important to note that a hypointense fracture line is not always observed. Fracture lines usually become visible when the healing process has started.

Non-displaced stress fractures are generally treated using conservative therapy which involves decreased activity and immobilization.

Report checklist
1. Where is the bone marrow edema within the metatarsal shaft?
2. Is there a hypointense fracture line? Is it displaced?
3. Is there periosteal edema?
4. Are there additional stress fractures?

Suggested Reading

Ashman CJ, Klecker RJ, Yu JS. Forefoot pain involving the metatarsal region: differential diagnosis with MR imaging. Radiographics. 2001;21:425–40.

Burge AJ, Gold SL, Potter HG. Imaging of sports-related midfoot and forefoot injuries. Sports Health. 2012;4:518–34.

Nattiv A, Kennedy G, Barrack MT, et al. Correlation of MRI grading of bone stress injuries with clinical risk factors and return to play: a 5-year prospective study in collegiate track and field athletes. Am J Sports Med. 2013;41:1930–41.

Case 6.2

Indication A 28-year-old male with chronic lateral hindfoot pain.

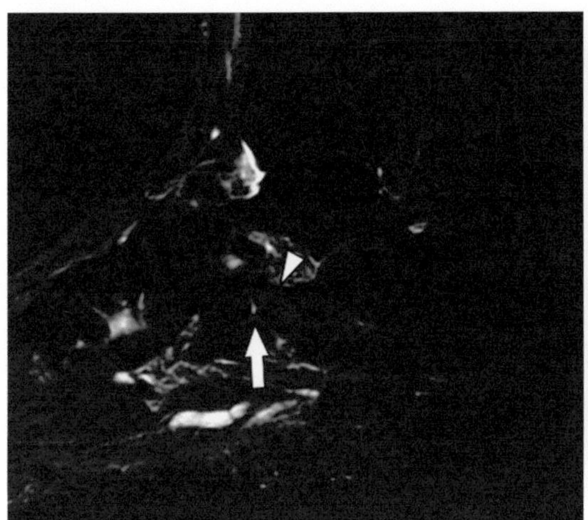

Sagittal STIR

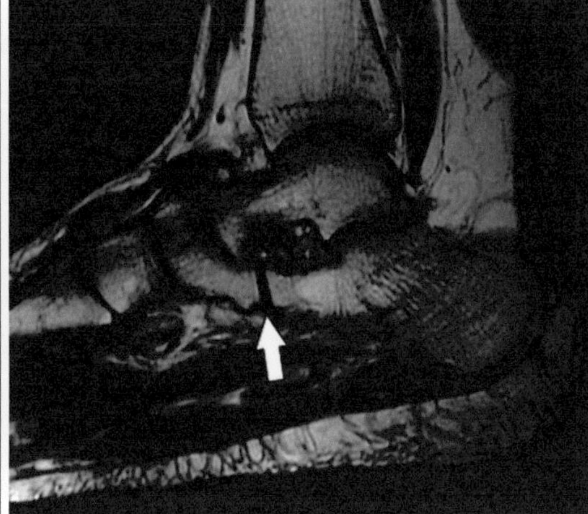

Sagittal T1

Findings

There is abnormal elongation of the anterior calcaneal process with irregularity at its articulation
(arrows) with the lateral aspect of the navicular.
There is no bony fusion. Minimal bone marrow
edema is seen at the anterior calcaneal process
(arrowhead).

Impression/Recommendation

Non-osseous calcaneonavicular coalition.

Discussion: Tarsal Coalition

Tarsal coalition is characterized as abnormal
fusion between two or more tarsal bones due to
failure of proper segmentation. These abnormal
unions may be fibrous (syndesmosis), cartilaginous (synchondrosis), or osseous (synostosis).
The incidence is less than 1% and is bilateral in
up to 50% of patients. The most common types of
tarsal coalitions are calcaneonavicular or talocalcaneal (typically middle facet), seen in about
90% of cases. Rarely, the calcaneocuboid or
cuboid-navicular joints may also be involved.
Although patients may be asymptomatic and are
often incidentally discovered on imaging performed for other reasons, the majority of patients
usually present with hindfoot or midfoot pain and
ankle stiffness.

Plain radiographs are very helpful in diagnosing osseous tarsal coalitions; however, they are
less accurate and more difficult to appreciate
non-osseous coalitions (fibrous or cartilaginous).
MRI is useful in distinguishing between osseous
and non-osseous coalitions and in detecting other
associated abnormalities. MRI also allows better
visualization of the extent of involvement for pre-
surgical planning.

Calcaneonavicular coalitions typically occur
between the anterior calcaneal process and the
posterolateral aspect of the navicular. This is best
seen on the sagittal plane which demonstrates an
elongated anterior process of the calcaneus termed
the "anteater's nose." Talocalcaneal coalitions
most commonly occur at the middle facet of the
subtalar joint and the sustentaculum tali. The normal middle facet usually has an upward or straight
appearance on a coronal plane, while in a coalition
this often results in a downward sloping middle
facet *(see supplementary images)*. In osseous
coalitions, there is marrow continuity across the
coalition. Although it is not that essential to differentiate between a fibrous and cartilaginous
coalition, a fibrous coalition usually demonstrates
low signal intensity on both T1- and T2-weighted
images at the junction of the bones. In cartilaginous coalition, there is typically intermediate

signal on T1 and high signal intensity on the T2-weighted fat-suppressed images. There may be associated bone marrow edema and subchondral cystic changes across the coalition.

Treatment of coalitions usually starts with conservative management which includes NSAIDs and orthotics. Surgery can be performed in cases where the patient does not respond to conservative management. This can involve resection of the coalition with fat placed in the interval.

Supplementary Images

Report checklist

1. Where is the location of the coalition?
2. Is the coalition osseous or non-osseous?
3. Is there bone marrow edema or subchondral cystic changes across the coalition?
4. Are there degenerative changes at the posterior subtalar joint? Osteochondral lesions at the talar dome?

Suggested Reading

Lawrence DA, Rolen MF, Haims AH, Zayour Z, Moukaddam HA. Tarsal coalitions: radiographic, CT, and MR imaging findings. HSS J. 2014;10(2):153–66.

Newman JS, Newberg AH. Congenital tarsal coalition: multimodality evaluation with emphasis on CT and MR imaging. Radiographics. 2000;20:321–32.

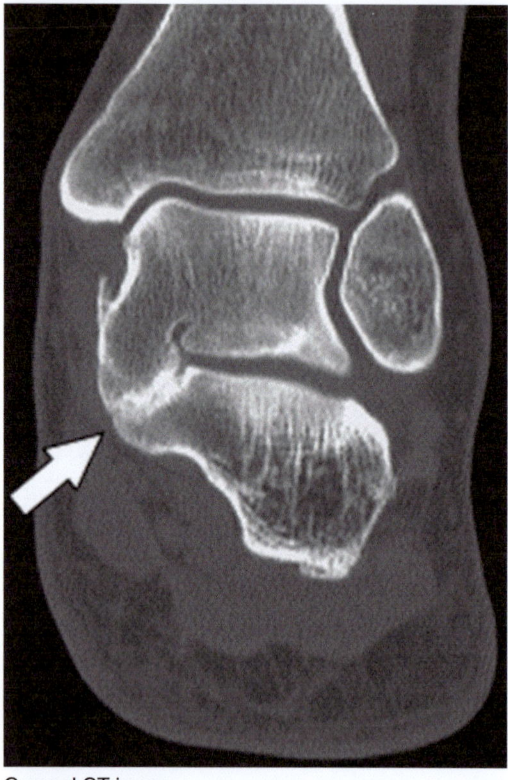

Coronal CT image

Non-osseous tarsal coalition. There is downsloping of the middle facet (arrow) of the subtalar joint

Case 6.3

Indication A 30-year-old female with chronic medial foot pain that is aggravated with physical activity.

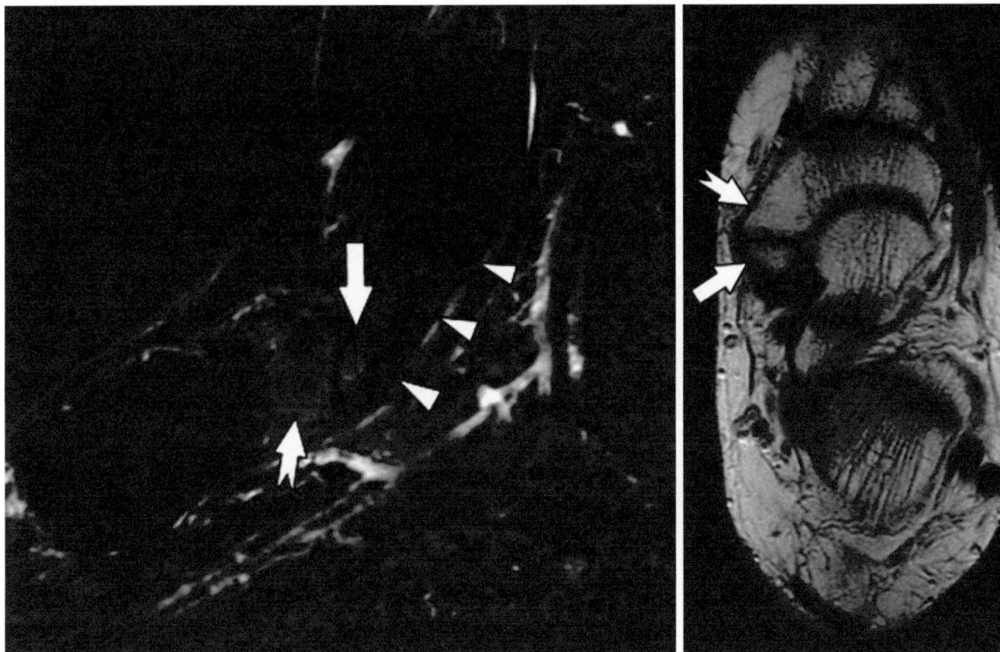

Sagittal STIR   Axial T1

Findings
There is moderate bone marrow edema within a type 2 accessory navicular (arrows) as well as within the adjacent medial navicular tuberosity (notched arrows). There is no significant fluid within the synchondrosis or subchondral cystic changes. The posterior tibialis tendon is intact without tendinosis or tenosynovitis (arrowheads).

Impression/Recommendation
Bone marrow edema across a type 2 accessory navicular, likely the cause of the patient's medial foot pain.

Discussion: Accessory Navicular Bone
An accessory navicular bone is an anatomic variant, in which the tuberosity of the navicular bone develops from a secondary ossification center. It is seen in about 4–21% of the population and is usually discovered incidentally. There are three types of accessory navicular: Type 1 is a 4–6 mm ossicle lying within the posterior tibial tendon. Type 2 accessory navicular is the most common type and is a triangular or heart-shaped 9–15 mm ossicle adjacent to the navicular tuberosity connected by a 1–2 mm cartilaginous or fibrous synchondrosis. Most of the fibers of the distal posterior tibialis tendon insert directly onto the accessory ossicle. Type 3 is also referred to as a cornuate navicular and represents a prominent navicular tuberosity which is essentially a type 2 accessory navicular that is completely fused to the navicular.

Type 2 accessory navicular is the most symptomatic of the 3 types and may serve as a cause of medial foot pain, especially in young athletes, which has been termed painful accessory navicular syndrome. Patients usually present with chronic or acute on chronic medial foot pain that is aggravated by walking or weight-bearing.

MRI findings associated with a symptomatic type 2 accessory navicular include bone marrow edema in the accessory navicular bone and the navicular tuberosity, suggesting chronic stress-related injury. There can be overlying soft tissue edema. The presence of fluid in the synchondrosis and subchondral cysts on either side of the synchondrosis may suggest chronic instability. Additionally, thickening of the distal posterior tibial tendon may be present due to tendinosis or tenosynovitis.

In symptomatic cases, patients are usually treated conservatively with NSAIDs and orthotics. Surgery may be considered in cases that fail conservative management which involves fusion of the ossicle or excision of the ossicle with reinsertion of the posterior tibial tendon.

Report checklist

1. What is the degree of bone marrow edema in the type 2 accessory navicular (mild, moderate, or severe)?
2. Is there bone marrow edema in the medial navicular tuberosity?
3. Is there fluid in the synchondrosis or subchondral cystic changes?
4. Is there tendinosis or tenosynovitis within the distal fibers of the posterior tibial tendon?

Suggested Reading

Choi YS, Lee KT, Kang HS et al. MR imaging findings of painful type II accessory navicular bone. Correlation with surgical and pathologic studies. Korean J Radiol. 2004;5:274–9.

Mosel LD, Kat E, Voyvodic F. Imaging of the symptomatic type II accessory navicular bone. Australas Radiol. 2004;48(2):267–71.

Case 6.4

Indication A 28-year-old female with forefoot pain at the 2nd MTP joint.

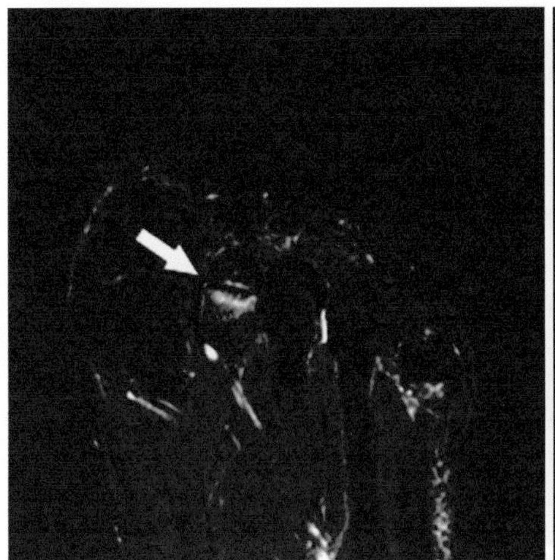
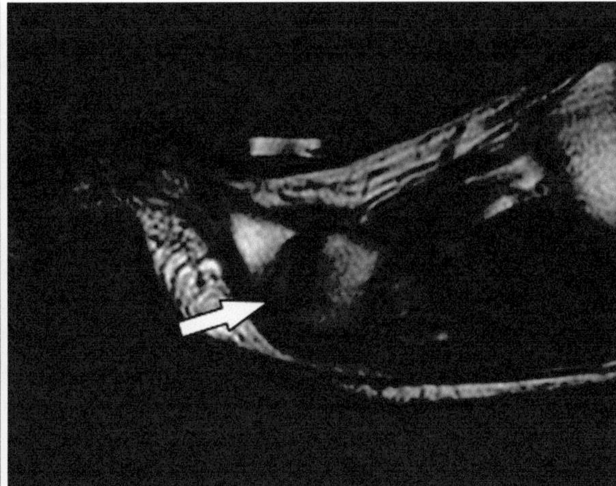

Axial T2 fat saturated   Sagittal T1

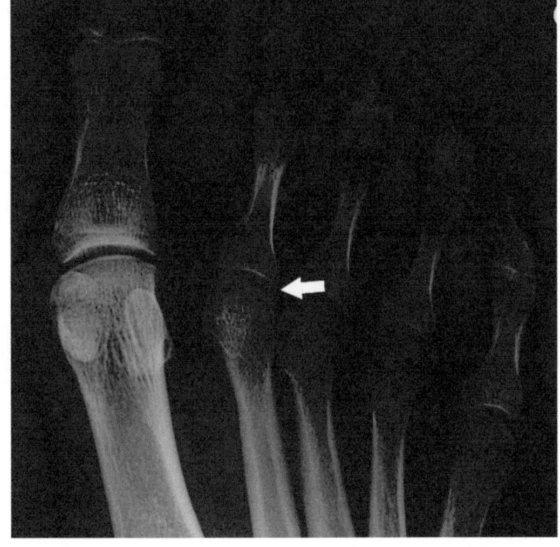

Findings

There is flattening of the subchondral bone at the 2nd metatarsal head with surrounding bone edema (arrows). There are no reciprocal osseous changes at the base of the 2nd proximal phalanx. There is no joint effusion, intra-articular loose bodies or secondary osteoarthritis. The plantar plate is intact.

Impression/Recommendation

Osteonecrosis of the 2nd metatarsal head (Freiberg's infraction).

Discussion: Freiberg's Infraction

Freiberg's infraction also known as Freiberg's disease is an osteochondrosis of the metatarsal head most commonly involving the 2nd (65%) or the 3rd (25%) metatarsal heads. Pathologically, it is characterized by microvascular infarction and trabecular fracture at the head of the metatarsal with resultant collapse of the subchondral bone and eventually secondary joint osteoarthritis. It most commonly affects women in the second or third decades and is thought to be related to chronic repetitive trauma. Patients usually present with localized pain and tenderness at the metatarsal head. Freiberg's infraction can be bilateral in up to 10% of cases.

Early in the disease, radiographs are usually normal; however, MRI may show bone marrow edema in the metatarsal head seen as diffuse high signal on the fluid-sensitive sequences. This may be accompanied with a subtle subchondral fracture line seen as a linear hypointense line on both the T1- and T2-weighted images. The lack of bone marrow edema at the proximal phalanx helps to exclude osteoarthritis as an etiology. As the disease progresses, there can be flattening of the metatarsal head, osseous fragmentation, and finally intra-articular loose bodies with secondary osteoarthritis.

Treatment is usually nonoperative which includes cast immobilization and non-weight-bearing. Rarely do patients need surgical treatment.

Report checklist

1. Which metatarsal head is involved?
2. What is the degree of bone marrow edema? Can a subchondral fracture line be visualized?
3. Is there collapse of the articular surface or osseous fragmentation?
4. Are there reciprocal changes at the phalangeal side of the joint?
5. Are there intra-articular loose bodies? Joint effusion? Secondary changes of osteoarthritis?
6. How is the plantar plate?

Suggested Reading

Cerrato RA. Freiberg's disease. Foot Ankle Clin. 2011;16(4):647–58.

Torriani M, Thomas BJ, Bredella MA, et al. MRI of metatarsal head subchondral fractures in patients with forefoot pain. AJR Am J Roentgenol. 2008;190(3):570–5.

Case 6.5

Indication A 34-year-old male with chronic ankle pain after a twisting injury 6 months prior. Radiographs show a cortical defect at the lateral talar dome.

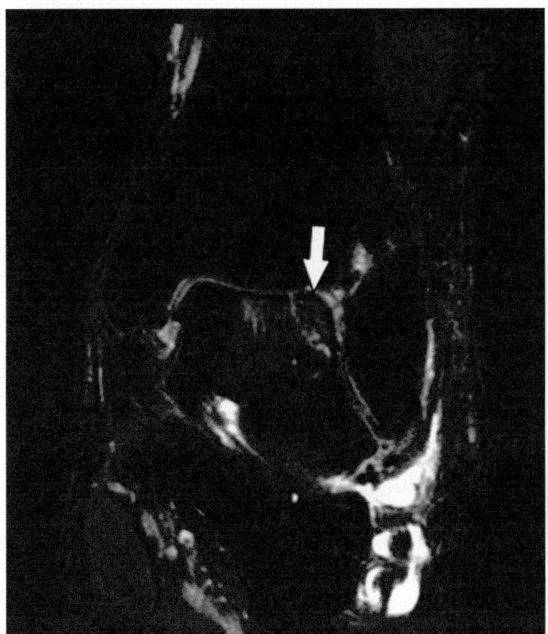

Coronal T2 fat saturated

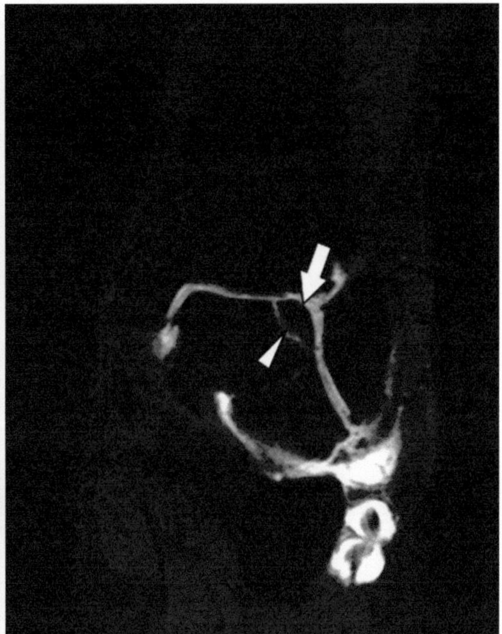

Coronal T1 fat saturated (MR arthrogram)

Findings

There is a 6 × 7 mm osteochondral lesion (arrows) at the lateral talar dome. There is bone marrow edema, both within the osteochondral fragment and the underlying talus. Intra-articular contrast extends beneath the osteochondral fragment (arrowhead) which suggests an unstable osteochondral fragment.

Impression/Recommendation

Unstable, non-displaced osteochondral lesion of the talus.

Discussion: Osteochondral Lesion of the Talus

Osteochondral lesions of the talus (OLT) are lesions that involve both the subchondral bone and the overlying articular cartilage of the talus. The term OLT is preferred, although the condition has also been called osteochondritis dissecans (OCD) or osteochondral defect. OLT can

occur from an ankle inversion injury or from repeated trauma. They involve the medial or lateral aspect of the talar dome with equal frequency. Patients usually present with chronic ankle pain and instability.

A small cortical defect can sometimes be seen on plain radiographs; however, the majority of these lesions are radiographically occult and are only seen on MRI. An MRI classification scheme has been developed for staging OLT with the primary goal to differentiate a stable *(see supplementary images)* from an unstable lesion. This is important as the treatment approach will differ. The four-stage classification appears on MRI as follows:

- Stage I: focal bone marrow edema at the talar dome with normal overlying cartilage
- Stage II: focal bone marrow edema at the talar dome with a partial tear of the overlying cartilage
- Stage IIa: as stage II, but with associated subchondral cysts

- Stage III: a completely separated osteocartilaginous fragment within its site of origin
- Stage IV: an osseous defect at the talar dome with a displaced intra-articular loose body.

MRI signs that suggest an unstable osteochondral fragment include fluid signal or intra-articular contrast partially or completely surrounding the osteochondral fragment and/or cystic changes underneath an osteochondral fragment. The presence of low signal intensity in the osteochondral fragment on all pulse sequences is a sign of osteonecrosis.

Without treatment, unstable osteochondral lesions usually progress and eventually are displaced into the joint as a loose body. Thus, most unstable lesions are treated surgically.

Supplementary Images

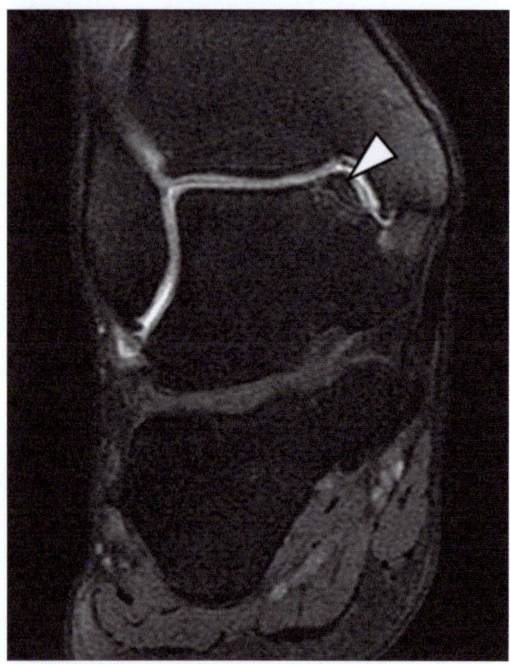

Coronal T1 fat saturated (MR arthrogram)

Stable OLT. There is a 7 mm osteochondral lesion at the medial talar dome. Intra-articular contrast does not extend beneath the osteochondral fragment, indicating a stable lesion

Report checklist

1. What is the location and size of the osteochondral lesion (OLT)?
2. Is the overlying articular cartilage intact?
3. What is the stability of the osteochondral fragment? (Unstable lesions have contrast/fluid at the donor site and/or cystic changes underneath the lesion)
4. What is the viability of the bone fragment (fragmentation, osteonecrosis)?
5. Is the osteochondral fragment displaced into the joint and where is it located?

Suggested Reading

Griffith JF, Wang YX, Lodge SJ, et al. Small field-of-view surface coil mr imaging of talar osteochondral lesions. Foot Ankle Int. 2010;31(6):517–22.

Laffenêtre O. Osteochondral lesions of the talus: current concept. Orthop Traumatol Surg Res. 2010;96:554–66.

Verhagen RA, Maas M, Dijkgraaf MG, et al. Prospective study on diagnostic strategies in osteochondral lesions of the talus. Is MRI superior to helical CT? J Bone Joint Surg Br. 2005;87(1):41–6.

Case 6.6

Indication A 37-year-old male runner with chronic posterior ankle pain not responding to conservative measures.

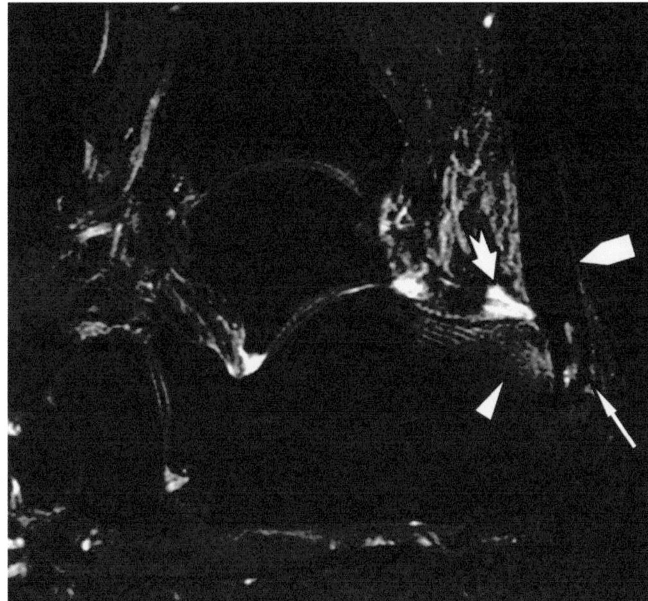

Sagittal STIR

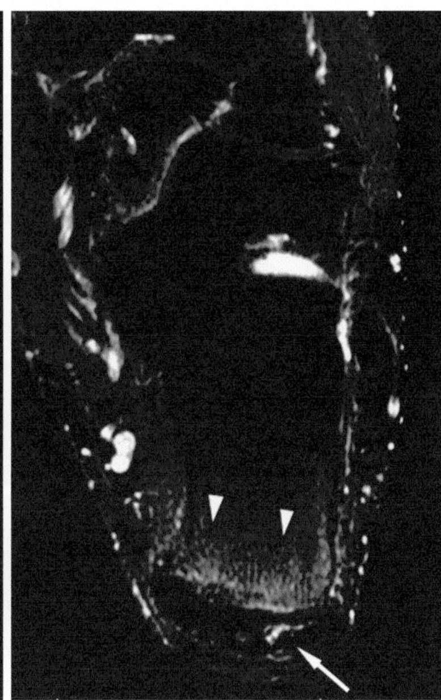

Axial T2 fat saturated

Findings

There is moderate thickening of the distal Achilles tendon (block arrow) as its insertion on the calcaneus compatible with moderate tendinosis. This is associated with mild peritendinous edema within the surrounding soft tissues and within Kager's fat pad. There is also reactive bone marrow edema in the posterosuperior aspect of the calcaneus (arrowheads). There are small linear high signal abnormalities within the distal tendon substance suggesting low-grade partial-thickness interstitial tearing (thin arrows). There is however no full-thickness tear. There is mild fluid distention of the retrocacaneal bursa (notched arrow) compatible with retrocalcaneal bursitis.

Impression/Recommendation

Moderate insertional Achilles tendinosis and mild retrocalcaneal bursitis. There is no full-thickness tendon tear.

Discussion: Insertional Achilles Tendinopathy

Achilles tendon abnormalities are classified as either insertional or noninsertional *(please refer to Case 6.7 for further discussion on noninsertional Achilles tendinopathy)*. Insertional Achilles tendinopathy is characterized as inflammation and irritation of the Achilles tendon at the distal calcaneal insertion and is usually related to chronic overuse injury commonly seen in runners or with improper fitting shoes.

MRI will depict distal tendon thickening at its insertion with increased signal intensity within the tendon substance. This is usually accompanied by peritendinous edema representing peritendinitis (paratenonitis) as well as distension and inflammatory changes of the retrocalcaneal bursa and/or retroachilles bursa. Reactive bone marrow edema at the posterosuperior aspect of the calcaneus is commonly seen in more advanced disease. Small focal areas of interstitial partial-thickness tendon tearing (fascicular tears) can also be seen; however, this can progress to full-thickness tear if not appropriately treated.

Haglund's deformity is a bony prominence of the posterosuperior calcaneal tuberosity best detected on the sagittal images or lateral radiographs. Although there are many asymptomatic patients with this deformity, it is believed that this prominence results in impingement of the deep fibers of the Achilles tendon which can cause fraying with chronic overuse and associated retrocalcaneal bursitis, termed Haglund's syndrome *(see supplementary images)*.

Most insertional tendinopathies are treated conservatively with rest, NSAIDS, and pain injections. In persistent or severe cases, surgery may be necessary.

Supplementary Images

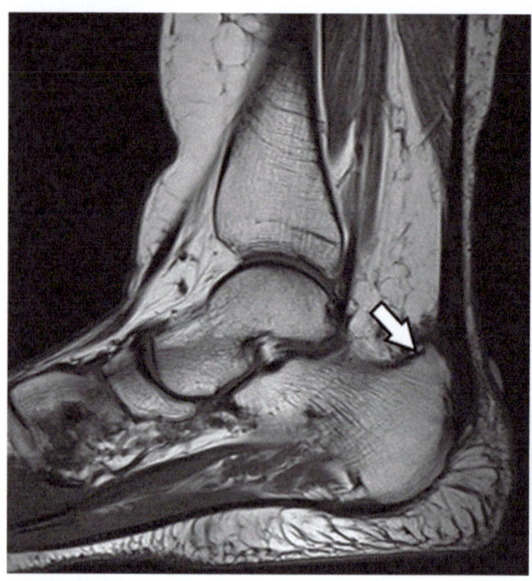

Sagittal T1

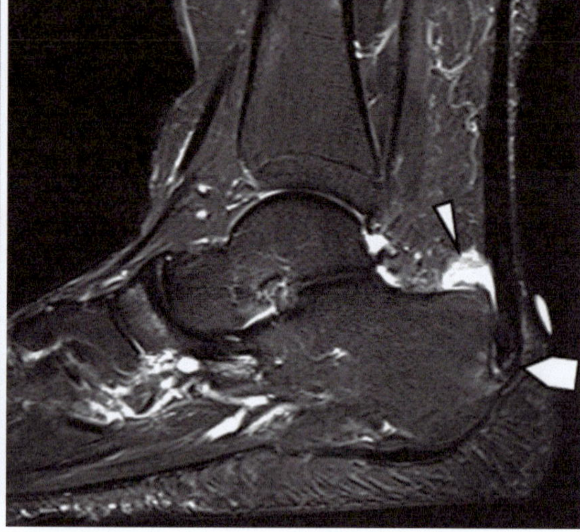

Sagittal STIR

There is focal bony prominence (Haglund's deformity) at the posterosuperior calcaneal tuberosity (arrow) associated with insertional Achilles tendinosis (block arrow) and retrocalcaneal bursitis (arrowhead). The triad is called Haglund's syndrome

Report checklist
1. What is the degree of Achilles tendinosis (mild, moderate, severe)?
2. Where is the abnormality located along the Achilles tendon (at the insertion or in the midtendon substance)?
3. Is there a focal tendon tear? Is it partial-thickness or complete?
4. Is there surrounding soft tissue edema (peritendinitis/paratenonitis)?
5. Is there reactive bone barrow edema at the calcaneus?
6. Is there Haglund's deformity or Haglund's syndrome?

Suggested Reading

Chang CD, Wu JS. Magnetic resonance imaging findings in heel pain. Magn Reson Imaging Clin N Am. 2017:25(1):79–93.

Pierre-Jerome C, Moncayo V, Terk MR. MRI of the Achilles tendon: a comprehensive review of the anatomy, biomechanics, and imaging of overuse tendinopathies. Acta Radiol. 2010;51:438–54.

Schweitzer ME, Karasick D. MR imaging of disorders of the Achilles tendon. AJR Am J Roentgenol. 2000;175(3):613–25.

Case 6.7

Indication A 30-year-old male athlete presented with sudden posterior ankle pain 2 weeks ago while playing basketball. Now has difficulty weight-bearing and weak plantar flexion. Evaluate Achilles tendon.

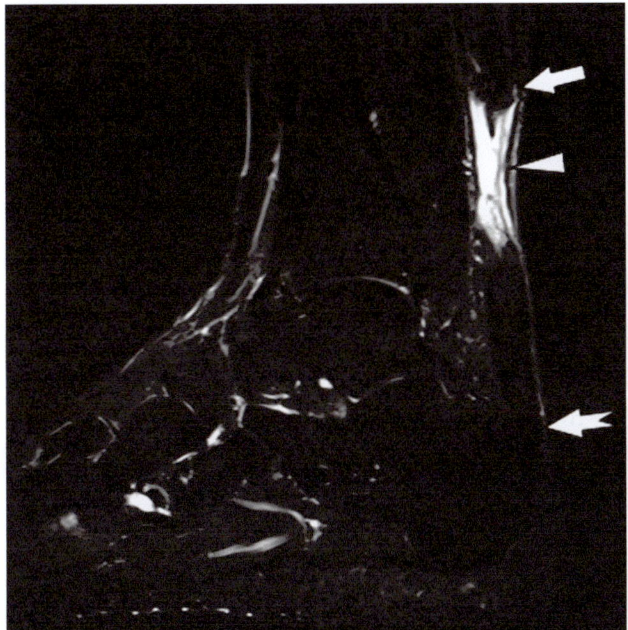

Sagittal STIR

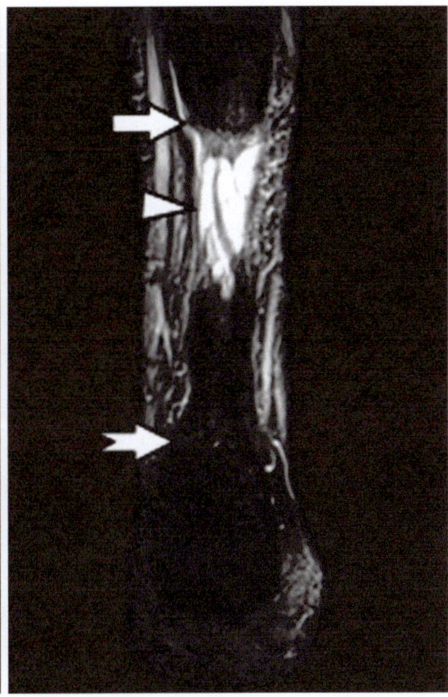

Coronal T2 fat saturated

Findings

There is a complete rupture of the Achilles tendon 5 cm from its distal attachment on the calcaneus with retraction of the proximal tendon end (arrow). The tendon gap (arrowheads) between the torn fibers measures 4 cm. The torn tendon edges are thickened and frayed. The Achilles tendon insertion (notched arrow) is intact. The plantaris tendon is normal and intact (not shown).

Impression/Recommendation

Complete rupture of the Achilles tendon at its mid-substance with 4 cm of tendon gap.

Discussion: Noninsertional Achilles Tendinopathy/Tear

The Achilles tendon is approximately 15 cm in length and formed from the fusion of the aponeurosis of the soleus and the medial and lateral heads of the gastrocnemius muscles. The Achilles tendon does not have a true synovial sheath but instead is covered by a richly vascularized thin membrane referred to as the paratenon. On MRI, the normal Achilles should be homogeneously hypointense on all imaging sequences with smooth contours. The normal average anteroposterior thickness is 6 mm with a concave anterior border. The plantaris tendon is seen in about 90% of individuals which usually inserts directly on the calcaneus medially; however, it can also blend in with the Achilles tendon more proximally.

Achilles tendon abnormalities are usually related to chronic overuse and microtrauma and injuries are classified as either insertional or more commonly noninsertional *(please refer to Case 6.6 for further details on insertional Achilles tendinopathy)*. Noninsertional Achilles tendinosis and tears most commonly occur at a relatively watershed hypovascular area 4–6 cm above its insertion on the calcaneus. Achilles tendinosis is the earliest form of injury, which is evident by fusiform thickening of the tendon with increased anteroposterior and cross-sectional diameters as well as convex anterior border, suggestive of hypoxic tendinosis *(see supplementary images)*. Focal areas of intermediate intrasubstance signal abnormalities within the tendon suggest mucoid degeneration. This may be associated with paratenonitis (peritendinitis) which is evident as high signal intensity on the T2-weighted sequences around the Achilles tendon and within Kager's fat pad.

Presence of fluid signal in the tendon substance indicates a partial tear. The signal may be linear and longitudinal which suggests partial-thickness interstitial tearing. Partial tears may also be transverse in orientation, and the distinction between these two should be mentioned in the report. Complete tears show a fluid-filled gap, complete discontinuity, and retraction of the tendon fibers. Accurate description of these tears is important for surgical planning. The report should accurately describe the location and distance of the tear from the distal calcaneal insertion best evaluated on the sagittal plane. The level of proximal tendon retraction and the gap between the torn tendon edges should be measured. The status of the torn tendon stump should be evaluated describing whether there is fraying and thickening. One should also evaluate the status of the plantaris tendon. Muscle atrophy in subacute to chronic cases can be evident which usually starts in the soleus muscle, and hence a large field of view on the sagittal sequences is often required.

Tendinosis and peritendinitis are usually treated conservatively with rest and NSAIDs. In cases of complete Achilles tendon tears, this usually requires surgical repair.

Supplementary Images

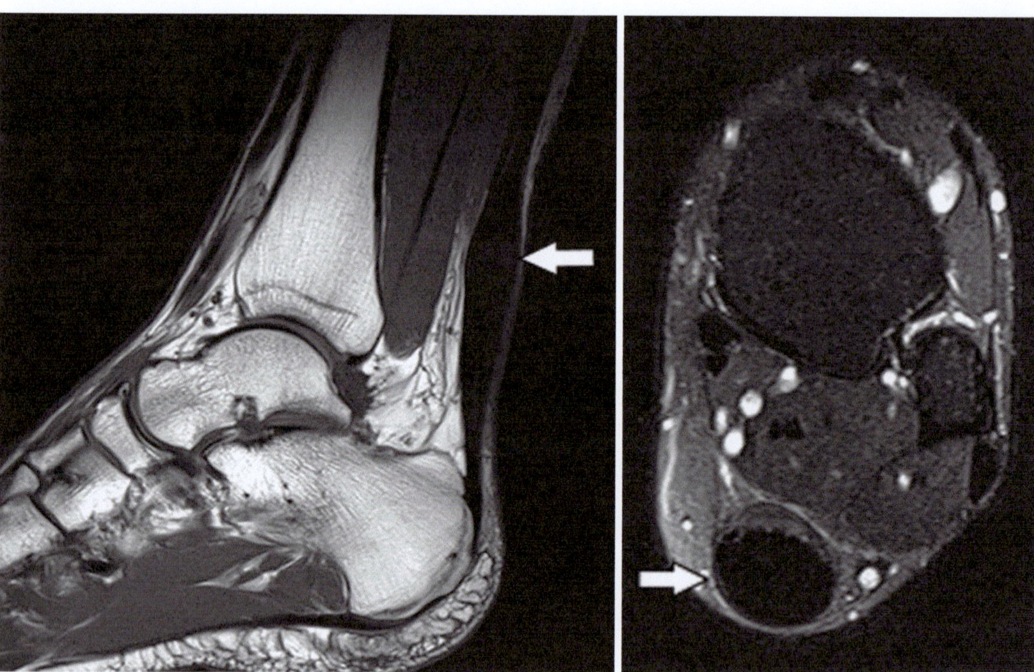

There is fusiform thickening (arrows) of the Achilles tendon at its watershed zone about 4–6 cm from its calcaneal insertion compatible with mid-substance tendinosis. There is no focal tendon tear

Report checklist

1. What is the degree of Achilles tendinosis (mild, moderate, severe)?
2. Where is the abnormality located along the Achilles tendon (at the calcaneal insertion or tendon mid-substance)?
3. Is there a focal tendon tear? Is it partial-thickness or complete?
4. If there is a full-thickness tear, what is the distance of the tear from the calcaneal insertion? What is distance of the tendon gap between the torn ends?
5. How is the plantaris tendon? Do you see it attached along the medial calcaneus?

Suggested Reading

Haims AH, Schweitzer ME, Patel RS, et al. MR imaging of the Achilles tendon: overlap of findings in symptomatic and asymptomatic individuals. Skeletal Radiol. 2000;29:640–5.

Schweitzer ME, Karasick D. MR imaging of disorders of the Achilles tendon. AJR Am J Roentgenol. 2000;175:613–25.

Case 6.8

Indication A 54-year-old female with pes planus deformity and chronic medial ankle pain. MRI performed to evaluate the posterior tibial tendon.

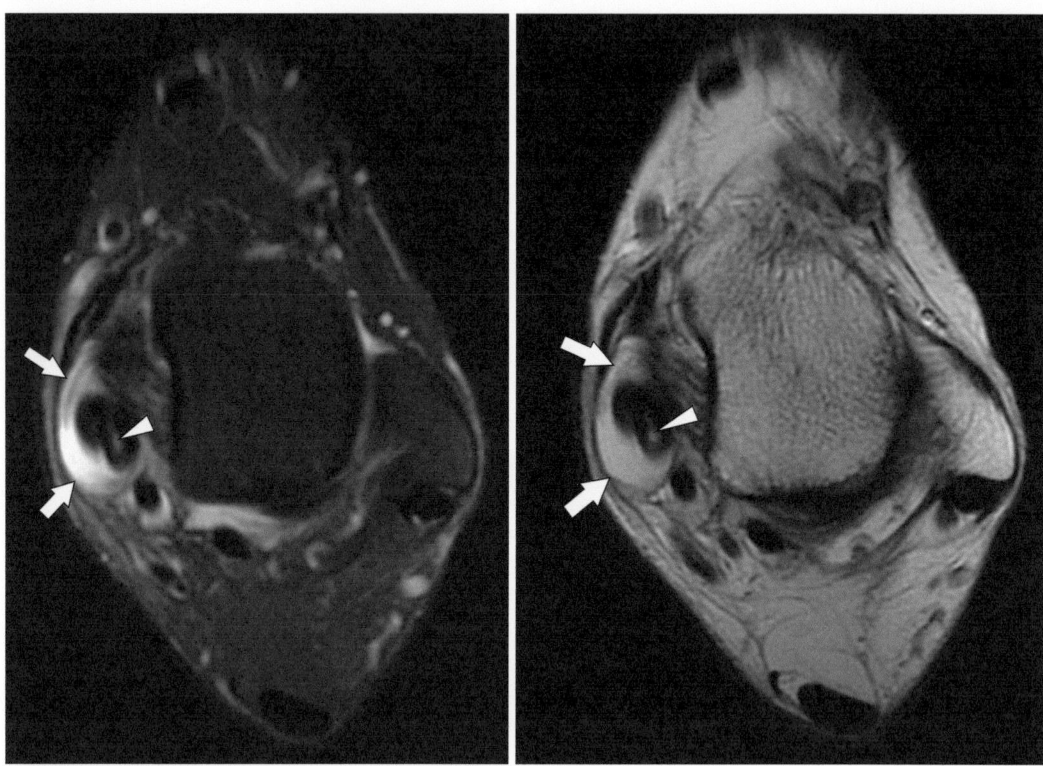

Axial T2 fat saturated

Axial PD

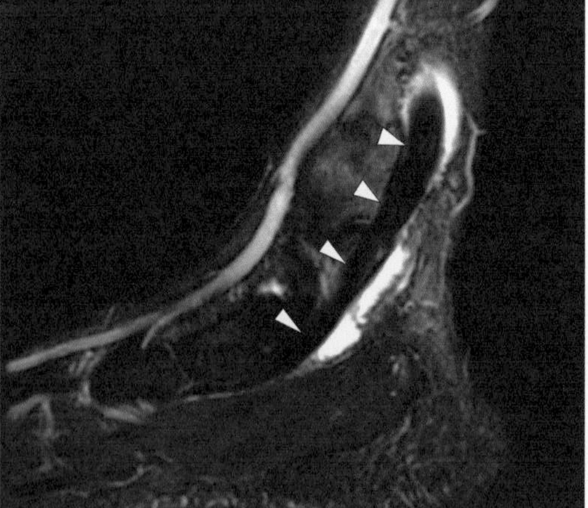

Sagittal STIR

Findings

There is severe tenosynovitis of the posterior tibialis tendon with a large amount of fluid in the tendon sheath (arrows). The PTT is markedly thickened, and there is intermediate signal in the substance of the tendon consistent with a longitudinal split tear (arrowheads) extending over a distance of 3 cm from the level of the medial malleolus to the tendon insertion on the navicular. There is also mild tenosynovitis of the flexor digitorum tendon. The spring ligament is intact (not shown). The sinus tarsi contains normal fatty signal.

Impression/Recommendation

Longitudinal split tear of the tibialis posterior tendon and severe tenosynovitis.

Discussion: Posterior Tibial Tendon Dysfunction

The posterior tibial tendon (PTT) is the primary inverter of the foot and also maintains the longitudinal arch of the foot. Failure of the PTT is referred to clinically as PTT dysfunction, which ranges from tendinosis to complete rupture resulting in progressive flatfoot deformity. PTT injury is the most common cause of acquired adult flatfoot deformity. The PTT may be injured due to several reasons; chronic degeneration is the most common etiology; other causes include acute trauma, systemic disorders like rheumatoid arthritis, seronegative spondyloarthropathies, and chronic steroid use. It is seen more commonly in women and often presents in the sixth decade. Patients usually complain of medial ankle pain and flattening of the medial arch.

The PTT originates from the tibialis posterior muscle and courses posterior to the medial malleolus which then inserts onto the medial aspect of the navicular with smaller tendon slips inserting onto the cuneiforms and the bases of the 2nd–4th metatarsals. The PTT is the largest and most medial of the three flexor tendons, with an oval shape and twice the diameter of the adjacent flexor digitorum longus (FDL) tendon. There is a zone of hypovascularity beginning at approximately the level of the medial malleolus and extending distal to it. This portion of the tendon is at increased risk for ruptures.

On MRI, the normal PTT should have uniform low signal intensity on all pulse sequences. A trace amount of fluid in the tendon sheath can be a normal finding if the fluid is less than 2 mm in thickness and does not surround more than 50% of the circumference of the tendon sheath on axial images. Tenosynovitis is present when the fluid in the tendon sheath is circumferential about the tendon or is thicker than 2 mm in thickness. Tendinosis is seen as abnormal intrinsic signal within the tendon.

Tears of the PTT have been classified into three types based on MRI findings. Type 1 tears are seen as thickening of the tendon (greater than twice the size of the FDL tendon) with increased intrasubstance signal and are referred to as hypertrophic tendinosis. Partial-thickness interstitial longitudinal tears are often seen. Type 2 tears have an attenuated tendon that is smaller than the adjacent FDL tendon and is referred to as atrophic tendinosis. Type 3 tear is a complete rupture, seen on MRI as disruption of the tendon with a fluid-filled gap and retraction of the torn tendon ends.

With chronic rupture of the PTT and failure of the medial longitudinal arch of the foot, there is increased force transmitted on other static stabilizers of the arch such as the spring ligament, deltoid ligament complex, and the sinus tarsi. The spring ligament (also known as the plantar calcaneonavicular ligament) is a ligamentous structure that originates from the undersurface of the sustentaculum tali and inserts on the inferior surface of the navicular bone. With depression of the longitudinal arch, increased force on the spring ligament usually leads to tearing of this ligament *(see supplementary images)*. Other MRI findings seen in acquired flatfoot deformity include hindfoot valgus, uncovering of the medial talar head, calcaneofibular abutment, and pes planus deformity.

Conservative treatment of PTT dysfunction involves support of the medial longitudinal arch with orthoses, physical therapy, and analgesics. However, if conservative measures fail, surgery may be required, which may involve osseous stabilization or primary repair of the PTT.

Supplementary Images

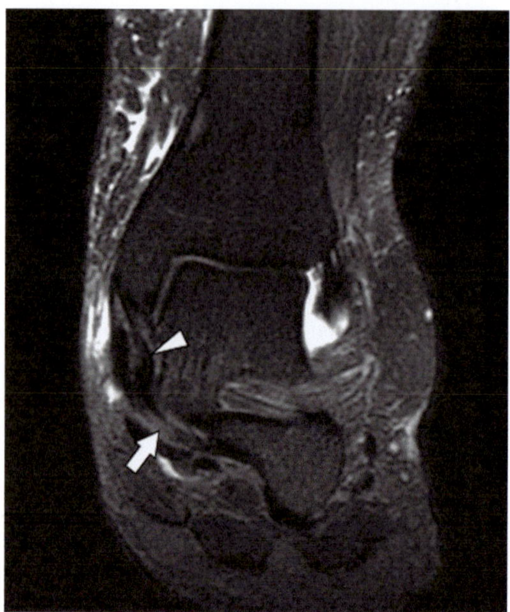

Coronal T2 fat saturated

There is high signal intensity and attenuation of the spring ligament (arrow) suggesting a partial tear. There is also thickening and intermediate signal in the tibiospring ligament (arrowhead), a component of the deltoid ligament complex

Report checklist

1. Is there tendinosis of the PTT?
2. Is there a longitudinal split tear or complete tear of the PTT?
3. Where is the location of the tear? What is the craniocaudal length of the tear?
4. Is there an associated tenosynovitis?
5. How are the remainder flexor tendons?
6. How are the spring ligament, deltoid ligament complex, and the sinus tarsi? Is there pes planus on standing radiographs (if present)?

Suggested Reading

Arnoldner MA, Gruber M, Syré S, et al. Imaging of posterior tibial tendon dysfunction--Comparison of high-resolution ultrasound and 3T MRI. Eur J Radiol. 2015;84:1777–81.

Lin YC, Kwon JY, Ghorbanhoseini M, Wu JS. The hindfoot arch: what role does the imager play? Radiol Clin North Am. 2016;54:951–68.

Case 6.9

Indication A 48-year-old female with chronic lateral ankle pain and tenderness over the peroneal tendons. Evaluate for injury to the peroneal tendons.

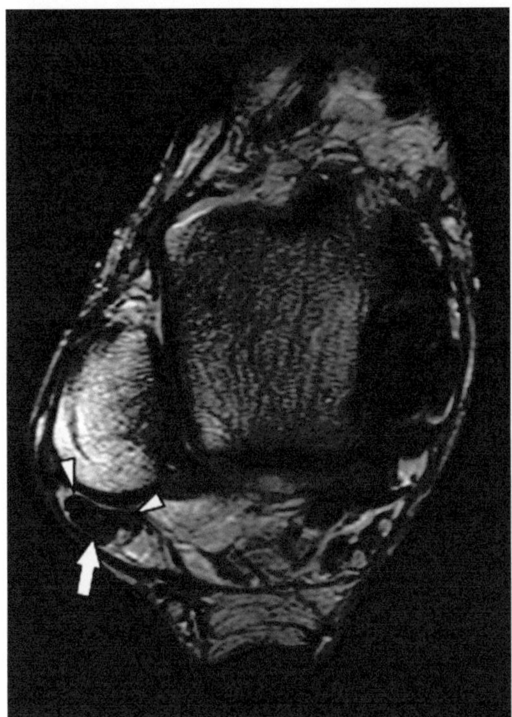

Axial PD

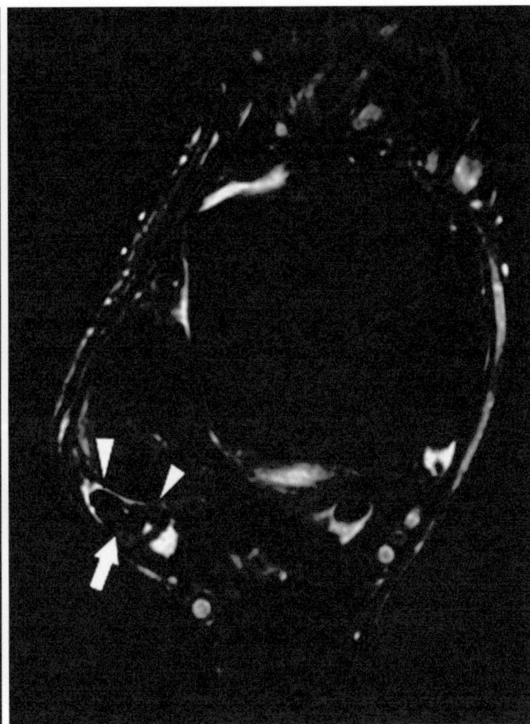

Axial T2 fat saturated

Findings

There is thinning and flattening of the peroneus brevis tendon at the level of the retromalleolar groove with a longitudinal split tear into two tendon slips (arrowheads) extending over a distance of approximately 3 cm (not shown). The peroneus brevis tendon at its attachment on the 5th metatarsal base is intact (not shown). There is a small amount of fluid in the common peroneal sheath. The superior peroneal retinaculum is intact. The peroneus longus tendon (arrow) is normal.

Impression/Recommendation

Longitudinal split tear of the peroneus brevis tendon over a 3 cm distance at the level of the retromalleolar groove.

Discussion: Peroneus Brevis Tendon Tear

The peroneal tendons are located in the lateral ankle and composed of the peroneus brevis (PB) and peroneus longus (PL) tendons. They act as plantar flexors and evertors of the foot and ankle. At the level of the ankle, the tendons run in a shallow fibro-osseous groove posterior to the distal fibula called the retromalleolar groove, with the PL tendon located posterolateral to the PB tendon. The PB inserts onto the lateral aspect of the 5th metatarsal base while the PL turns medially at the plantar aspect of the cuboid inserting on the plantar aspect of the medial cuneiform and base of the 1st metatarsal. They share a common peroneal sheath beginning above the lateral malleolus and extend to the level of the calcaneocuboid joint. The tendons are stabilized in the groove by the superior peroneal retinaculum, which is a thin band originating from the posterior ridge of the distal fibula and inserting on the lateral aspect of the calcaneus.

Injuries to the PB tendon can occur from an acute ankle sprain or more commonly due to overuse injuries. The PB tendon is located between the fibula and the PL tendon where it can become trapped and undergo degenerative tearing with chronic overuse. The most common type of PB tear is a longitudinal interstitial split tear, which usually begins at the level of the groove but can extend over long distances. This is evident on MRI as high signal intensity within the tendon on the fluid-sensitive sequences splitting the PB into two tendon slips with the PL insinuating between them.

Injuries to the peroneal tendons are usually associated with tenosynovitis *(see supplementary images),* which is diagnosed when there is circumferential fluid signal intensity surrounding the tendon or when the fluid diameter is greater than 2 mm. In patients with an acute injury, special attention should be made to the superior peroneal retinaculum (SPR) as concomitant injuries are common. This is evident by thickening of the retinaculum *(see supplementary image)* and surrounding edema as well as periosteal stripping of the SPR from its attachment on the lateral fibula or distal fibular avulsion fracture. It is important to differentiate a split PB tendon from an accessory peroneus quartus *(see supplementary images)* which is seen in 12–22% of people. In a split tear, the two hemitendons will reconstitute both distally and proximally into one tendon; however, an accessory peroneus quartus can be traced proximally to its myotendinous junction and distally to its attachment on the lateral calcaneus.

Treatment options include immobilization, NSAIDs, and physical therapy or surgical repair of the torn tendon.

Supplementary Images

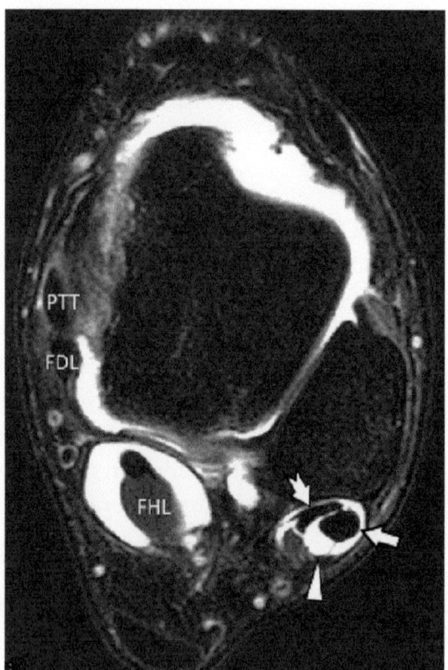

Axial T2 fat saturated

There is tenosynovitis of the common tendon sheath of the peroneus longus (arrow) and peroneus brevis (notched arrow). There is circumferential fluid (arrowhead) around the peroneal tendon sheath. There is also tenosynovitis of the flexor hallucis longus (FHL) and flexor digitorum longus tendons (FDL). The posterior tibialis tendon (PTT) is normal

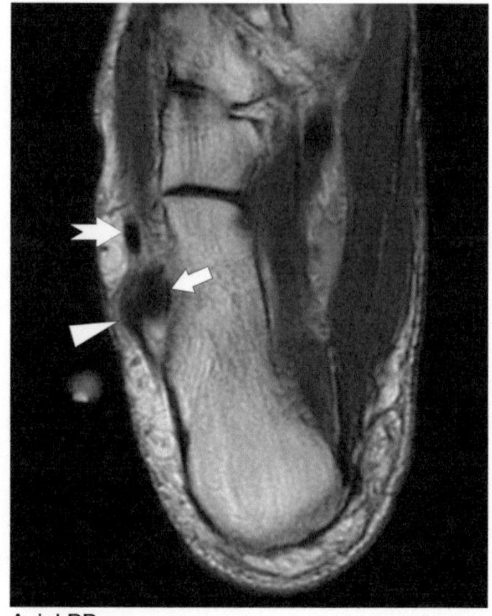

Axial PD

There is thickening of the distal portion of the peroneal retinaculum (arrowhead) adjacent to the peroneus longus tendon (arrow). The peroneus brevis tendon (notched arrow) is no longer bounded by the retinaculum distally (normal finding at this level)

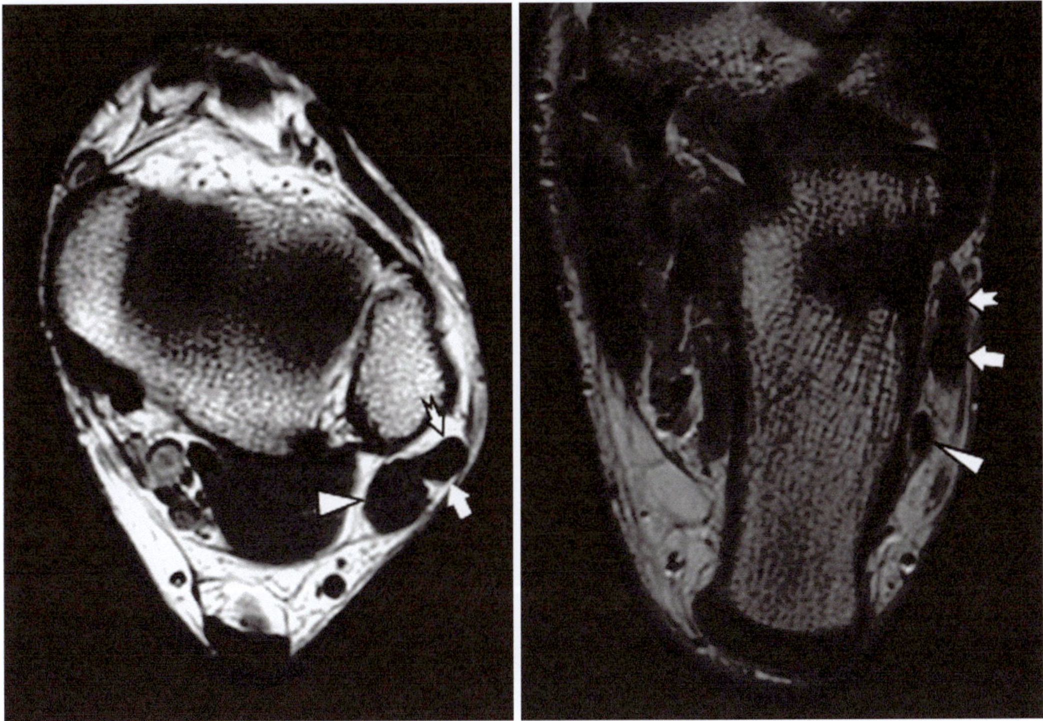

Axial PD   Axial PD

There is an accessory quartus muscle/tendon (arrowheads) next to the peroneus longus (arrows) and peroneus brevis (notched arrows) tendons. This should not be confused with a tear of either of the peroneal tendons

Report checklist

1. Is there a partial, complete, or split tear of the peroneus brevis tendon?
2. Where is the location of the tear? What is the craniocaudal length of the tear?
3. Is there an associated tenosynovitis?
4. Is there a tear of the superior peroneal retinaculum?
5. How is the peroneus longus tendon?
6. Could this be an accessory peroneus quartus tendon instead of a tear?

Suggested Reading

Lee SJ, Jacobson JA, Kim SM, et al. Ultrasound and MRI of the peroneal tendons and associated pathology. Skeletal Radiol. 2013;42(9): 1191–200.

Taljanovic MS, Alcala JN, Gimber LH, Rieke JD, Chilvers MM, Latt LD. High-resolution US and MR imaging of peroneal tendon injuries. Radiographics. 2015;35:179–99.

Wang XT, Rosenberg ZS, Mechlin MB, Schweitzer ME. Normal variants and diseases of the peroneal tendons and superior peroneal retinaculum: MR imaging features. RadioGraphics. 2005;25(3):587–602.

Case 6.10

Indication A 37-year-old woman with posterior heel pain for 3 months. Worse in the morning.

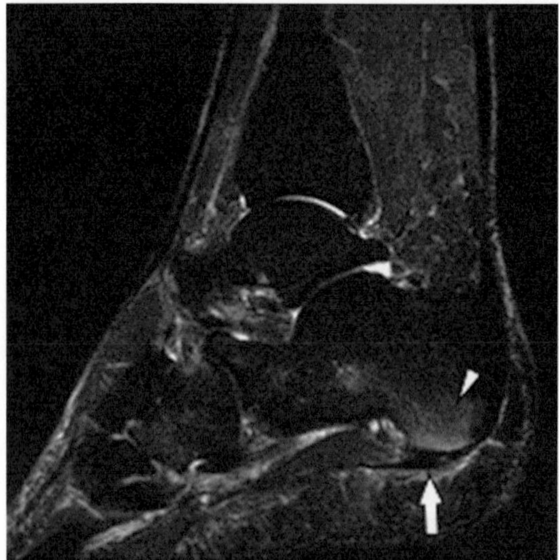

Sagittal STIR

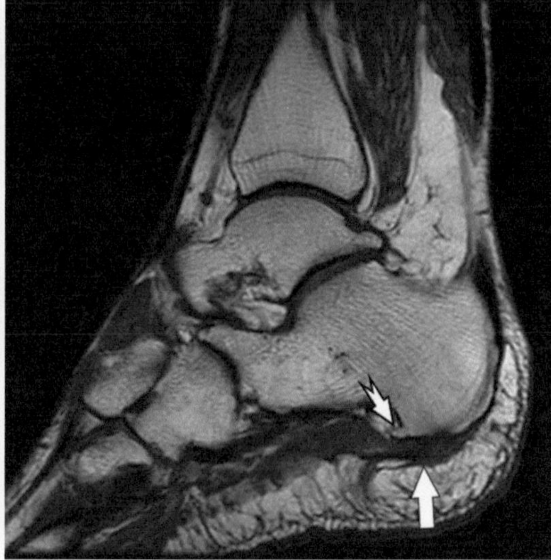

Sagittal T1

Findings

There is moderate fusiform thickening at the origin of the plantar fascia (arrows) with intrinsic high signal intensity as well as mild surrounding soft tissue edema both superficial and deep to the plantar fascia. The fascia measures 10 mm at its maximal thickness (normal is ≤4 mm). There is also reactive bone marrow edema at the plantar aspect of the calcaneus (arrowhead). There is no plantar fascia tear identified. A small plantar enthesophyte is noted (notched arrow).

Impression/Recommendation

Moderate acute on chronic plantar fasciitis.

Discussion: Plantar Fasciitis

The plantar fascia is a fibrous aponeurosis originating from the plantar calcaneal tuberosity coursing anteriorly along the plantar aspect of the foot and is composed of lateral, central, and medial bundles. At the level of the metatarsophalangeal joints, it fans out into five fascicles, one to each toe. The plantar fascia provides support to the longitudinal arch of the foot.

Plantar fasciitis is one of the most frequent causes of heel pain, which occurs due to a local inflammatory process often caused by chronic overuse. It usually involves the medial bundle at its origin from the calcaneus and is commonly seen in athletes, obese patients, and in patients with foot deformities. The mechanism of injury in these cases is repetitive microtrauma resulting in microtears adjacent to its attachment. On the other hand, plantar fasciitis can also be secondary to seronegative spondyloarthropathies such as reactive arthritis and ankylosing spondylitis. Patients with plantar fasciitis usually present with pain and tenderness at the medial tuberosity of the calcaneus. The pain is gradual in onset and is worse in the morning.

On MRI, the plantar fascia is best evaluated on the sagittal and coronal planes. The normal central and medial bundles are generally thicker than the lateral bundle. Any abnormalities seen on sagittal images are then confirmed in the coronal plane. In acute plantar fasciitis, there is usually abnormal fusiform thickening (>4 mm) at its origin with increased signal within the substance of the plantar fascia. This is usually associated with soft tissue edema both superficial and deep to the plantar aponeurosis. There may also be bone marrow edema at the plantar aspect of the calcaneus, which is reactive to the surrounding inflammatory changes. In more advanced cases, this may extend to cause either a partial or complete tear of the plantar fascia.

Chronic plantar fasciitis is usually seen as diffuse thickening of the plantar fascia origin but is dark on all pulse sequences with lack of surrounding soft tissue or bone marrow edema. In about 50% of cases, a plantar calcaneal enthesophyte (plantar spur) is present.

In approximately 90% of plantar fasciitis cases, the pain resolves with conservative therapy including nonsteroidal anti-inflammatory medications, pain injections, orthotics, physiotherapy, and immobilization with a cast. Surgical release of the medial attachment and spur resection may be required in cases that have failed conservative management.

Report checklist
1. What is the degree of plantar fascia thickening (mild, moderate, or severe)?
2. Where is the abnormal thickening (origin or distal)?
3. Is there surrounding soft tissue edema or reactive bone marrow edema at the calcaneus?
4. Is there an associated plantar fascia tear?
5. Is there a plantar enthesophyte/spur?

Suggested Reading

Chang CD, Wu JS. MR imaging findings in heel pain. Magn Reson Imaging Clin N Am. 2017;25:79–93.

Draghi F, Gitto S, Bortolotto C, et al. Imaging of plantar fascia disorders: findings on plain radiography, ultrasound and magnetic resonance imaging. Insights Imaging. 2017;8(1):69–78.

Theodorou DJ, Theodorou SJ, Farooki S, Kakitsubata Y, Resnick D. Disorders of the plantar aponeurosis: a spectrum of MR imaging findings. AJR Am J Roentgenol. 2001;176(1):97–104.

Case 6.11

Indication A 28-year-old male with lateral ankle pain and swelling after a twisting injury. MRI to rule out ligament injury.

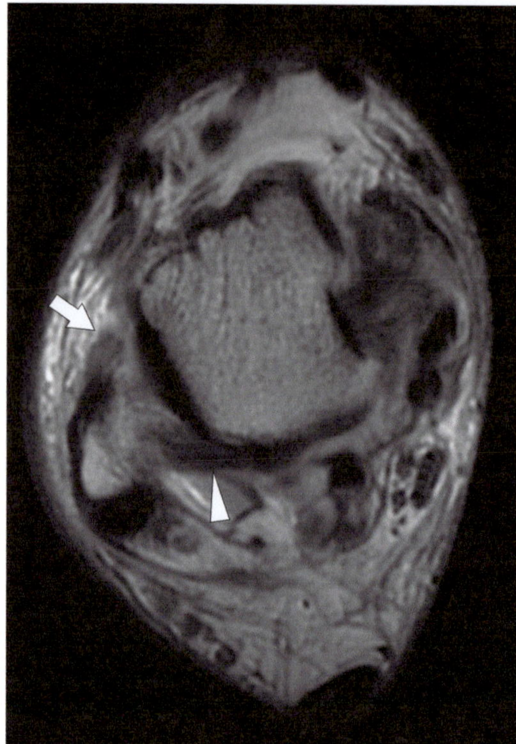

Axial PD

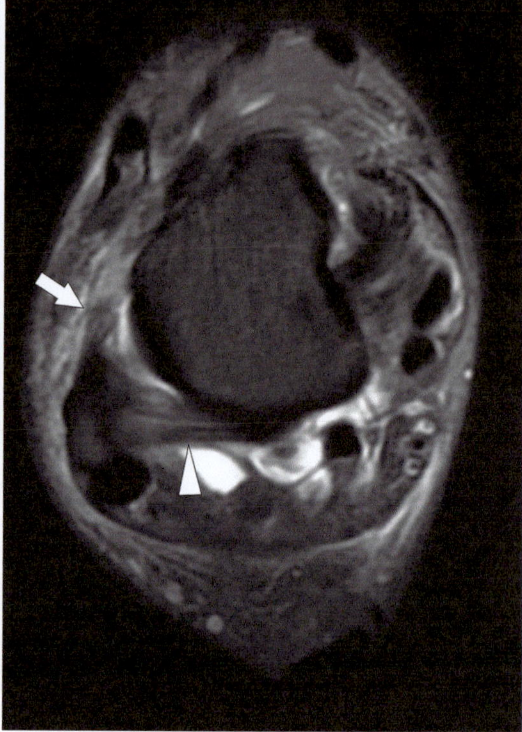

Axial T2 fat saturated

Findings

There is complete disruption of the anterior talofibular ligament (arrow) from its talar attachment. The ligament is thickened and with intermediate signal. There is adjacent soft tissue edema. The posterior talofibular (arrowhead) and calcaneofibular ligaments are intact. The syndesmotic ligaments are intact. The deltoid ligament complex is also intact.

Impression/Recommendation

Complete tear of the anterior talofibular ligament (ATFL).

Discussion: Lateral Collateral Ligament Complex Injury

Inversion injuries at the ankle are the most common type of mechanism of injury, and around 85% of ankle sprains involve the lateral liga-

ments. Most patients improve with conservative management and can return to their normal activities. MRI is usually reserved for patients who have persistent ankle pain or instability after an ankle injury. The lateral collateral ligament complex of the ankle consists of three individual ligaments: the anterior talofibular ligament (ATFL), the calcaneofibular ligament (CFL), and the posterior talofibular ligament (PTFL). The ATFL is the weakest of the lateral ligaments and is the most commonly injured ligament at the ankle. It appears as a thin hypointense band, best seen on the axial images, originating from the anterior margin of the lateral malleolus and runs anteromedially to insert onto the lateral talar process *(see supplementary images)*.

The CFL originates just below the ATFL from the tip of the fibula. From here, it runs obliquely downward deep to the peroneal tendons and attaches onto the lateral calcaneal surface. It is usually best seen on both axial and coronal images as a thin hypointense band deep to the peroneal tendons. It is common to not visualize the entire course of the CFL on the axial images due to its oblique orientation, and hence correlation with the coronal images is important to assess the entire ligament.

The PTFL has a broad fan-shaped origin from the concave surface of the lateral malleolus and extends horizontally to its insertion on the posterolateral talus. This ligament is the strongest of the lateral ligaments and is rarely injured. It is also best seen on axial and coronal images and has a normal striated appearance due to the presence of interspersed fat.

Injuries to the lateral collateral ligaments follow a predictable pattern. The ATFL ligament is the weakest and is usually the first to be injured, followed by injury to the CFL and finally, although very rare, the PTFL may be torn in very severe injuries. More commonly, the force is directed more superiorly with injury to the syndesmotic ligaments. On MRI, grade 1 sprain is seen as periligamentous edema surrounding the ligaments, otherwise is still intact. Grade 2 sprain is a partial-thickness tear and is recognized as thickening and irregularity with increased signal intensity within the ligament. Grade 3 sprain is a complete tear which is seen as complete disruption of the ligament and extravasation of joint fluid into the adjacent soft tissues. This may sometimes be accompanied by a distal fibular avulsion fracture which is best seen on a sagittal T1-weighted sequence. In chronic tears, the ligament may have different appearances and could either appear thickened due to scarring, thinned, or absent *(see supplementary images)*.

If injury extends to involve the syndesmotic ligaments, then this is considered a high ankle sprain. The syndesmosis consists of the anterior and posterior tibiofibular ligaments and the interosseous ligament which can be seen on axial and coronal planes as thin hypointense structures at the level of the tibial plafond. The anterior tibiofibular ligament has an oblique course from the anterior surface of the fibula extending superiorly and medially to the anterolateral tubercle of the tibia. Due to its oblique direction, the ligament needs to be followed on contiguous axial slices to appropriately assess the entire ligament. The posterior tibiofibular ligament arises from the posterior aspect of the distal fibula and extends horizontally to attach on the posterior aspect of the tibia. The anterior tibiofibular ligament is more important functionally and is also the most frequently injured ligament at the syndesmosis *(see supplementary images)*. Injury to the syndesmotic ligaments may also occur in isolation without the involvement of the ATFL and CFL and is considered a more severe type of ankle sprain and if managed inappropriately may result in chronic pain and ankle joint instability. In chronic injuries, there may be ossification at the syndesmotic interval, and this should not be mistaken for a neoplastic process.

Lateral collateral ligament injuries often lead to ankle joint instability. Adequate and timely treatment is important to avoid scarring and persistent laxity. Conservative treatment is employed for most cases and involves rest, ice, compression and elevation, and casting for immobilization.

Supplementary Images

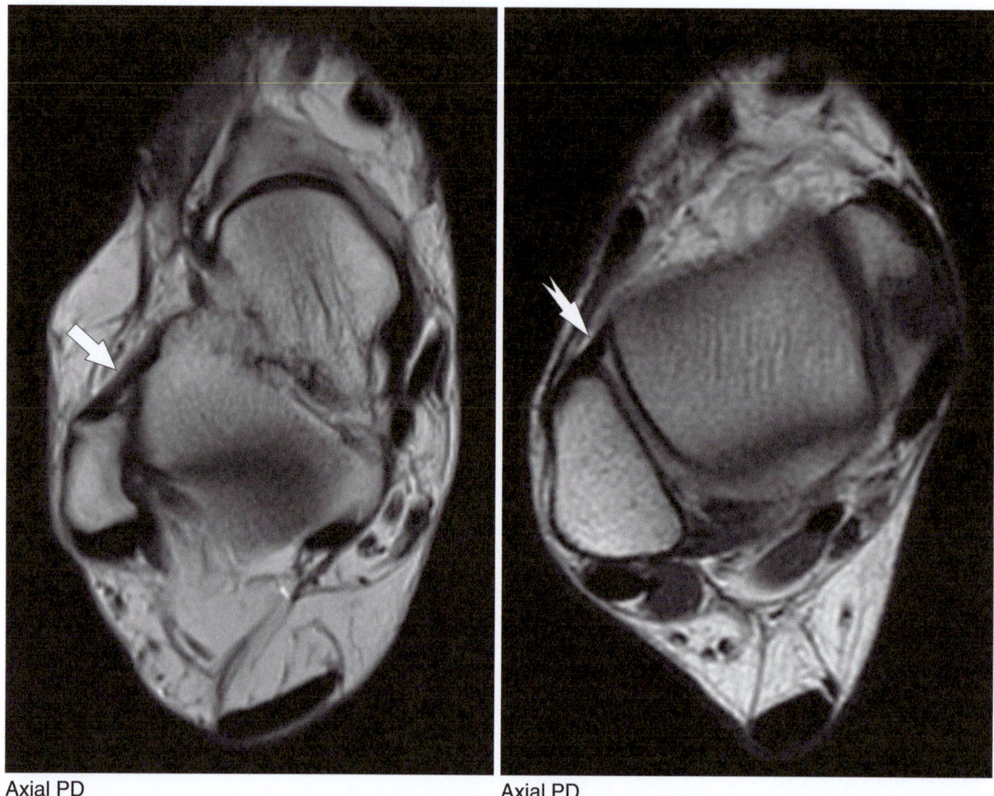

Axial PD

Axial PD

Normal appearance anterior talofibular (arrow) and anterior tibiofibular (notched arrow) ligaments

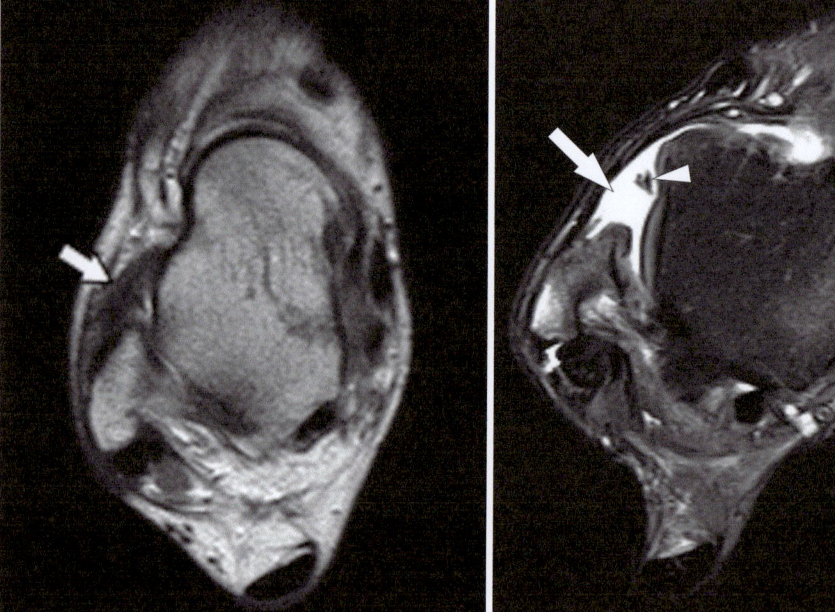

Axial PD

Axial T2 fat saturated

Chronic injury appearances of the ATFL. On the PD image, there is marked thickening of the ATFL (arrow). On the T2 fat saturated image in a different patient, there is absence of the ATFL, and fluid is seen in its expected location (arrow). There is a small loose body in the anterior aspect of the anterolateral gutter (arrowhead)

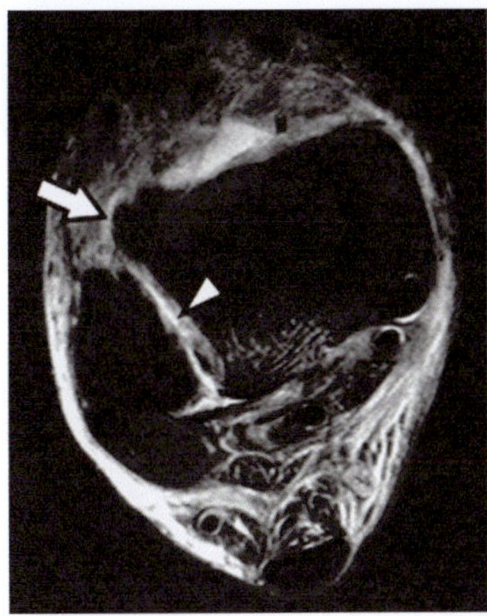
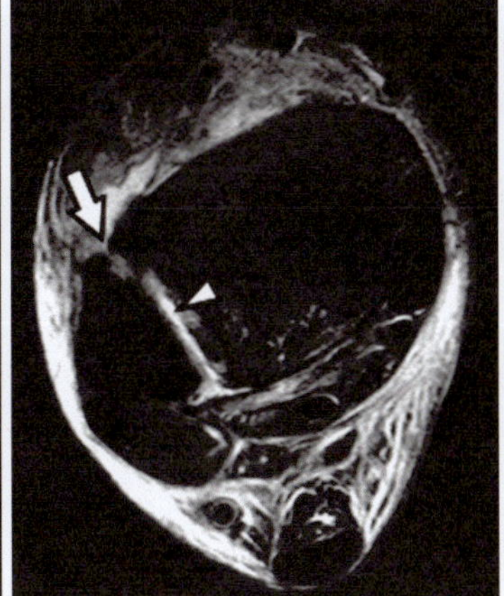
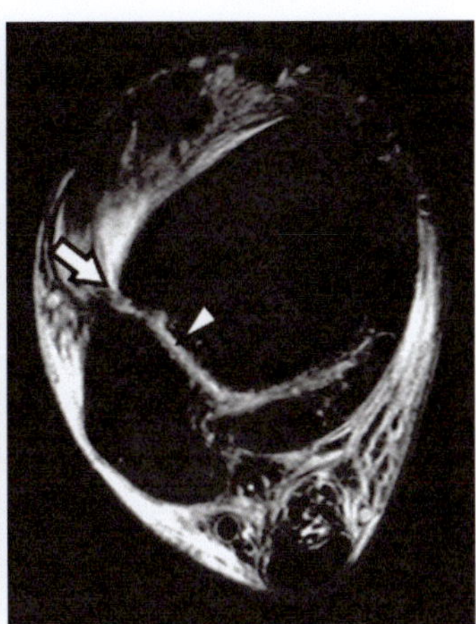

Axial T2 fat saturated

Axial T2 fat saturated

Axial T2 fat saturated

There is thickening and irregularity of the anterior tibiofibular ligament (arrows) with increased signal in the ligament as well as periligamentous soft tissue edema compatible with an acute grade 2 sprain. There is also fluid within the syndesmosis (arrowheads) which suggests tearing of the interosseous ligament. The posterior tibiofibular ligament is intact

Report checklist

1. Which ligaments are involved (ATFL, CFL, PTFL)?
2. What is the degree of injury (grade 1–3 sprain)?
3. Is there an associated avulsion fracture?
4. How are the syndesmotic ligaments?
5. Is there an associated injury of the medial deltoid ligament? An osteochondral lesion at the talar dome? Bone contusions or fractures?

Suggested Reading

Golanó P, Vega J, de Leeuw PA, Malagelada F, Manzanares MC, Götzens V, van Dijk CN. Anatomy of the ankle ligaments: a pictorial essay. Knee Surg Sports Traumatol Arthrosc. 2010;18:557–69.

Kreitner KF, Ferber A, Grebe P, et al. Injuries of the lateral collateral ligaments of the ankle: assessment with MR imaging. Eur Radiol. 1999;9:519–24.

Perrich KD, Goodwin DW, Hecht PJ, Cheung Y. Ankle ligaments on MRI: appearance of normal and injured ligaments. AJR Am J Roentgenol. 2009;193(3):687–95.

Case 6.12

Indication A 24-year-old male with recent fall. Complaining of medial ankle pain.

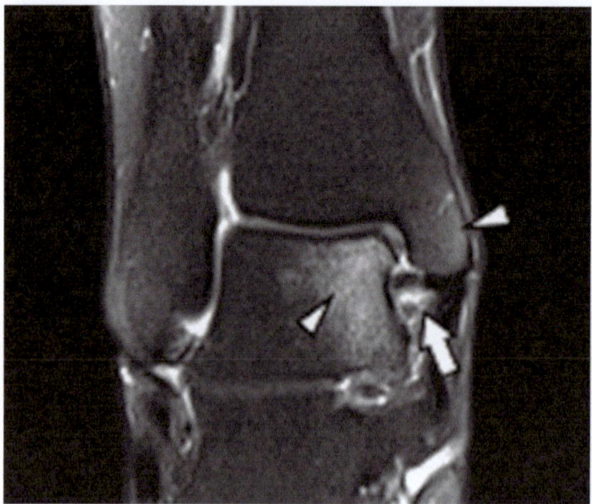

Coronal T2 fat saturated

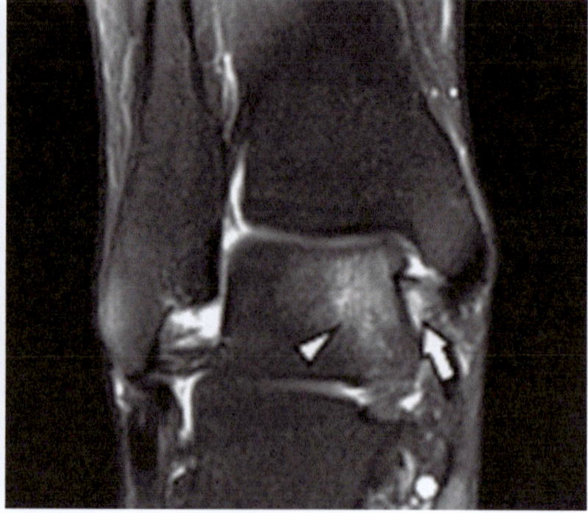

Coronal T2 fat saturated

Findings

There is increased signal intensity with loss of normal striations of the deep posterior tibiotalar ligament and small fluid-filled gaps (arrow) compatible with an acute grade 2 sprain. There is subchondral bone marrow edema within the medial malleolus and medial aspect of the talus compatible with bony contusions (arrowheads). No low signal fracture lines are seen. The superficial deltoid ligaments are intact. There are no osteochondral lesions at the talar dome. The spring ligament is normal.

Impression/Recommendation

Acute grade 2 sprain of the posterior tibiotalar (deep deltoid) ligament.

Discussion: Medial Ligament Complex Injury

The medial collateral ligament (deltoid ligament) is made up of five components classified into superficial and deep ligaments. The stronger deep ligaments consist of the smaller anterior component (anterior tibiotalar ligament) and a larger and stronger component (posterior tibiotalar ligament). These arise from the inner aspect of the medial malleolus and attach at the medial aspect of the talus. These ligaments are intra-articular, and of note, the posterior tibiotalar ligament is considered the most substantial component of the entire deltoid ligament complex. The superficial ligaments arise from the medial malleolus and consist of the tibiocalcaneal ligament that attaches on the sustentaculum tali, the tibionavicular ligament attaching to the medial navicular tuberosity, and the tibiospring ligament that attaches on the spring ligament.

The two ligaments of the deltoid complex seen on almost every MRI are the posterior tibiotalar ligament and tibiospring ligament, while the other three components can be variable in size or not visualized at all. The normal posterior tibiotalar ligament demonstrates striated fibers due to the interposition of fatty tissues and should not be mistaken for pathology. The tibiospring ligament is seen as a thin low signal intensity band running between the medial malleolus and the spring ligament. Therefore, one should look for these two ligaments on every MRI ankle exam (*see supplementary images*).

Injury to the deltoid ligament can be seen in patients with inversion injuries which are associated with lateral ligament injury and fibular fractures. The deep tibiotalar ligaments are most frequently injured in these types of injury due to crushing between the medial malleolus and medial aspect of the talus. Moreover, these are low-grade injuries and will appear as edematous changes and hemorrhage within the substance of the ligament evident as increased signal intensity with loss of normal striations (grade 1 sprain). High-grade injuries can either have partial (grade 2 sprain) or full-thickness tear (grade 3 sprain) demonstrated by fluid-filled gaps. The superficial ligaments are less commonly injured but when it does occur more frequently at the proximal attachment shown as thickening and ill definition of the ligament with surrounding soft tissue edema. Medial ligamentous injuries usually occur in conjunction with other injuries such as malleolar fractures and osteochondral injuries at the talar dome.

The majority of low-grade sprains of the deltoid ligament are treated conservatively with rest and cast. In high-grade injuries, surgical repair may be performed.

Supplementary Images

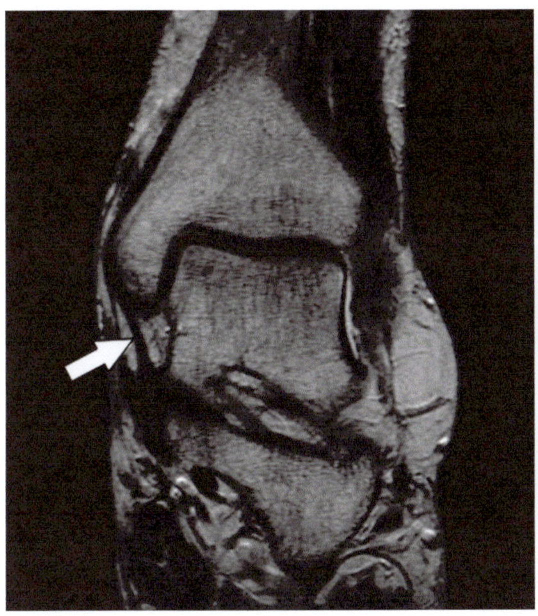

Coronal PD

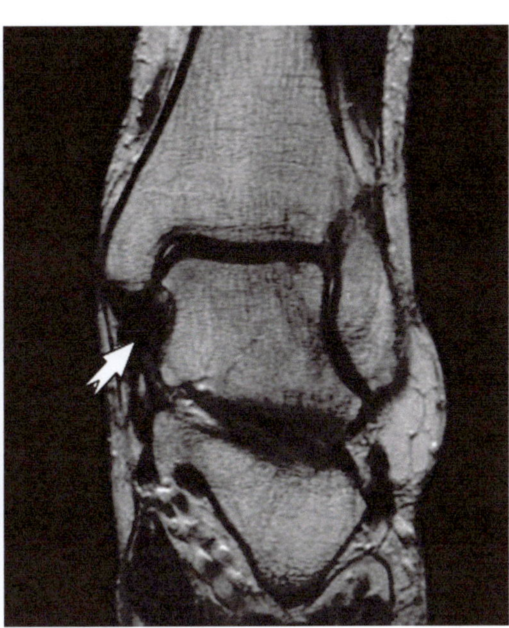

Coronal PD

Normal appearance of the tibiospring (arrow) and posterior tibiotalar (notched arrow) ligaments. These two ligaments of the deltoid complex should be visible on all MRI exams, whereas the other three components of the deltoid complex (anterior tibiotalar, tibiocalcaneal, and tibionavicular) are not always visualized on MRI, even in normal patients

Report checklist
1. Which ligaments are involved (deep or superficial components of the deltoid ligament)?
2. What is the degree of injury (grade 1–3 sprain)?
3. Are there bony contusions at the medial talus or medial malleolus?
4. Is there an associated injury of the lateral collateral ligaments? An osteochondral lesion at the talar dome?
5. Is there injury to the spring ligament?

Suggested Reading

Chhabra A, Subhawong TK, Carrino JA. MR imaging of deltoid ligament pathologic findings and associated impingement syndromes. Radiographics. 2010;30(3):751–61.

Mengiardi B, Pfirrmann CW, Vienne P, Hodler J, Zanetti M. Medial collateral ligament complex of the ankle: MR appearance in asymptomatic subjects. Radiology. 2007;242(3):817–24.

Mengiardi B, Pinto C, Zanetti M. Medial collateral ligament complex of the ankle: MR imaging anatomy and findings in medial instability. Semin Musculoskelet Radiol. 2016;20(1):91–103.

Perrich KD, Goodwin DW, Hecht PJ, Cheung Y. Ankle ligaments on MRI: appearance of normal and injured ligaments. AJR Am J Roentgenol. 2009;193(3):687–95.

Case 6.13

Indication A 28-year-old male with midfoot pain and swelling after a fall. Unable to weight bear. Suspect Lisfranc ligament injury.

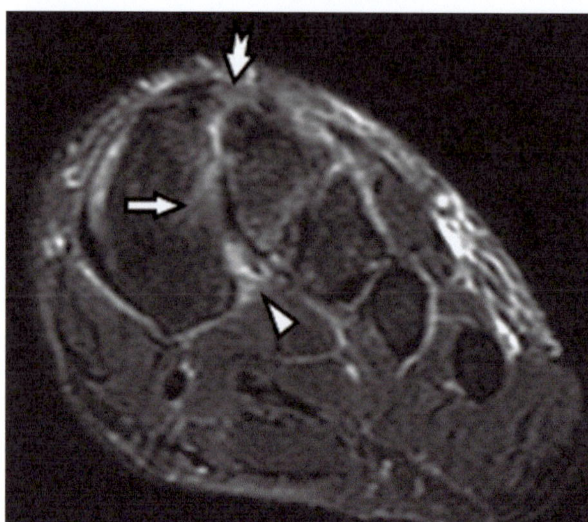

Coronal T2 fat saturated

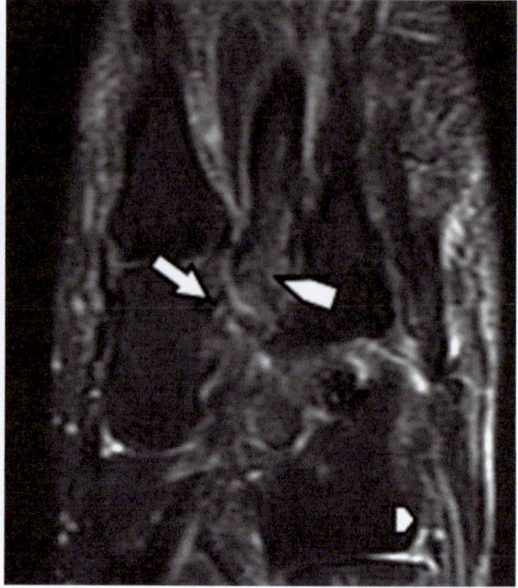

Axial T2 fat saturated

Findings

There is irregularity and periligamentous edema surrounding all three bundles of the Lisfranc ligament complex (dorsal, notched arrow; interosseous, arrow; plantar, arrowhead), best in the coronal plane. This is associated with bone marrow edema at the base of the 2nd metatarsal base representing bone contusions (block arrow). There is no fracture seen. Alignment at the base of the 2nd metatarsal and intermediate cuneiform remains preserved.

Impression/Recommendation

Sprain of the Lisfranc ligament complex.

Discussion: Lisfranc Ligament Injury

The Lisfranc (tarsometatarsal) joint is a complex osseous and ligamentous structure that provides midfoot stabilization. It is formed by the articulation of the base of the metatarsals with the tarsal bones. There are many ligaments at this joint, which includes the intercuneiform and intermetatarsal ligaments; however, the Lisfranc ligament complex (first interosseous ligament) is the strongest and thickest. It arises from the lateral aspect of the medial cuneiform and inserts on the medial aspect of the 2nd metatarsal base and is formed of

three obliquely oriented bundles (dorsal, interosseous, and plantar bundles). The dorsal ligament arises from the dorsum of the medial cuneiform and inserts at the dorsal aspect of the 2nd metatarsal base. The interosseous ligament is the most functionally important, connecting the medial cuneiform and 2nd metatarsal base. The plantar Lisfranc ligament originates from the plantar aspect of the medial cuneiform with separate attachments to the plantar surface of the 2nd and 3rd metatarsal bases *(see supplementary images).*

Injuries to the Lisfranc ligament are not uncommon and usually occur from high-velocity trauma like in a motor vehicle accident and can result in homolateral or divergent injuries. In a homolateral injury, the 1st–5th or 2nd–5th metatarsals are displaced laterally. In a divergent injury, the 1st metatarsal is dislocation medially, while the 2nd–5th metatarsals are displaced laterally. A lower velocity injury may result in a midfoot sprain, and patients usually present with pain and tenderness at the tarsometatarsal joints. These injuries can have a normal radiographic appearance, and the clinical diagnosis is often challenging. In these cases, MRI is helpful as it is more sensitive for evaluating bony contusions, soft tissue, and ligamentous injuries and should be performed once there is suspicion for an injury. MRI may demonstrate bone marrow edema at the base of the metatarsals and cuneiforms representing bony contusions with or without associated fractures. Injury to the Lisfranc ligament may show ligament elongation with periligamentous edema representing a mild sprain. It is important to note that the Lisfranc ligament may appear normal on MRI even in the presence of a significant injury, and hence any thickening, irregularity, or edema about the ligament should be considered suspicious for a significant injury. More severe injuries would demonstrate partial or complete discontinuity of the Lisfranc ligament. The three bundles of the Lisfranc ligament complex are injured in a predict-

able sequential manner from dorsal to plantar. Particular attention should be made to the interosseous component, as if this portion fails, then there can be loss of normal alignment between the medial cortex of the 2nd metatarsal and intermediate cuneiform. In addition, there can be superior elevation of the 2nd metatarsal base with the intermediate cuneiform. A missed diagnosis can have devastating consequences if left untreated. A midfoot sprain can lead to ligament rupture, rapid osteoarthritis, flattening of the longitudinal arch, foot deformity, and chronic pain.

Sprain can be treated conservatively with rest and immobilization. However, rupture of the interosseous ligament with malalignment is treated surgically.

Supplementary Images

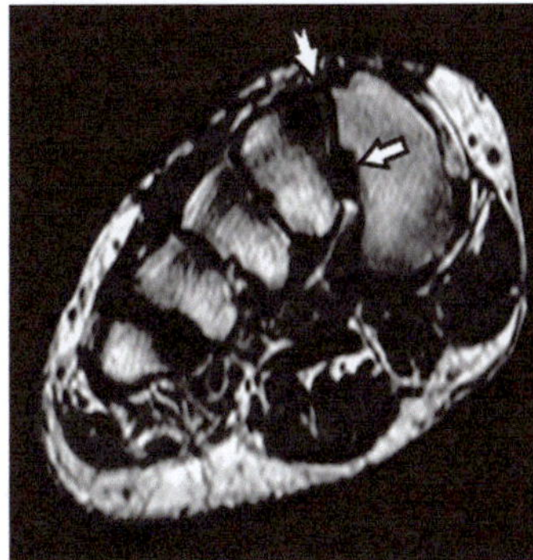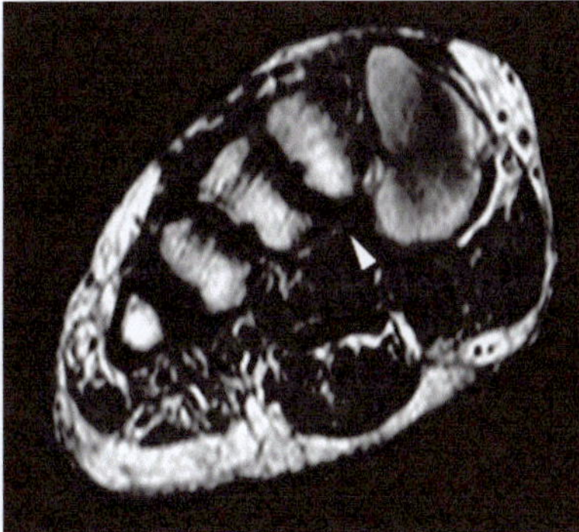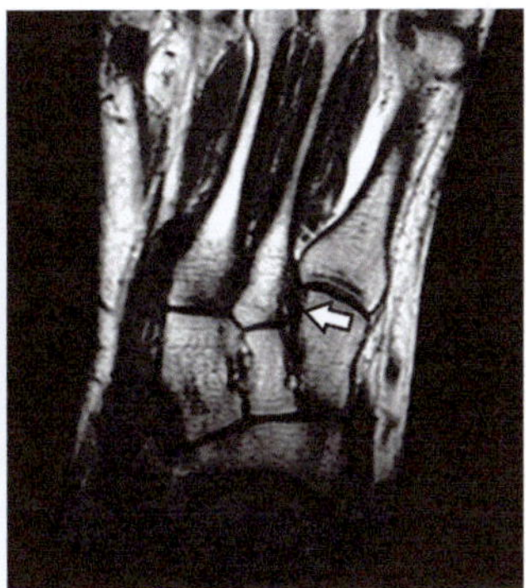

Coronal T1   Coronal T1   Axial T1

Normal MRI appearance of the Lisfranc ligament complex demonstrating the three bundles: dorsal (notched arrow), interosseous (arrow), and plantar (arrowhead)

Report checklist
1. What is the degree of injury (sprain, partial-thickness tear, or complete disruption)?
2. Location of the Lisfranc ligament injury (dorsal, interosseous, or plantar bundles)
3. Is there associated bone marrow contusions or fractures?
4. Is there loss of normal alignment between the 2nd metatarsal base and intermediate cuneiform?
5. How is the alignment of the other TMT joints? Is there a homolateral or divergent injury?
6. If this is a subacute or chronic injury, is there osteoarthritis and/or midfoot malalignment?

Suggested Reading

Castro M, Melão L, Canella C, et al. Lisfranc joint ligamentous complex: MRI with anatomic correlation in cadavers. AJR Am J Roentgenol. 2010;195(6):W447–55.

Macmahon PJ, Dheer S, Raikin SM, et al. MRI of injuries to the first interosseous cuneometatarsal (Lisfranc) ligament. Skeletal Radiol. 2009;38(3):255–60.

Raikin SM, Elias I, Dheer S, Besser MP, Morrison WB, Zoga AC. Prediction of midfoot instability in the subtle Lisfranc injury: comparison of magnetic resonance imaging with intraoperative findings. J Bone Joint Surg Am. 2009;91(4):892–9.

Case 6.14

Indication A 24-year-old football player with pain and tenderness at the 1st MTP joint.

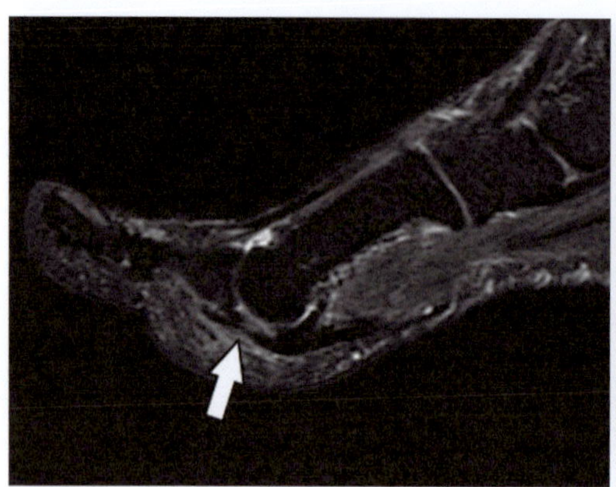

Sagittal STIR

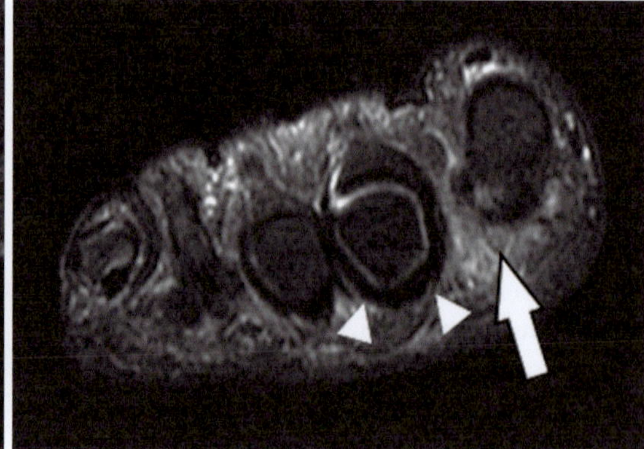

Coronal T2 fat saturated

Findings

There is increased signal intensity and attenuation at the distal insertion of the plantar plate of the 1st MTP joint (arrows) seen mainly on the lateral side with surrounding soft tissue edema compatible with a partial-thickness tear. The medial aspect of the plantar plate is intact. There is a small 1st MTP joint effusion. There is no bony contusion or focal chondral defect. [Note the normal U-shaped configuration of the plantar plate at the 2nd MTP joint (arrowheads)].

Impression/Recommendation

Partial-thickness tear of the plantar plate at the great toe "turf toe."

Discussion: Plantar Plate Injuries

The metatarsophalangeal (MTP) joints are stabilized by the plantar plate which is a fibrocartilaginous structure at the plantar aspect of the joint extending from the metatarsal head to the base of the proximal phalanx. On MRI, the normal plantar plate is seen as a hypointense structure that is best seen on the sagittal images as a linear hypointense structure while having a U-shaped biconcave appearance on the short axis (coronal) images. At the great toe, the anatomy is slightly more complex due to the presence of the sesamoids, where there is the attachment of the abductor and adductor hallucis muscles in addition to the presence of a plantar plate (also termed the sesamoid-phalangeal ligaments) as well as the intersesamoid ligament. The plantar plates blend with the collateral ligaments on either side of the joint. The collateral ligaments are seen as thin hypointense structures originating from the metatarsal head and attaching at the lateral aspect of the base of the proximal phalanges. The intersesamoid ligament is seen as a small dark ligament on the coronal images between the medial and lateral sesamoids. A common imaging pitfall is the presence of a small focal area of intermediate signal at the insertion of the plantar plate on the proximal phalanx. This is a normal finding representing the normal articular cartilage undermining the plantar plate and should not be mistaken for a tear. It usually measures about 2–3 mm; however, if this signal is greater, then the reader should begin questioning a plantar plate sprain or tear.

Injuries to the plantar plate can occur following an acute traumatic event related to a hyperextension injury at the MTP joints, most commonly involving the great toe in high-level athletes, and are commonly referred to as "turf toe." Alternatively, the plantar plates at the lesser MTP joints (2nd–5th) are usually injured from chronic repetitive trauma and abnormal weight-bearing stress, most frequently involving the 2nd MTP joint. Clinically, patients present with limited joint movement, pain, and swelling at the plantar aspect of the MTP joints. Injuries to the plantar plates could result in a low-grade sprain, partial-thickness tear, or a complete tear. The tears more commonly occur at the distal insertion of the plantar plate on the phalanx. Proximal tears at the metatarsal head are relatively uncommon.

On MRI, plantar plate injuries are seen as high signal intensity within the substance of the plantar plate as well as within the surrounding soft tissues. With higher-grade injuries, there is usually thinning and attenuation of the plantar plate suggesting partial-thickness tears or complete disruption of the ligament fibers with retraction proximally, which is best evaluated on the sagittal plane. Tears may involve the medial or lateral aspect of the plantar plate or alternatively extend through its whole thickness and extend into the collateral ligaments. This can be associated with bone marrow contusions at either the metatarsal head or base of the proximal phalanx, focal chondral defects, or joint effusion and synovitis. At the great toe, there may also be proximal retraction of the sesamoids in cases of complete disruption. With time, there is instability at the MTP joint, and there may be dorsal subluxation of the proximal phalanx *(see supplementary images)*.

Most plantar plate injuries are treated conservatively with immobilization or use of a walking boot. Surgery is usually reserved for patients with large complete tears or in cases of joint instability.

Report checklist

1. What is the degree of injury (sprain, partial-thickness tear, or complete disruption)?
2. Location of the plantar plate injury (distal attachment or proximal origin)
3. Does it involve the medial or lateral aspect of the plantar plate? Or does it extend along its whole thickness?
4. How are the collateral ligaments?
5. Is there proximal retraction of the plantar plate or the sesamoids?
6. Are there focal bony contusions? Joint effusion? Or chondral defects?
7. Is there MTP joint subluxation?

Suggested Reading

Crain JM, Phancao JP, Stidham K. MR imaging of turf toe. Magn Reson Imaging Clin N Am. 2008;16:93–103.

Nery C, Baumfeld D, Umans H, Yamada AF, MR imaging of the plantar plate normal anatomy, turf toe, and other injuries. Magn Reson Imaging Clin N Am. 2017;25(1):127–44.

Supplementary Images

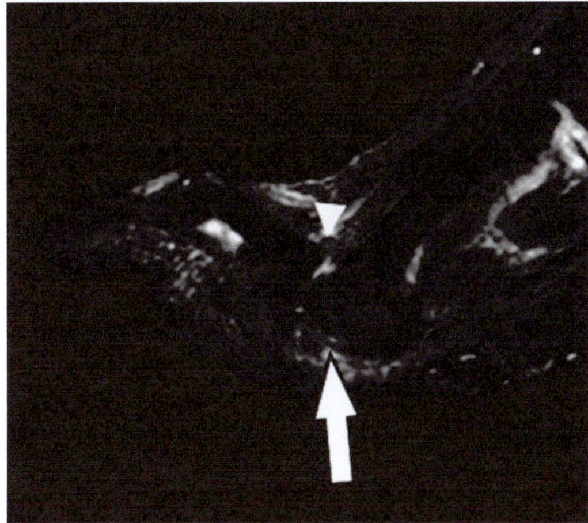

Sagittal STIR

There is a complete tear of the plantar plate at the 2nd MTP joint at its distal attachment on the 2nd proximal phalanx with proximal retraction of about 7 mm (arrow). Note mild dorsal subluxation of the 2nd proximal phalanx (arrowhead)

Case 6.15

Indication A 33-year-old female with posterior ankle pain and decreased range of motion.

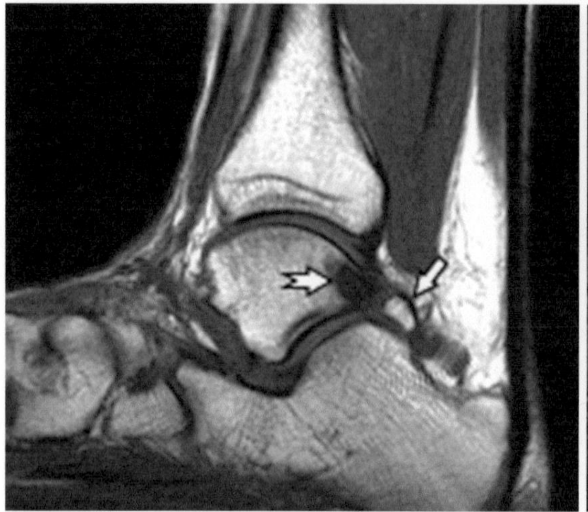

Sagittal T1

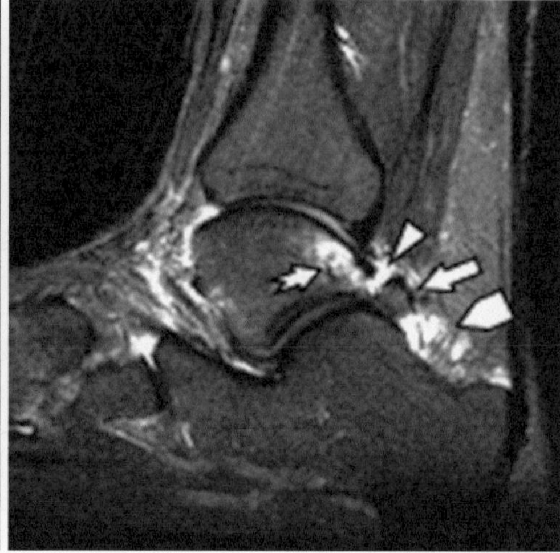

Sagittal STIR

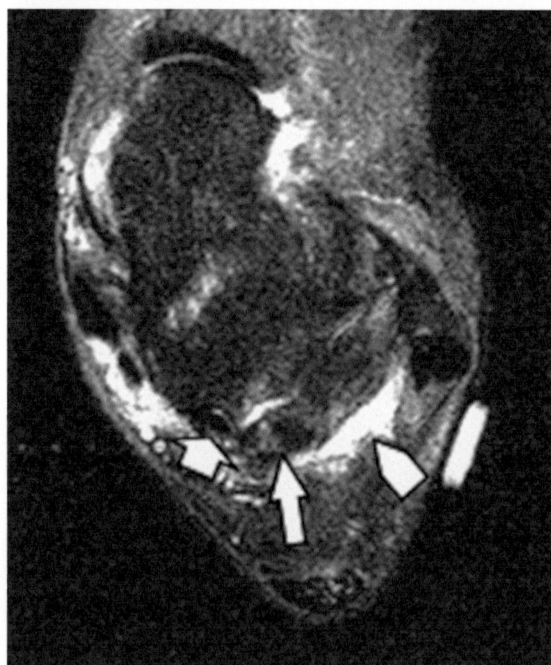

Axial T2 fat saturated

Findings

There is an oval ossific structure posterior to the talus consistent with an os trigonum (arrow). This is associated with bone marrow edema and subchondral cystic changes at the posterior aspect of the talus (notched arrows) as well as fluid within the synchondrosis (arrowhead). Mild synovitis is seen at the posterior joint recess (block arrow). The flexor hallucis longus tendon (short arrow) is normal without tenosynovitis.

Impression/Recommendation

Os trigonum syndrome/posterior impingement syndrome.

Discussion: Posterior Impingement Syndrome

Posterior impingement syndrome of the ankle is also known as "os trigonum syndrome" and refers to a group of abnormalities that most commonly results from repetitive plantar flexion of the foot leading to posterior ankle pain and decreased range of motion. The condition can be related to either osseous or soft tissue abnormalities. Several osseous variants at the posterior ankle increase the likelihood of developing posterior impingement. The lateral tubercle of the talus may be elongated, referred to as "Stieda's process." An accessory ossicle of the lateral tubercle of the talus may remain unfused, termed an os trigonum which articulates with the lateral tubercle via a synchondrosis. These osseous variants and the surrounding soft tissues may become compressed between the posterior aspect of the distal tibia and the calcaneus leading to chronic irritation and synovitis at the posterior joint recess. Alternatively, posterior impingement can be soft tissue related, often secondary to prior ankle sprain with scarring and thickening of the posterior ligaments, mainly of the posterior talofibular ligament as well as the intermalleolar ligament. Rarely, intra-articular loose bodies in the posterior joint recess may cause posterior impingement.

On MRI, there can be bone marrow edema at the posterior talus and/or os trigonum (if present). The presence of hyperintense signal and subchondral cysts along the margins of the synchondrosis is a nonspecific finding and could indicate a degree of stress-related changes; however, the presence of fluid signal intensity along the synchondrosis indicates instability. This can be associated with thickening and hyperintense signal within the posterior intermalleolar and the posterior talofibular ligament as well as synovitis at the posterior joint recess or in the posterior subtalar joint. In fact, the presence of bone marrow edema at the posterior talus or os trigonum with posterior ankle synovitis should suggest the diagnosis of posterior ankle impingement. Some cases may have associated tenosynovitis of the flexor hallucis longus tendon.

Posterior ankle impingement usually improves with conservative treatment and rest. However, in refractory chronic ankle pain, arthroscopic debridement of scar tissue with resection of the os trigonum may be performed.

> **Report checklist**
> 1. Is there an os trigonum or Stieda's process?
> 2. Is there bone marrow edema at the posterior talus or os trigonum?
> 3. Is there fluid signal in the synchondrosis to suggest instability at the synchondrosis?
> 4. Is there thickening of the posterior ankle ligaments?
> 5. Is there synovitis of the posterior joint recess or posterior subtalar joint?
> 6. Are there loose bodies?
> 7. Is there tenosynovitis of the flexor hallucis longus tendon?

Suggested Reading

Berman Z, Tafur M, Ahmed SS, Huang BK, Chang EY. Ankle impingement syndromes: an imaging review. Br J Radiol. 2017;90(1070): 20160735.

Cerezal L, Abascal F, Canga A, Pereda T, García-Valtuille R, Pérez-Carro L, Cruz A. MR imaging of ankle impingement syndromes. AJR Am J Roentgenol. 2003;181(2):551–9.

Case 6.16

Indication A 44-year-old male with past history of ankle sprain. Now presents with chronic lateral ankle pain and instability.

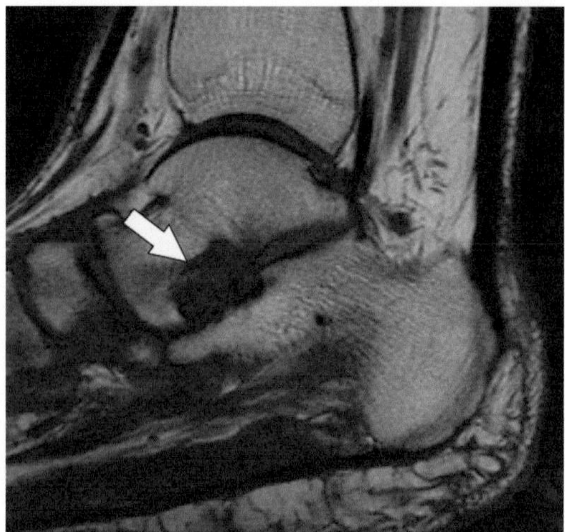

Sagittal T1

Findings

There is low T1 signal intensity obliterating the sinus tarsi (arrow) with lack of visualization of the normal sinus tarsi ligaments. These findings could be seen with sinus tarsi syndrome in the appropriate clinical context. There are no associated changes in the adjacent bony structures.

Impression/Recommendation

Sinus tarsi syndrome.

Discussion: Sinus Tarsi Syndrome

The sinus tarsi is a cone-shaped region located between the calcaneus and talus which is narrow medially and broader laterally. The sinus tarsi is occupied mainly by fat; however it also contains two ligaments which provide stability to the subtalar joint – the cervical ligament at the anterior aspect of the sinus tarsi and the interosseous ligament seen medially. There are also small neurovascular structures traversing this space.

Sinus tarsi syndrome is a clinical diagnosis characterized by lateral ankle pain and the sensation of hindfoot instability. It is most commonly seen in patients who have had an ankle inversion injury and is almost always associated with tears of the lateral ankle ligaments. It is thought that after an ankle sprain there is damage to the nerves and vascular engorgement within the sinus tarsi with secondary inflammation and fibrosis. Other uncommon causes include ganglion cysts within the sinus tarsi and arthropathies as gout.

On MRI, the sinus tarsi is best evaluated on a sagittal T1- and T2-weighted images. The typical appearance of the sinus tarsi is diffusely bright signal on the T1-weighted images due to the presence of abundant fat. The ligaments can be seen as hypointense linear structures traversing through the normal fat *(see supplementary images)*. The presence of minimal fluid or edema is commonly seen on MRI and is considered a normal finding.

As stated earlier, the diagnosis of sinus tarsi syndrome is mainly clinical, and caution should be made in making this diagnosis solely by MRI findings. With that said, imaging findings seen in patients with sinus tarsi syndrome include indistinctness or disruption of the ligaments and diffuse infiltration of the fat within the sinus tarsi with synovitis and fibrosis evident as diffuse low signal on the T1-weighted images and low or bright signal on the T2-weighted images depending if the fat is replaced predominantly by inflammatory tissue or fibrosis. In more advanced cases, there may be degenerative changes within the subtalar joint with subchondral cystic changes and bone marrow edema.

Sinus tarsi syndrome is not an independent pathology and is usually secondary to an underlying chronic pathology of the hindfoot or midfoot which should always be sought for when one is suspicious of this diagnosis. The most common underlying disorders are lateral ligament tears, posterior tibial tendinopathy, and spring ligament tears.

Treatment of sinus tarsi syndrome ranges from conservative management as rest and physical therapy, steroid injections or subtalar joint synovectomy.

Supplementary Images

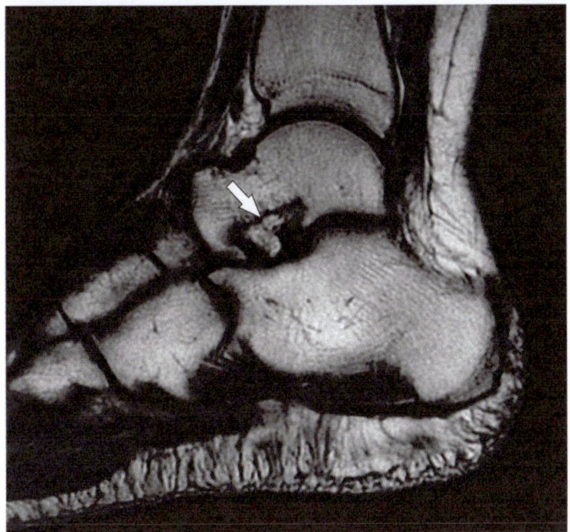

Sagittal T1

Normal appearance of the sinus tarsi (arrow)

> **Report checklist**
> 1. Is there obscuration of the normal fat in the sinus tarsi?
> 2. Are there ganglion cysts or focal masses within the sinus tarsi?
> 3. Is there any underlying bone marrow edema or subchondral cystic changes at the roof of the sinus tarsi or in the calcaneus?
> 4. How are the lateral ankle ligaments? The spring ligament? The posterior tibialis tendon?

Suggested Reading

Lee KB, Bai LB, Park JG, et al. Efficacy of MRI versus arthroscopy for evaluation of sinus tarsi syndrome. Foot Ankle Int. 2008;29(11): 1111–6.

Lektrakul N, Chung CB, Lai Ym, et al. Tarsal sinus: arthrographic, MR imaging, MR arthrographic, and pathologic findings in cadavers and retrospective study data in patients with sinus tarsi syndrome. Radiology. 2001;219(3): 802–10.

Case 6.17

Indication A 38-year-old female with pain and numbness at the second web space.

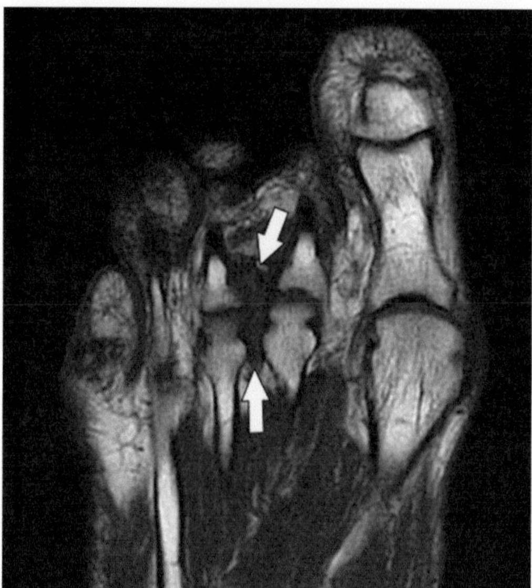

Axial T1

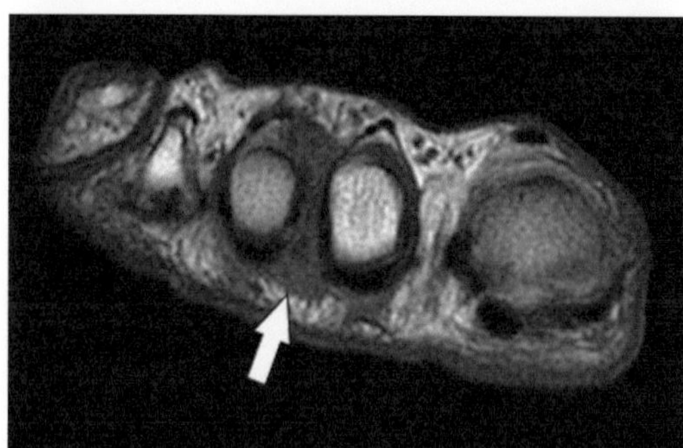

Coronal T1

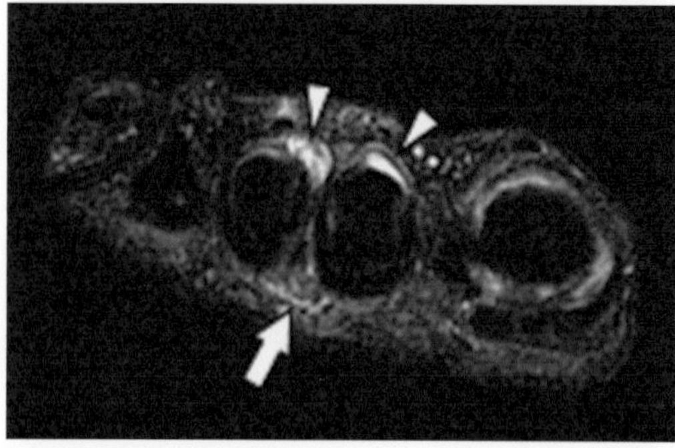

Coronal T2 fat saturated

Findings

There is a well-defined soft tissue mass within the 2nd intermetatarsal space projecting into the plantar subcutaneous fat (arrows) demonstrating isointense to hypointense signal on the T1-weighted images and low signal on the T2-weighted images compatible with Morton's neuroma. There is fluid in the 2nd and 3rd MTP joints (arrowheads).

Impression/Recommendation

Morton's neuroma.

Discussion: Morton's Neuroma

Morton's neuromas are not neoplasms but instead represent nerve degeneration and perineural fibrosis of the common digital nerves as it passes between the metatarsal heads. It develops from repetitive irritation and entrapment of the nerve leading to mass-like enlargement. They are most commonly seen in middle-aged women and are thought to be related to poorly fitting shoes and high heels. It is most commonly seen at the 2nd and 3rd intermetatarsal spaces, and patients usually present with pain and numbness at the intermetatarsal spaces radiating to the toes.

Morton's neuromas are commonly seen in asymptomatic individuals; however, those lesions are usually small, measuring less than 5 mm. The best sequence to identify these lesions is a coronal T1-weighted non-fat-suppressed sequence which provides high contrast between the lesion and the adjacent fat. On the short axis (coronal) images, a neuroma appears as a well-defined oval or dumbbell-shaped mass located between the distal margins of the metatarsal heads projecting inferiorly into the plantar subcutaneous fat. It demonstrates intermediate to hypointense signal on the T1-weighted images and relatively low signal on the T2-weighted images. One should always look at the T2-weighted fat-suppressed images to make sure that the lesion does not demonstrate high fluid signal to suggest intermetatarsal bursitis *(see supplementary images)* or ganglion cysts which are also common in this location. Morton's neuromas can have associated intermetatarsal bursitis, and it is common to see both processes on MRI. Gadolinium contrast is not necessary for making the diagnosis of Morton's neuromas; however, it can be helpful at times. Enhancement of Morton's neuromas can be variable but typically there is avid enhancement.

Treatment of Morton's neuromas usually starts with conservative management which includes footwear modification and rest. Injection with anesthetic such as lidocaine or bupivacaine can confirm that the Morton's neuroma is the site of the pain and injection with long-acting steroids, and low-percentage alcohol can help provide longer-term relief. Surgical resection is generally reserved for large neuromas and in patients who have not responded adequately to conservative treatment or injections.

Supplementary Images

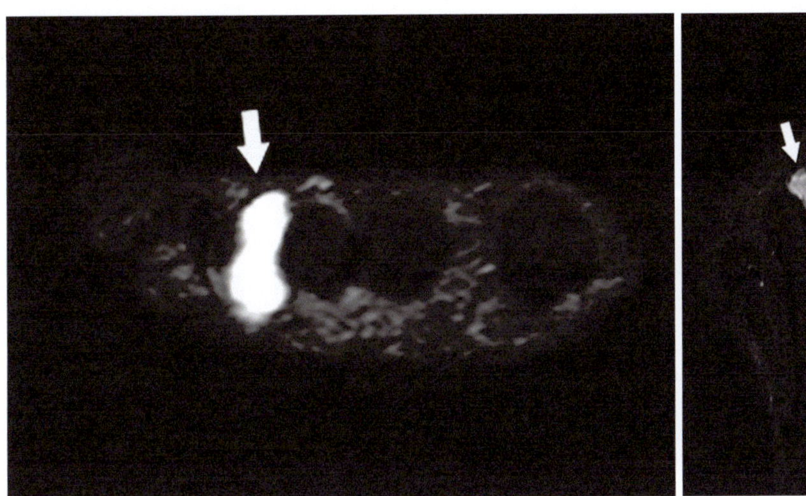

Intermetatarsal bursitis. There is a dumbbell shaped T2 bright fluid-filled structure (arrows) between the 3rd and 4th metatarsal heads

Report checklist
1. What is the size and location of the Morton's neuroma?
2. Is the lesion low signal on T1-weighted images and extends into the plantar soft tissues?
3. Is there associated intermetatarsal bursitis?
4. Is there a Morton's neuroma in the other intermetatarsal spaces?

Suggested Reading

Fazal MA, Khan I, Thomas C. Ultrasonography and magnetic resonance imaging in the diagnosis of Morton's neuroma. J Am Podiatr Med Assoc. 2012;102:184–6.

Sharp RJ, Wade CM, Hennessy MS, Saxby TS. The role of MRI and ultrasound imaging in Morton's neuroma and the effect of size of lesion on symptoms. J Bone Joint Surg (Br). 2003;85:999–1005.

Case 6.18

Indication A 28-year-old male runner with right calf pain for 2 weeks after a marathon race. Evaluate for fracture or muscle injury.

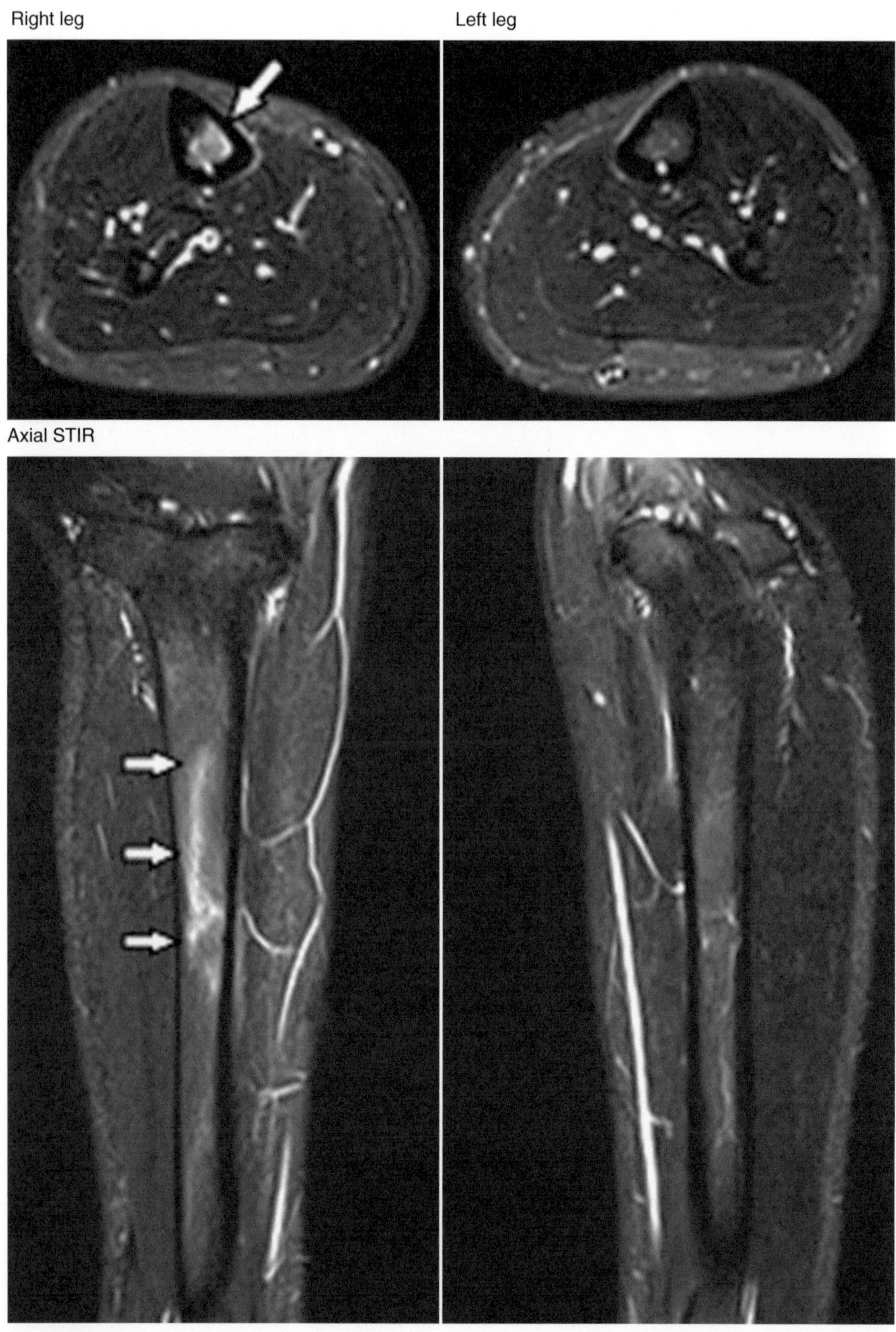

Findings

There is ill-defined bone marrow edema at the medial aspect of the right tibia with associated periosteal edema (arrows). There is no underlying fracture or suspicious osseous lesion. The surrounding muscles of the calf are normal in morphology without strain or fatty atrophy. The left lower leg is normal.

Impression/Recommendation

Right medial tibial stress syndrome. Limited weight-bearing is recommended as patient is at increased risk for a stress fracture.

Discussion: Medial Tibial Stress Syndrome

Medial tibial stress syndrome, also known as "shin splints," is an overuse injury of the tibia. It is characterized by vague, diffuse leg pain approximately 4 cm above the medial malleolus, which may extend up to 12 cm proximally. This injury is classically seen in runners and hikers. It is a stress reaction of the periosteum, bone, and/or fascia along the posteromedial tibia; this is caused by excessive traction at the periosteal-fascial junction at the insertion of the soleus muscle.

On MRI, medial tibial stress syndrome demonstrates hyperintense periosteal edema along the medial tibial border on the fluid-sensitive sequences. In more advanced cases, there may also be bone marrow edema in the medullary cavity, and later on, a clear stress fracture line may develop as a linear hypointense line.

Most cases of medial tibial stress syndrome are managed conservatively. Rest and limited weight-bearing are essential to prevent progression to a stress fracture. Additionally, nonsteroidal anti-inflammatory drugs, cushioned insoles, and casting may be tried. Surgery is rarely needed in these cases.

Report checklist

1. Where is the location of periosteal bone marrow edema?
2. Does the bone marrow edema involve the medullary cavity?
3. Is there a stress fracture line?
4. Is there a strain of the calf muscles?
5. Is there a contralateral injury or elsewhere along the same bone?
6. Could this be an underlying lesion (look for T1 signal replacing normal fat signal and sharp margins)?

Suggested Reading

Bergman AG, Fredericson M, Ho C, et al. Asymptomatic tibial stress reactions: MRI detection and clinical follow-up in distance runners. AJR Am J Roentgenol. 2004;183(3): 635–8.

Kijowski R, Choi J, Shinki K, et al. Validation of MRI classification system for tibial stress injuries. AJR Am J Roentgenol. 2012;198(4): 878–84.

Case 7.1

Indication A 64-year-old male known to have prostate cancer with right hip pain.

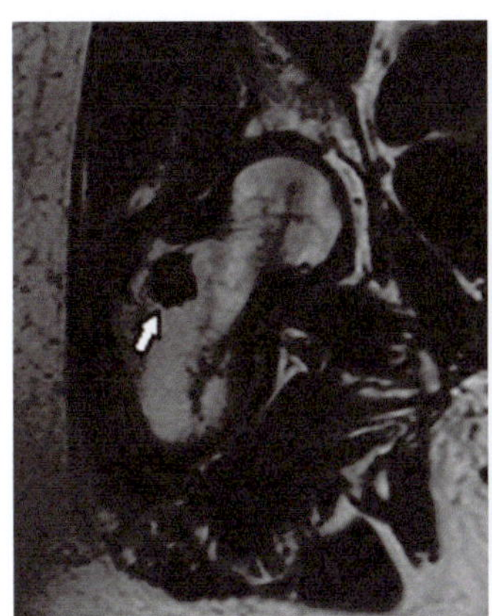
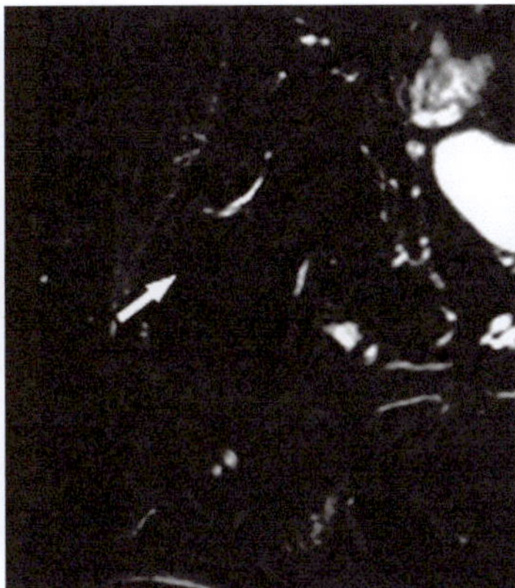
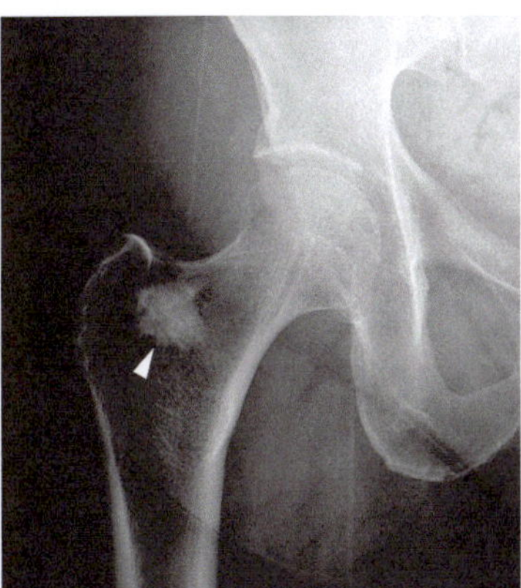

Coronal T1   Coronal T2 fat saturated

Findings

There is a 1.3 cm lesion (arrows) in the right greater trochanter which has uniform low signal on both T1- and T2-weighted sequences. The lesion corresponds to a sclerotic lesion with spiculated borders (arrowhead) on the prior radiographs. There is no perilesional edema or additional similar lesions.

Impression/Recommendation

1.3 cm sclerotic lesion with MR characteristics compatible with a bone island.

Discussion: Bone Island (Enostosis)

A bone island or enostosis is technically not a true neoplasm. It is a hamartoma where normal tissue (cortical bone) is in an ectopic location (medullary cavity of the bone). They are very common and often seen as an incidental finding. They are typically periarticular in location but can occur in nearly any bone. The most common locations are the pelvis, proximal femurs, and ribs. They are rare in the spine, especially the cervical spine. Bone islands should be asymptomatic, and symptomatic ones should raise the possibility of an alternate diagnosis.

© Springer Nature Switzerland AG 2020

T. M. Hegazi, J. S. Wu, *Musculoskeletal MRI*, https://doi.org/10.1007/978-3-030-26777-3_7

On imaging, bone islands will appear as a well-defined oval lesions, typically less than 1 cm. Bone islands can have a "brush border" margin with radiating spicules that should be uniformly dense. On MRI, bone islands are low signal on all pulse sequences. Occasionally they can have mild surrounding edema, especially if large. Bone islands usually have low or no uptake on bone scintigraphy; however, large bone islands can have some uptake. Giant bone islands are >2 cm *(see supplementary images).* Patients with osteopoikilosis (an autosomal dominant disorder) can have multiple bone islands, typically in the pelvis. Genetic testing has shown that these patients can have LEMD3 and EXT1 gene mutations. The main diagnostic dilemma is whether a sclerotic bone lesion is a bone island which would require no workup or is an osteoblastic metastasis, such as from prostate cancer. Recent studies have shown that bone island typically have higher Hounsfield unit (HU) than untreated sclerotic metastasis with lesions with >885 HU having a 92% accuracy for being a bone island. Moreover, bone island should not grow rapidly, and a sclerotic metastasis should be considered if the lesion grows >25% in 6 months or > 50% in 1 year. If prostate cancer metastasis is suspected, these patients will typically have a PSA > 10 ng/mL. Lastly sclerotic metastasis is unlikely to have the spiculated borders and tend to have smooth borders. It is important to check for a history of a pre-existing malignancy, especially in ones that can lead to sclerotic metastasis such as prostate, carcinoid, or treated breast cancer.

Bone islands are classic "don't touch" lesions and do not require treatment. However, if there is high concern for an alternative diagnosis, follow-up imaging in 3–6 months to establish stability can be helpful. In growing or inconclusive lesions, core needle biopsy can be helpful.

Supplementary Images

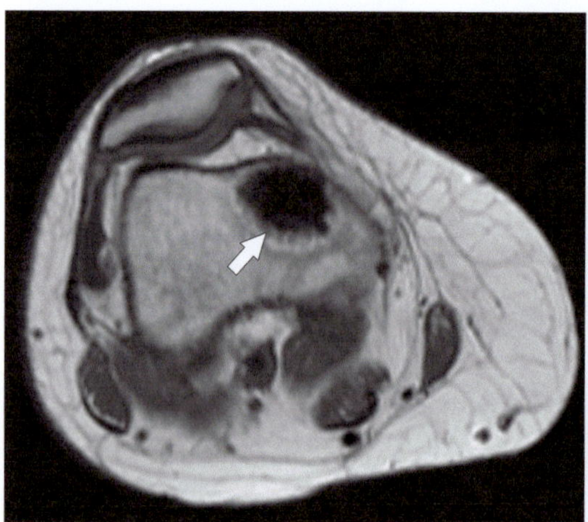

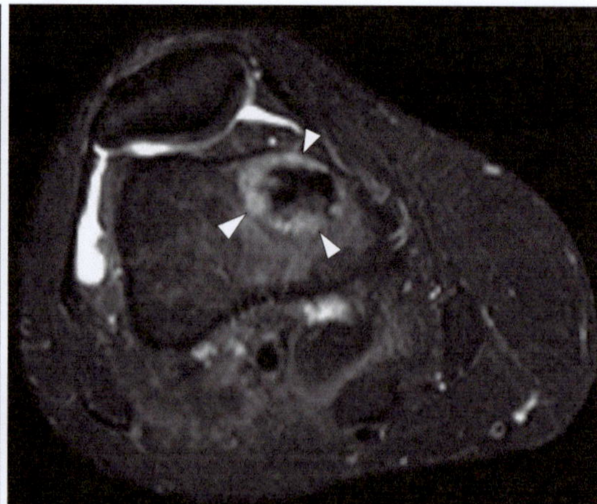

Giant bone island (arrow) with perilesional edema (arrowheads)

Report checklist
1. What is the size and location of the lesion?
2. Is the lesion uniformly low signal on all MRI pulse sequences? (Large lesions can have perilesional edema)
3. Is there a smooth or spiculated border?
4. Does the patient have a pre-existing malignancy that can cause sclerotic metastasis (prostate, carcinoid, treatment cancers)?
5. Are there multiple lesions?

Suggested Reading

Bernard S, Walker E, Raghavan M. An Approach to the Evaluation of Incidentally Identified Bone Lesions Encountered on Imaging Studies. AJR Am J Roentgenol. 2017;208:960–70.

Vanel D, Ruggieri P, Ferrari S, Picci P, Gambarotti M, Staals E, Alberghini M. The incidental skeletal lesion: ignore or explore?. Cancer Imaging. 2009;9:S38–43.

Case 7.2

Indication A 33-year-old female with knee pain. Radiographs show a sclerotic lesion in the distal femur.

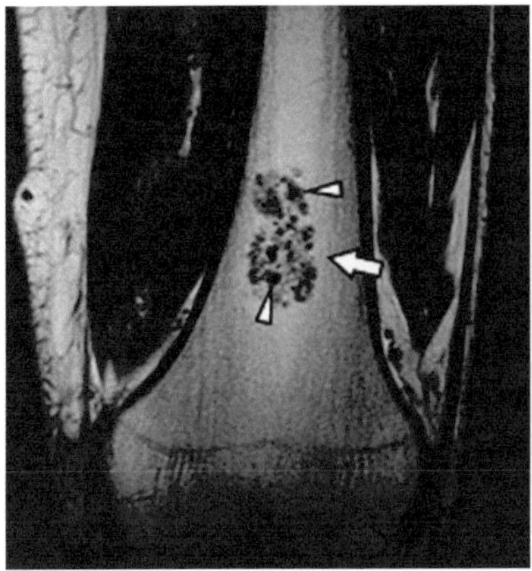
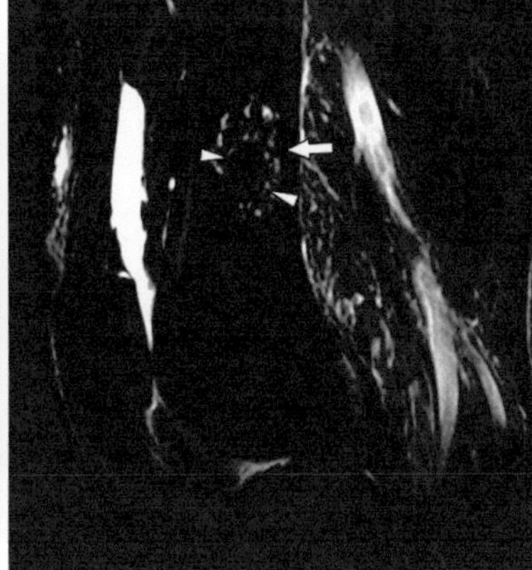
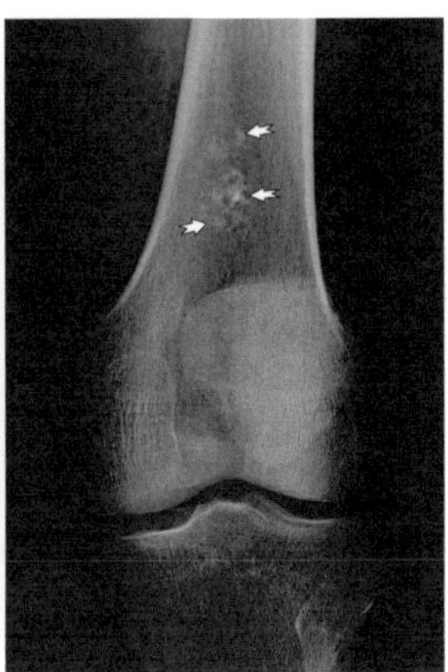

Coronal T1   Sagittal T2 fat saturated

Findings

There is a 3.5 × 2.5 cm lobulated intramedullary lesion (arrows) in the distal femur. The lesion has heterogeneous low T1 signal and high T2 signal with punctate foci (arrowheads) of low T1 and T2 signal corresponding to the calcifications (notched arrows) seen on the prior radiographs. There is no cortical breakthrough, endosteal scalloping, or soft tissue component to suggest a more aggressive lesion.

Impression/Recommendation

Well-defined intramedullary lesion with nonaggressive imaging characteristics most compatible with an enchondroma.

Discussion: Enchondroma

Enchondromas are very common and represent 10–25% of all benign bone tumors. They are most commonly diagnosed in the second to fourth decades of life. This tumor arises from mature hyaline cartilaginous rests which have been displaced into medullary bone often near the physeal scar. The most common locations are the proximal humerus, distal femur, and tubular bones of hands and feet. Enchondromas are often asymptomatic and discovered incidentally.

Painful lesions should raise suspicion for degeneration to a chondrosarcoma, especially if the lesion was previously asymptomatic. However, it can be hard to determine if symptoms are due to the lesion or other causes such as osteoarthritis.

On imaging, enchondromas typically have a central metaphyseal location. They have a well-defined border with stippled "arcs and rings" chondroid-type calcified matrix centrally. Lesions in the small tubular bones of the hands/feet can be expansile and lack chondroid matrix calcifications. Conversely, some lesions can be entirely calcified. Mild endosteal scalloping of the cortex can occur due to the lobular growth pattern but should be less than 1/3 of the cortical thickness and less than 1 cm in length. If the endosteal scalloping is more than this, a chondrosarcoma should be considered. Enchondromas can be confused with bone infarcts; however, bone infarcts tend to have a well-outlined margin and peripheral calcifications. Also, bone infarcts should not have endosteal scalloping or bone expansion. On MRI, enchondromas appear as lobulated low T1 and high T2 signal lesions due to their high water content. There can be foci of low signal due to calcifications. A helpful feature is chemical shift artifact at the periphery of lesion due to the interface of the water content in the hyaline cartilage with the surrounding fat.

Occasionally enchondromas can give rise to a chondrosarcoma, especially in lesions located in the central skeleton (ribs, pelvis, scapula, sternum) and in large lesions. The true rate of malignant transformation of enchondromas into chondrosarcoma is difficult to assess as it is virtually impossible to determine the true incidence of enchondromas, but it is estimated to be <1%. Features that can favor chondrosarcoma over an enchondroma include endosteal cortical scalloping >1/2 thickness (best distinguishing feature); pain, especially in a previously asymptomatic lesion; growing lesion, especially after skeletal maturity; periosteal reaction; centrally located lesions; large size (>5 cm); soft tissue component; epiphyseal location; lucent areas in densely calcified lesions; and older patients.

Small asymptomatic enchondromas do not require any treatment. However, symptomatic lesions or large lesions with suspicious imaging findings should be followed by imaging or treated. Curettage and bone grafting for large or suspicious lesions can be performed, and recurrence is low. With the wide use of MRI, enchondromas are frequently encountered in everyday clinical practice.

Report checklist
1. What is the size and location of the lesion?
2. Does the lesion have imaging features of a chondroid lesion (lobulated border, stippled central calcifications, chemical shift artifact)?
3. Is there endosteal scalloping, periosteal reaction, or soft tissue component to suggest a more aggressive cartilage tumor requiring treatment?
4. Is the lesion in the appendicular skeleton (long bones, hands, feet) or centrally located? (Central lesions are more likely to be chondrosarcomas.)

Suggested Reading

Chung BM, Hong SH, Yoo HJ, Choi JY, Chae HD, Kim DH. Magnetic resonance imaging follow-up of chondroid tumors: regression vs. progression. Skeletal Radiol. 2018;47:755–61.

Douis H, Parry M, Vaiyapuri S, Davies AM. What are the differentiating clinical and MRI-features of enchondromas from low-grade chondrosarcomas? Eur Radiol. 2018;28:398–409.

Case 7.3

Indication A 19-year-old male with knee pain. Radiographs show a lucent lesion in the distal femur.

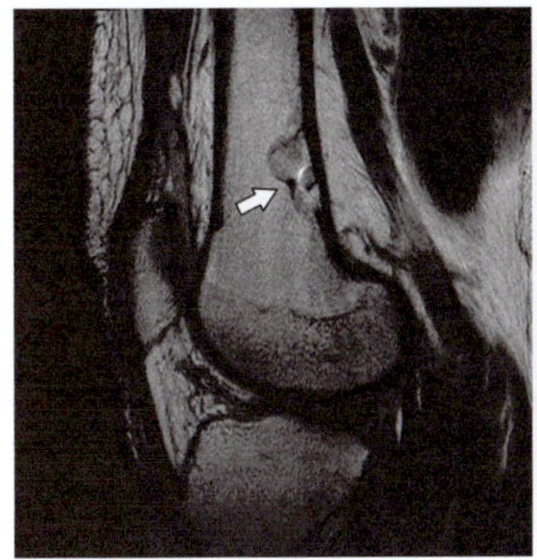
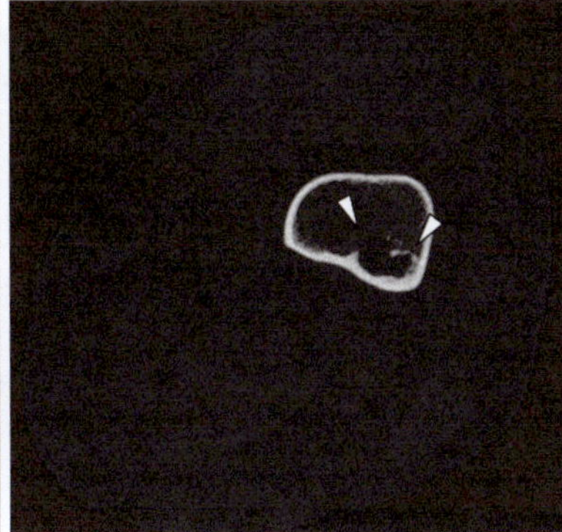
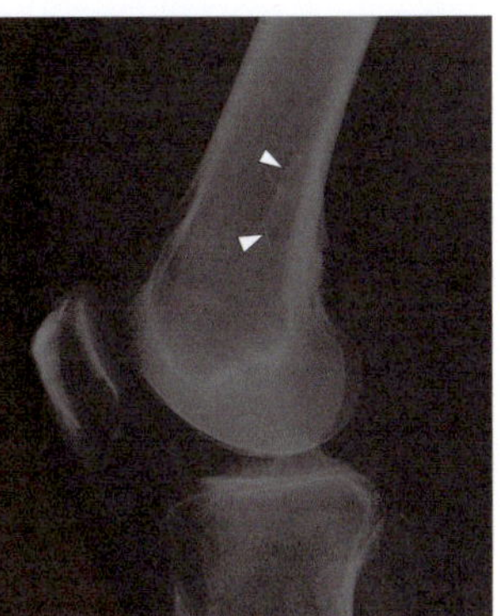

Sagittal PD   Axial CT

Findings

There is a 2.5 cm lesion (arrow) in the distal femoral metaphysis posteriorly. The lesion is cortically based and has a thin low signal sclerotic rim. There is heterogeneous signal intensity on PD-weighted image with areas of fluid and fat signal. There is no perilesional edema or fracture. This lesion correlates with the lesion on the prior radiographs and CT where there is a thin sclerotic rim (arrowheads).

Impression/Recommendation

Well-defined cortically based lesion with nonaggressive imaging characteristics most compatible with a non-ossifying fibroma (NOF).

Discussion: Non-ossifying Fibroma (NOF)

Non-ossifying fibromas (NOF) are benign developmental defects comprised of fibroblastic spindle cells, interlacing collagen, and xanthomatous/multinucleated giant cells. NOF are identical pathologically to fibrous cortical defects (FCD), and together the two lesions are classified as fibrous xanthomas. The terms FCD and NOF are often used interchangeably. However, FCD is smaller and is centered in the cortex, whereas a NOF tends to be larger and extends into the medullary cavity. There is no agreed upon cutoff size between FCD and NOF, though an upper limit of 3 cm has been suggested for FCD. NOF is an extremely common lesion, present in 30% of the normal population during the first two decades. However, they are rarely seen on radiographs after age 20 as the lesion will involute and typically completely disappear with age. A new lesion that occurs in adulthood is unlikely to be an NOF. NOFs may occur due to traumatic injury to the physeal plate at the site of a tendon or ligament insertion, but in general the cause is not completely understood. NOFs are typically asymptomatic, except for large lesions which can result in a pathologic fracture.

NOF are classic "don't touch" lesions, and it is important to not suggest biopsy for lesions with classic imaging and clinical features. NOF should contact the cortex and are typically longer than they are wide. On MRI there is low-intermediate signal on T1 and variable signal on T2. There should be a low signal thin rim of sclerosis, and the lesion should not have perilesional edema unless there is an associated fracture. A CT or radiograph can be helpful to show the peripheral sclerotic rim.

NOFs are typically not treated unless they are large and at risk for pathologic fracture. Large lesions can be treated with curettage and packing.

Small asymptomatic lesions can be left alone or followed with serial radiographs, if unchanged at 3 months, then every 6–12 months, until regress or become symptomatic. If NOFs are multiple, they can be associated with certain familial syndromes such as neurofibromatosis (von Recklinghausen's disease) or Jaffe-Campanacci syndrome.

Report checklist
1. What is the size and location of the lesion?
2. What is the age of the patient and is this a new lesion in an adult? (NOF should not occur as a new lesion in an adult patient)
3. Does the lesion contact the cortex?
4. Is there a thin low signal sclerotic rim?
5. Is there perilesional edema or fracture?
6. Are there multiple lesions to suggest a familial syndrome?

Suggested Reading

Herget GW, Mauer D, Krauß T, El Tayeh A, Uhl M, Südkamp NP, Hauschild O. Non-ossifying fibroma: natural history with an emphasis on a stage-related growth, fracture risk and the need for follow-up. BMC Musculoskelet Disord. 2016;17:147.

Jee WH, Choe BY, Kang HS, Suh KJ, Suh JS, Ryu KN, Lee YS, Ok IY, Kim JM, Choi KH, Shinn KS. Nonossifying fibroma: characteristics at MR imaging with pathologic correlation. Radiology. 1998;209:197–202.

Case 7.4

Indication A 27-year-old woman with lateral distal thigh pain. Radiographs show bony exostosis from the lateral femur. MRI performed to assess cartilage cap.

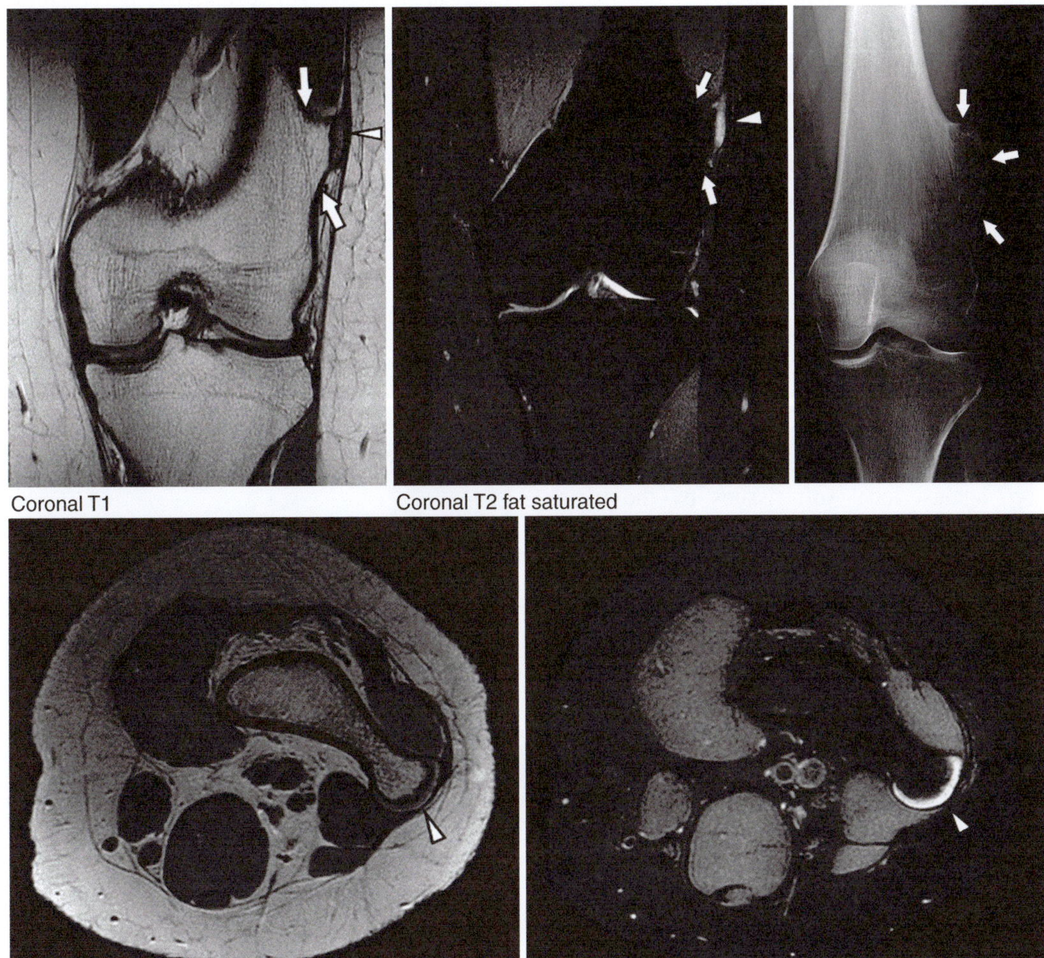

Findings

There is an exophytic mass (arrows) arising from the lateral distal femoral metaphysis, extending away from the knee joint. The lesion has a broad base and measures 3.2 × 1.2 × 1.8 cm. There is continuity of the marrow cavity of the host bone with the lesion. There is a thin T2 bright cartilaginous cap (arrowheads) that measure 2 mm in thickness. There is no marrow edema in the lesion or mass effect on the adjacent neurovascular structures.

Impression/Recommendation

Sessile osteochondroma from the femur with thin cartilage cap. No signs of malignant degeneration.

Discussion: Osteochondroma

Osteochondroma is a very common benign bone tumor and is seen in 3–5% of the population. It is hypothesized to represent growth plate cartilage displaced to the metaphysis and is most commonly seen in the femur, tibia, and humerus. If multiple, as seen in multiple hereditary exostoses (MHE), the pelvic bones are commonly involved. These tumors are often asymptomatic and discovered incidentally on imaging. Clinical symptoms are often related to mechanical irritation of adjacent tissues. Neurovascular compression can lead to paresthesias and pseudoaneurysms (especially in the popliteal fossa), and an adventitial bursitis can result from pressure against local soft tissues by the tumor. Pedunculated osteochondromas can develop a fracture at the base.

On imaging, a key feature of an osteochondroma is continuity of the marrow cavity of the host bone with the lesion. The cortices of the host bone and osteochondroma should also be continuous. Osteochondromas can be sessile (base is broader than the width) or pedunculated (base more narrow than main tumor). Osteochondroma often point away from the joint, due to local mass effect from surrounding muscles. Another characteristic feature is the cartilage cap on the surface of the tumor. The cap is the thickest during childhood and shrinks with age. If the cap is greater than 2 cm thick in adults and 3 cm in children, then suspicion for malignant transformation of the cap into a chondrosarcoma should be raised. However, the average thickness of the cap in secondary chondrosarcomas is 5–6 cm (*see supplementary images*). Also, cartilage cap growth after skeletal maturity can suggest malignant transfor-

mation. CT and US can be unreliable for measuring the cap thickness. MRI is best, and the hyaline cartilage cap will be bright on T2 due to high water content and will typically enhance. MRI is also excellent for evaluating complications of osteochondromas such as neurovascular compression, adventitial bursitis, and fracture.

Treatment of osteochondromas depends on symptoms. Many small tumors do not require treatment. Resection of lesions that cause mechanical injury of adjacent soft tissues maybe needed. Lesions with malignant transformation typically require more extensive surgery.

Supplementary Images

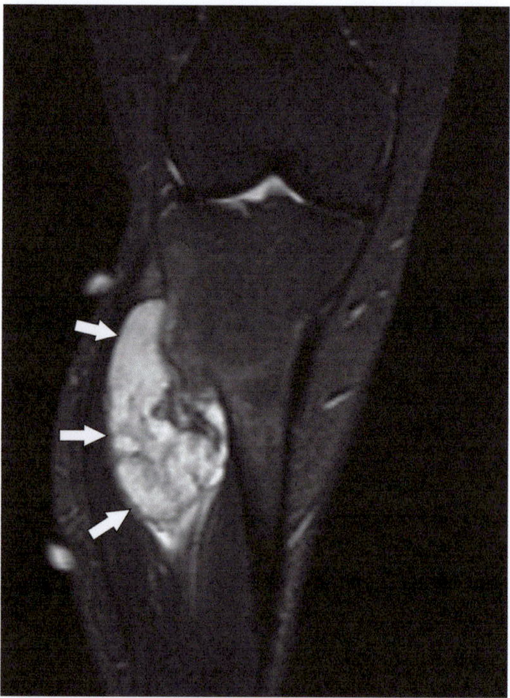

Coronal T2 fat saturated

Malignant transformation of the cartilage cap in an osteochondroma to a chondrosarcoma. The cartilage cap (arrows) is thickened measuring 4.5 cm and is hyperintense on the T2-weighted sequences

Report checklist

1. What is the size and location of the lesion?
2. Is there continuity of the host bone marrow cavity with the lesion?
3. Is the osteochondroma sessile or pedunculated? If pedunculated, is there a fracture at the base?
4. Is there a cartilaginous cap and, if so, how thick? Caps >2cm , especially if increased in size after skeletal maturity should raise concern for malignant transformation)
5. Is there mechanical injury of adjacent soft tissues (neurovascular impingement, adventitial bursitis)?
6. Are there additional lesions to suggest the presence of multiple hereditary exostoses (MHE)?

Suggested Reading

Gavanier M, Blum A. Imaging of benign complications of exostoses of the shoulder, pelvic girdles and appendicular skeleton. Diagn Interv Imaging. 2017;98:21–8.

Kok HK, Fitzgerald L, Campbell N, Lyburn ID, Munk PL, Buckley O, Torreggiani WC. Multimodality imaging features of hereditary multiple exostoses. Br J Radiol. 2013;86:20130398.

Case 7.5

Indication A 19-year-old man with right thigh pain and swelling, worsening over the past 3months.

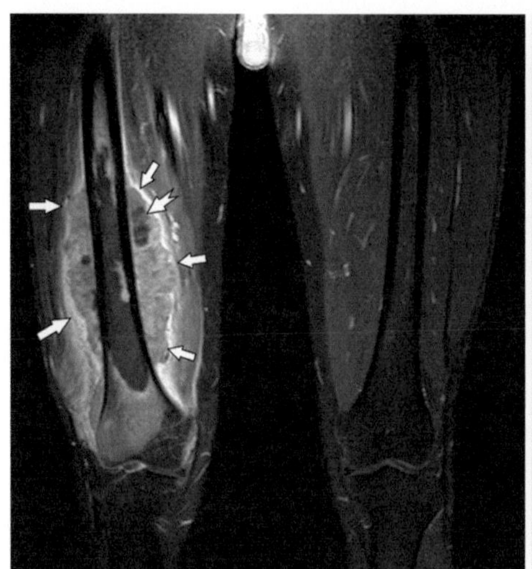

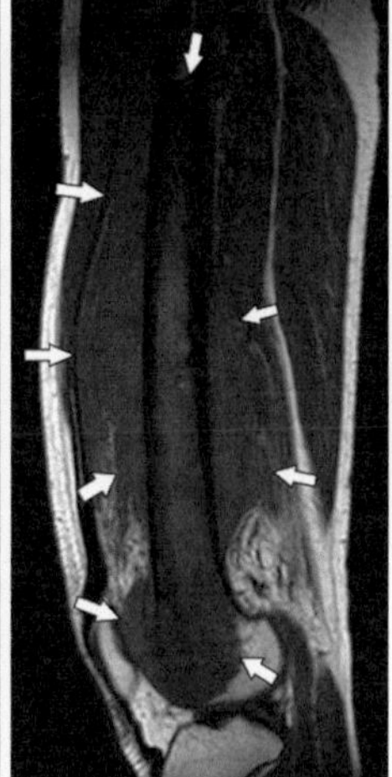

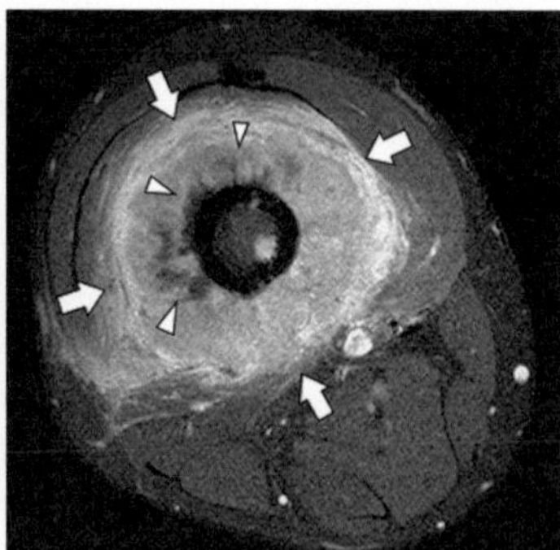

Axial T1 fat saturated post contrast

Coronal T1 fat saturated post contrast   Sagittal T1

Findings

There is a large mass (arrows) centered in the right distal femur which contains a large soft tissue component and has associated aggressive spiculated periosteal reaction (arrowheads). The soft tissue mass component permeates through the cortical bone without frank bony destruction. The lesion has signal intensity that is isointense to skeletal muscle on the T1-weighted images and heterogeneous signal on the T2-weighted images and has solid enhancement. The marrow abnormality measures 27.5 cm in the craniocaudal dimension. The soft tissue mass component measures 15.3 × 8.5 × 9.3 cm. The mass extends into the anterior knee joint. There is no reactive effusion. The mass contacts the posterior neurovascular bundle without encasement. There is a 3.0 × 1.5 area of nonenhancement (notched arrow) in the proximal medial aspect of the mass suggestive of tumor necrosis.

Impression/Recommendation

Large aggressive bone lesion in the distal femur concerning for osteosarcoma or lymphoma. Tissue sampling recommended.

Discussion: Osteosarcoma

Conventional osteosarcoma is an intramedullary malignant neoplasm that produces osseous matrix. It is most common in the young adult and is the second most common primary tumor of bone (#1 malignant bone tumor is myeloma) and represents 20% of all primary bone malignancies. About 30% of osteosarcomas occur in patients over age 40 (often with predisposing conditions such as Paget's disease or irradiated bone). Osteosarcomas are most common in the distal femur (40%), proximal tibia, and proximal humerus and usually metaphyseal in location. Patients often complain of dull aching pain, especially at night, limited range of motion, and a palpable mass. Lab tests can show elevated alkaline phosphatase and lactic acid dehydrogenase.

On imaging osteosarcomas typically appear as a focal lesion with mixed lucency and sclerosis. There is often a wide zone of transition with aggressive features (cortical breakthrough, soft tissue mass). There is typically aggressive periosteal reaction (disorganized, sunburst, Codman's triangle). A helpful diagnostic feature of osteosarcomas and other round blue cell tumors (lymphoma, Ewing sarcoma) is extension of the tumor from the medullary cavity through the cortex into the extramedullary soft tissue without frank cortical destruction. Other tumors with large soft tissue components such as a plasmacytoma or renal cell metastasis *(see supplementary images)* will have cortical destruction. Since the mass replaces the bone marrow, the mass is typically isointense or hypointense to skeletal muscle on T1-weighted sequences. There will be heterogeneous, often hyperintense, signal on T2-weighted sequences and solid internal enhancement after the administration of gadolinium contrast. Osseous matrix will appear as very low signal on T1- and T2-weighted images; however, the degree of dense bone matrix can be variable or absent. Comparison to radiographs or CT can be extremely helpful to assess the degree of osseous matrix. Contrast administration is important as it can highlight areas of necrosis which should be avoided during targeted biopsy in order to increase diagnostic yield. When describing the mass, it is also important to include useful features for preoperative planning. These include the size and exact location of the mass, intra-articular or neurovascular involvement, and skip lesions.

Treatment of conventional osteosarcoma is with preoperative chemotherapy to reduce vascularity and size of the mass followed by surgical resection. Clinicians seek >90% tumor necrosis prior to surgery, and preservation of joint function is of high priority.

Supplementary Images

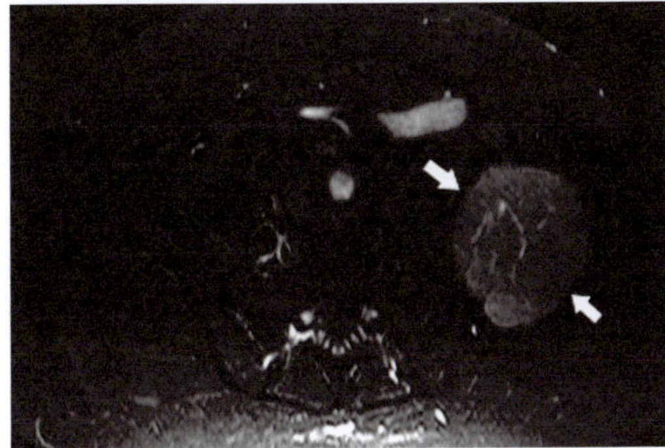

Axial T2 fat saturated

Plasmacytoma in the left iliac bone. There is a large soft tissue mass (arrows) emanating from the left iliac bone. The cortices are not visualized due to destruction by the tumor

Report checklist

1. What is the size and exact location of the lesion?
2. Does the lesion have aggressive imaging features (soft tissue component, periosteal reaction)?
3. Is there osteoid matrix? (Compare to radiographs or CT if available)
4. Is there soft tissue extension of the lesion from the medullary cavity with an intact cortex? (If so, think of Ewings, osteosarcoma, lymphoma)
5. Are there areas of nonenhancement suggesting tumor necrosis?
6. Is there intra-articular extension or involvement of the neurovascular structures which could affect surgery?
7. Are there skip lesions?

Suggested Reading

Saifuddin A, Sharif B, Gerrand C, Whelan J. The current status of MRI in the pre-operative assessment of intramedullary conventional appendicular osteosarcoma. Skeletal Radiol 2019;48:503–16.

Yarmish G, Klein MJ, Landa J, Lefkowitz RA, Hwang S. Imaging characteristics of primary osteosarcoma: nonconventional subtypes. Radiographics. 2010;30(6):1653–72.

Case 7.6

Indication A 29-year-old male with right hip pain and limited range of motion. Radiographs show a calcified lesion in the right ischiofemoral region.

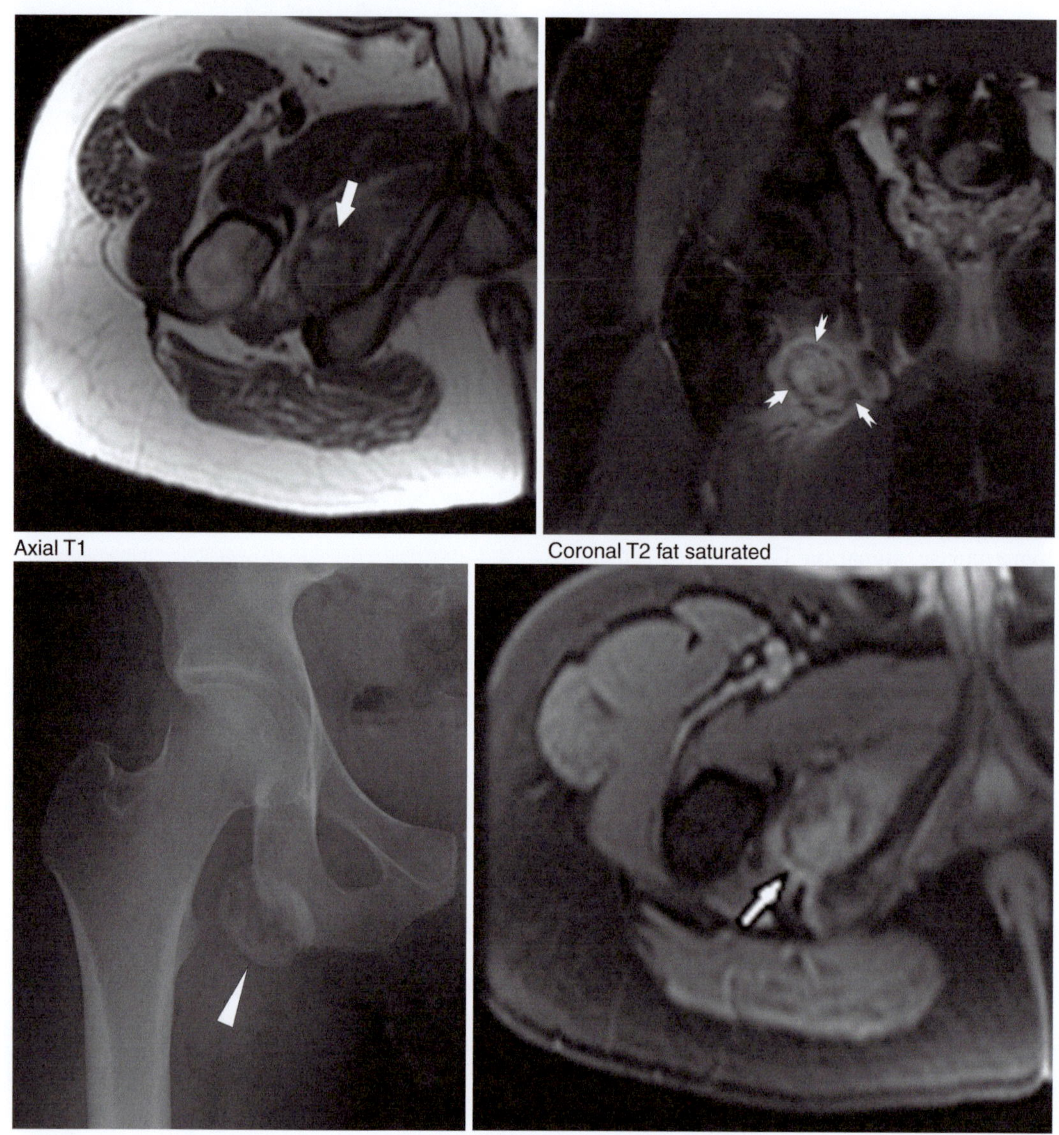

Axial T1

Coronal T2 fat saturated

Axial T1 fat saturated post contrast

Findings

There is a 3.7 × 3.5 × 3.0 cm mass (arrows) in the right adductor compartment adjacent to the ischial tuberosity. The mass is hypointense on T1-weighted images and hyperintense on T2-weighted images. There is a peripheral ring of low signal (notched arrows) on all sequences compatible with calcification as seen on the prior radiographs (arrowhead). The lesion demonstrates heterogeneous but solid internal enhancement after gadolinium contrast administration. There is perilesional edema and enhancement in the adjacent muscles.

Impression/Recommendation

Well-defined lesion with peripheral calcification as described suggestive of myositis ossificans. Correlation with prior history of trauma is recommended. Also, follow-up radiographs are recommended to document further ossification.

Discussion: Myositis Ossificans

Myositis ossificans (MO) is a form of heterotopic ossification where there is abnormal formation of mature lamellar bone in the soft tissues, usually following trauma. However, the patient is often unable to recall any precipitating trauma. MO can also occur in certain nontraumatic conditions, including burns, paraplegia, surgery, traumatic brain injury, hemophilia, polio, ankylosing spondylitis, and diffuse idiopathic skeletal hyperostosis (DISH). MO commonly occurs in the upper and lower extremities, usually in the lateral muscles. Patients may be asymptomatic or present with pain, swelling, or an elevated erythrocyte sedimentation rate (ESR).

Imaging of MO is highly dependent on the stage. Early on, a nonspecific soft tissue mass is often seen in the muscle. Ossification develops 3–8 weeks after onset, beginning peripherally and progressing centrally. During the early stage of calcification formation, MO forms faint irregular densities; but with time, a rim of mature lamellar bone and central osteoid matrix can develop. The MRI appearance is variable depending on the stage of development and, earlier on, can mimic a sarcoma as there may be enhancement following contrast administration. Differentiation from an osteochondroma or surface osteosarcoma may also be difficult if the area of ossification is adherent to the adjacent bone. CT can be helpful in demonstrating a plane of soft tissue between the mass and the bony cortex. Myositis ossificans may be difficult to distinguish from an osteosarcoma even on biopsy specimens.

Treatment with nonsurgical options using indomethacin, bisphosphonates (prophylaxis), and radiation are typically favored over surgical intervention. However, surgical excision may be necessary in very symptomatic cases.

Report checklist

1. What is the size and location of the lesion?
2. Has there been a history of trauma and/or does the patient have predisposing conditions for MO formation?
3. Are there calcifications in a peripheral location within the lesion? Compare to prior studies if available. Recommend CT or radiographs to assess for peripheral calcifications if no prior studies if suspected
4. Is the mass adherent to the bone? If so, consider a surface osteosarcoma or osteochondroma

Suggested Reading

Walczak BE, Johnson CN, Howe BM. Myositis ossificans. J Am Acad Orthop Surg. 2015;23:612–22.

Wang H, Nie P, Li Y, Hou F, Dong C, Huang Y, Hao D. MRI findings of early myositis ossificans without calcification or ossification. Biomed Res Int. 2018;2018:4186324.

Case 7.7

Indication A 76-year-old woman with thigh swelling and pain.

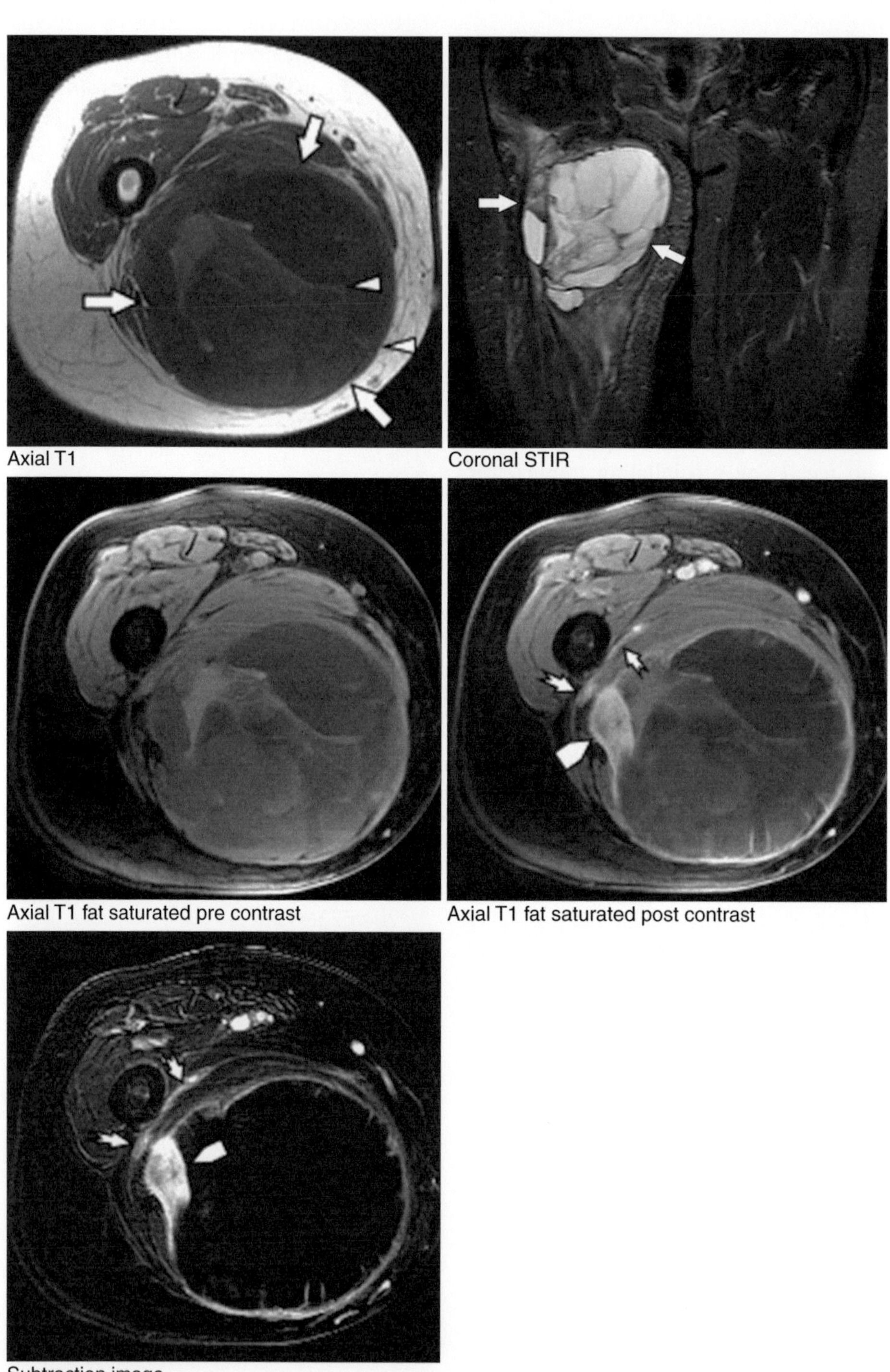

Axial T1

Coronal STIR

Axial T1 fat saturated pre contrast

Axial T1 fat saturated post contrast

Subtraction image

Findings

There is a 9.7 (AP) × 11.4 (TV) × 13.3 cm (CC) lesion (arrows) in the posterior compartment of the thigh situated between and displacing the adductor magnus as well as the semimembranosus, semitendinosus, and biceps femoris muscles. The majority of the lesion is composed of multiple fluid locules with areas of layering intermediate T1 signal (arrowheads) consistent with blood products. Following the administration of gadolinium, there is a 3.9 (AP) × 1.6 (TV) × 1.2 (CC) cm enhancing component (block arrows) about the lateral margin of the mass as well as septal and peripheral enhancement. There is reactive edema within the muscles of the posterior compartment as well as within the fascial planes of the adductor muscles. As for the neurovascular structure, the sciatic nerve (notched arrows) is draped around the lateral aspect of the mass; however, there appears to be a fat plane between the nerve and mass. No osseous involvement is seen.

Impression/Recommendation

Large thigh hematoma with 4 cm enhancing nodular component. Findings are suspicious for intra-tumoral hematoma. Percutaneous biopsy of the solid nodule is recommended to exclude malignancy.

Discussion: High-Grade Pleomorphic Sarcoma with Large Intra-Tumoral Hematoma

Hematomas arising in a sarcoma are fortunately uncommon (3% of sarcomas); however, they should be considered in any hematoma with atypical clinical and/or imaging features. The consequences of misdiagnosis of a sarcoma can be dire, delaying needed treatment at a time when early diagnosis is important. Hematomas can arise at sites of trauma, in patients with bleeding disorders or in patients on anticoagulation medication. However, they can also appear as a result of a soft tissue tumor with bleeding. Pleomorphic sarcoma and synovial sarcomas are the most common sarcomas to have intra-tumoral hematomas. The lesions can be misdiagnosed as simple hematomas without malignancy, and the average diagnostic delay is 6.7 months. The thigh and chest wall are the most common sites for intra-tumoral hematomas. Patients typically present with a rapidly enlarging mass with or without a history of trauma.

On MR imaging, hematomas can have variable MRI signal intensity depending on the amount and stage of blood products present within it. Subacute hemorrhage can be hyperintense on both T1-weighted images and fat saturated T1 sequences. Hematomas are typically hyperintense on T2; however, there can be low T2 signal areas from hemosiderin deposition. A low signal hemosiderin rim can be present and accentuated on gradient echo sequences. Fluid-fluid levels can be present as the result of the various stages of bleeding within the lesion. It is extremely important to give contrast for suspected intra-tumoral hematomas. Classic hematomas should have only peripheral enhancement, often a thin smooth peripheral rim. When there is a thick wall or nodular enhancing components, a necrotic tumor or tumor with adjacent hematoma should be considered. A soft tissue abscess is also in the differential, and clinical symptoms of infection should be assessed.

Suspected intra-tumoral hematomas should undergo biopsy and the enhancing components sampled after aspiration of the hematoma. Fine needle aspiration with cytologic evaluation is typically not sufficient to diagnosis a sarcoma, and image-guided core needle biopsy is preferred. For nondiagnostic cases, open surgery biopsy may be needed. Depending on the sarcoma subtype, radiation or adjuvant chemotherapy maybe needed, followed by wide resection with margins clear of tumor.

Report checklist
1. What is the size and exact location of the mass?
2. What is the relationship of the mass to the neurovascular structures, bone, and joint space?
3. Are there hemorrhagic products in the lesion? High signal on T1 and T1 fat sat sequences? Hemosiderin with blooming on GRE sequences? Fluid-fluid levels? Nonenhancement on post-contrast images?
4. Is there a thickened enhancing rim or nodular areas of enhancement? These should be described and targeted biopsy during biopsy
5. Is there a history of trauma to the area or is the patient on anticoagulation or has a bleeding disorder?
6. Could this be an abscess?

Suggested Reading

Allen AH. Large Undifferentiated pleomorphic sarcoma of the posterior thigh. Am J Case Rep. 2019;20:318–322.

Baheti AD, O'Malley RB, Kim S, Keraliya AR, Tirumani SH, Ramaiya NH, Wang CL. Soft-tissue sarcomas: an update for radiologists based on the revised 2013 World Health Organization Classification. AJR Am J Roentgenol. 2016;206:924–32.

Hoshi M, Naoto Oebisu, Ieguchi NM, Ban Y, Takami M, Nakamura H. Clinical features of soft tissue sarcoma presenting intra-tumour haematoma: case series and review of the literature. Int Orthop. 2017;41:203–9.

Case 7.8

Indication A 61-year-old male with thigh swelling.

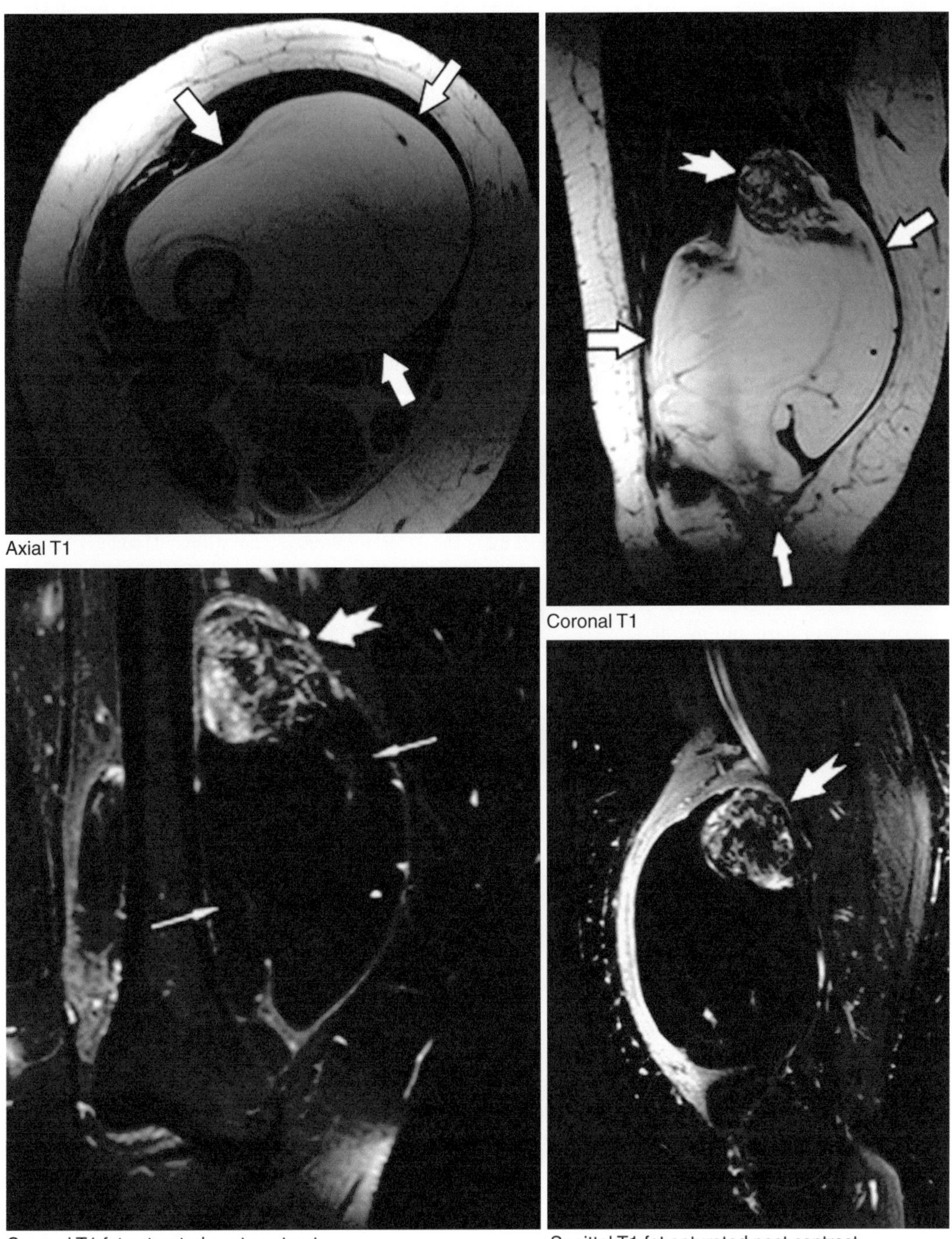

Axial T1

Coronal T1

Coronal T1 fat saturated post contrast

Sagittal T1 fat saturated post contrast

Findings

There is a very large 24.2 × 15.4 × 12.9 cm fatty mass (arrows) in the anteromedial aspect of the lower thigh. The mass is centered in the vastus medialis and encases the femur without bony invasion. The vast majority of the mass has increased signal on T1-weighted sequences and decreased signal on the fat saturated sequences consistent with fat. However, there is a 4.7 × 3.8 × 4.2 cm nodular component (arrowheads) at its superior aspect which contains non-fatty material. Following the administration of contrast, there is heterogeneous enhancement (notched arrows) of the nodular component as well as enhancement of some irregular septations (thin arrows) within the midportion of the mass, indicating that this is not a simple lipoma. There is no adjacent marrow edema in the femur or involvement of the neurovascular structures by the mass.

Impression/Recommendation

Large fatty mass with heterogeneously enhancing nodular component suggestive of an atypical lipoma/well-differentiated liposarcoma. Ultrasound-guided biopsy of the nodular component is recommended.

Discussion: Atypical Lipoma/Well-Differentiated Liposarcoma

Lipomas are the most common soft tissue tumor and contain tissue histologically identical to adipose fat. The incidence of lipomas is 2.1 per 100 individuals. Lipomas are often asymptomatic and are mostly cosmetic issues; however, large lesions can be painful and/or irritate adjacent structures (nerves, vessels, muscles). The main dilemma when encountering a lipoma is whether it is a simple lipoma or a liposarcoma. There are a variety of liposarcomas with the most common lesion being an atypical lipoma (ALT). However, the term well-differentiated liposarcoma is histopathologically the exact same lesion. The term ALT is used for lesions in the extremities, whereas well-differentiated liposarcoma is the term used for lesions within the trunk such as the retroperitoneal, medi-astinum, and scrotum. This distinction was made to reflect the low morbidity and low incidence of recurrence of tumors in the extremities, since wide excision is achievable, as opposed to that of retroperitoneal and mediastinal tumors, in which complete excision is difficult. This distinction was abandoned in the 2002 World Health Organization (WHO) classification, so both tumors are now considered to be the same entity. Some authors still reserve the term ALT for tumors that occur in the subcutaneous soft tissue. ALT/well-differentiated liposarcomas do not metastasize; however, they have a high local recurrence rate. High-grade liposarcomas (intermediate or high) can metastasize, typically to the lung.

MRI is by far the best imaging test for evaluating fatty soft tissue lesions as one can easily assess the amount of fatty and non-fatty tissue. Simple lipomas have the same signal intensity as subcutaneous fat on all MR pulse sequences *(see supplementary images)*. The classic lipoma is composed entirely of fat, without areas of nodularity or thickened septations. However, a substantial percentage of benign lipomas demonstrate non-fatty features. In a study by Kransdorf et al., 31% (11 of 35) of lipomas showed non-fatty content, which the authors attributed to fat necrosis and associated calcification, fibrosis, inflammation, and myxoid change. ALTs or well-differentiated liposarcoma will have non-fatty components, and features found to favor a diagnosis of well-differentiated liposarcoma over simple lipomas are lesion size greater than 10 cm, presence of thick (2 mm) septae (diffuse or focal), presence of globular and/or nodular non-fatty areas or masses, and lesion composition of less than 75% fat. The nodular non-fatty areas and thickened septa will typically enhance. Intermediate or high-grade liposarcomas will contain even less fat than ALTs and may even have no visible fat. Ultimately, if a fatty mass cannot be reported as a simple lipoma or other benign fat-containing mass, a liposarcoma needs to be considered, and biopsy should be recommended.

For ALT/well-differentiated liposarcoma or higher-grade liposarcomas, surgical resection is the definitive treatment. Thus, it is important to carefully describe the exact location of the lesion and whether there is involvement of adjacent neurovascular structures or muscles.

Supplementary Images

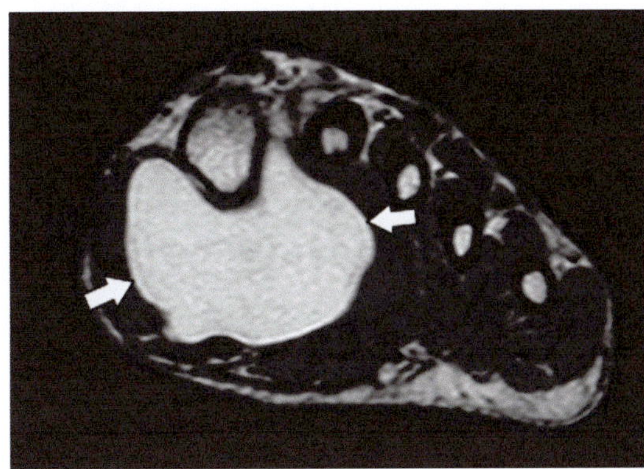

Coronal T1

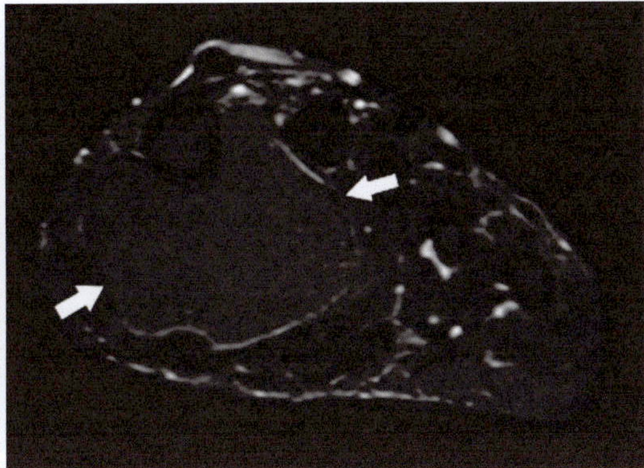

Coronal T1 fat saturated post contrast

Simple lipoma in the forefoot. There is a 3 cm fatty mass (arrows) inferior to the first metarsal shaft which shows complete and uniform fat saturated and no internal enhancement or septal/nodular areas

Report checklist

1. What is the size and exact location of the mass?
2. Is the mass entirely composed of fat and completely suppresses in signal on fat-suppressed sequences?
3. Are there non-fatty areas (nodules, large vessels, thickened septations, calcifications)? These should be described to aid in targeted biopsy
4. Is there involvement of the mass on adjacent soft tissue structures such as nerves, vessels, and muscles?

Suggested Reading

Coran A, Ortolan P, Attar S, Alberioli E, Perissinotto E, Tosi AL, Montesco MC, Rossi CR, Tropea S, Rastrelli M, Stramare R. Magnetic resonance imaging assessment of lipomatous soft-tissue tumors. In Vivo. 2017;31(3):387–95.

Wortman JR, Tirumani SH, Jagannathan JP, Tirumani H, Shinagare AB, Hornick JL, Ramaiya NH. Primary extremity liposarcoma: MRI features, histopathology, and clinical outcomes. J Comput Assist Tomogr. 2016;40:791–8.

Case 7.9

Indication A 37-year-old male with left upper arm pain and palpable mass. MRI for further evaluation.

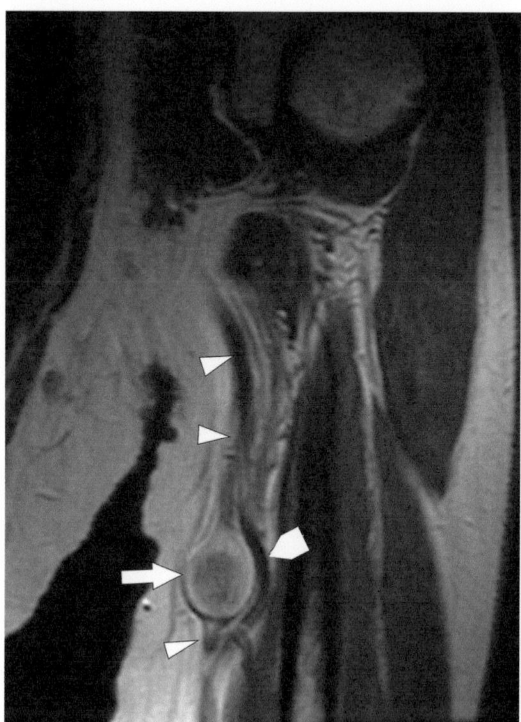

Coronal T1

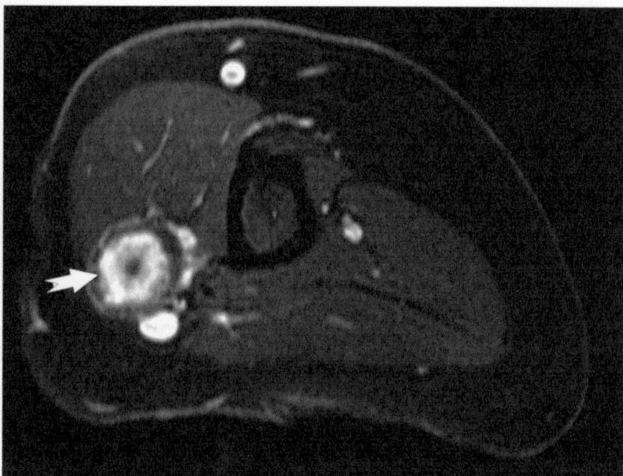

Axial T2 fat saturated

Findings

There is a 2.3 cm round mass (arrow) intimately associated with the median nerve (arrowheads) in the upper arm. The median nerve is seen to enter and exit the mass and causes mass effect on the adjacent vessels (block arrow). On T2-weighted images, the lesion (notched arrow) has hyperintense signal with a central foci of low signal (target sign). There is no perilesional edema and no additional masses are seen.

Impression/Recommendation

Well-defined soft tissue mass lesion in the upper arm most compatible with a peripheral nerve sheath tumor, schwannoma.

Discussion: Peripheral Nerve Sheath Tumor (PNST)

Peripheral nerve sheath tumors (PNSTs) are common and include both schwannomas and neurofibromas. Schwannomas are more common and usually sporadic. Neurofibromas are more likely to be multiple and can be associated with various syndromes, such as neurofibromatosis. Schwannomas arise from Schwann cells, whose role is to produce the myelin that covers the nerve; thus, they can be eccentrically located at surgery. Neurofibromas arise from the nerve substance itself and are harder to separate from normal nerve fibers at surgery. PNST are most commonly diagnosed in the young adult, and patients can have motor or sensory disturbances or both.

On imaging, PNSTs typically appear as a well-defined, smooth-bordered mass aligned along the nerve. They are typically isointense to muscle on T1W and hyperintense to fat on T2W images. In some cases, the lesions may have a "target sign" appearance on T2W images, with high signal peripherally and low signal centrally, corresponding to myxoid and fibrocollagenous content, respectively. The target appearance can be seen in both neurofibromas and schwannomas but is more commonly present in neurofibromas. Contrast enhancement can be variable. On occasion, the nerve from which the tumor arises becomes thickened immediately adjacent to the tumor, giving rise to a "tail sign." When the PNST enlarges, a surrounding rim of fat is maintained – this becomes especially apparent on lesions that arise within muscle and is termed the "split fat sign." Although the nerve is peripherally located in schwannomas and centrally located in neurofibromas, the two lesions can be difficult to distinguish at imaging. Moreover, it may be impossible to differentiate benign from malignant PNSTs. However, malignant PNSTs are typically larger, have ill-defined margins and central necrosis, and demonstrate rapid growth.

For small PNSTs that are asymptomatic, these lesions can be left alone or be followed by imaging. For symptomatic and large lesions (>5 cm), biopsy or surgical excision is the mainstay of treatment. If biopsy is being performed, conscious sedation should be considered as these lesions can be very painful at biopsy.

Report checklist
1. What is the size and location of the mass?
2. Is the mass associated with a nerve?
3. Are there imaging features of a PNST (target sign, tail sign, split fat sign)?
4. Are there multiple lesions and/or does the patient have neurofibromatosis?
5. Is the mass > 5 cm, has central necrosis, or has increased in size? If yes, raise the possibility of a malignant nerve sheath tumor and recommend biopsy

Suggested Reading

Demehri S, Belzberg A, Blakeley J, Fayad LM. Conventional and functional MR imaging of peripheral nerve sheath tumors: initial experience. AJNR Am J Neuroradiol. 2014;35:1615–20.

Soldatos T, Fisher S, Karri S, Ramzi A, Sharma R, Chhabra A. Advanced MR imaging of peripheral nerve sheath tumors including diffusion imaging. Semin Musculoskelet Radiol. 2015;19:179–90.

Wasa J, Nishida Y, Tsukushi S, Shido Y, Sugiura H, Nakashima H, Ishiguro N. MRI features in the differentiation of malignant peripheral nerve sheath tumors and neurofibromas. AJR Am J Roentgenol. 2010;194:1568–74.

Case 7.10

Indication A 29-year-old female with palpable mass at the dorsal aspect of the midfoot. It is not tender on examination.

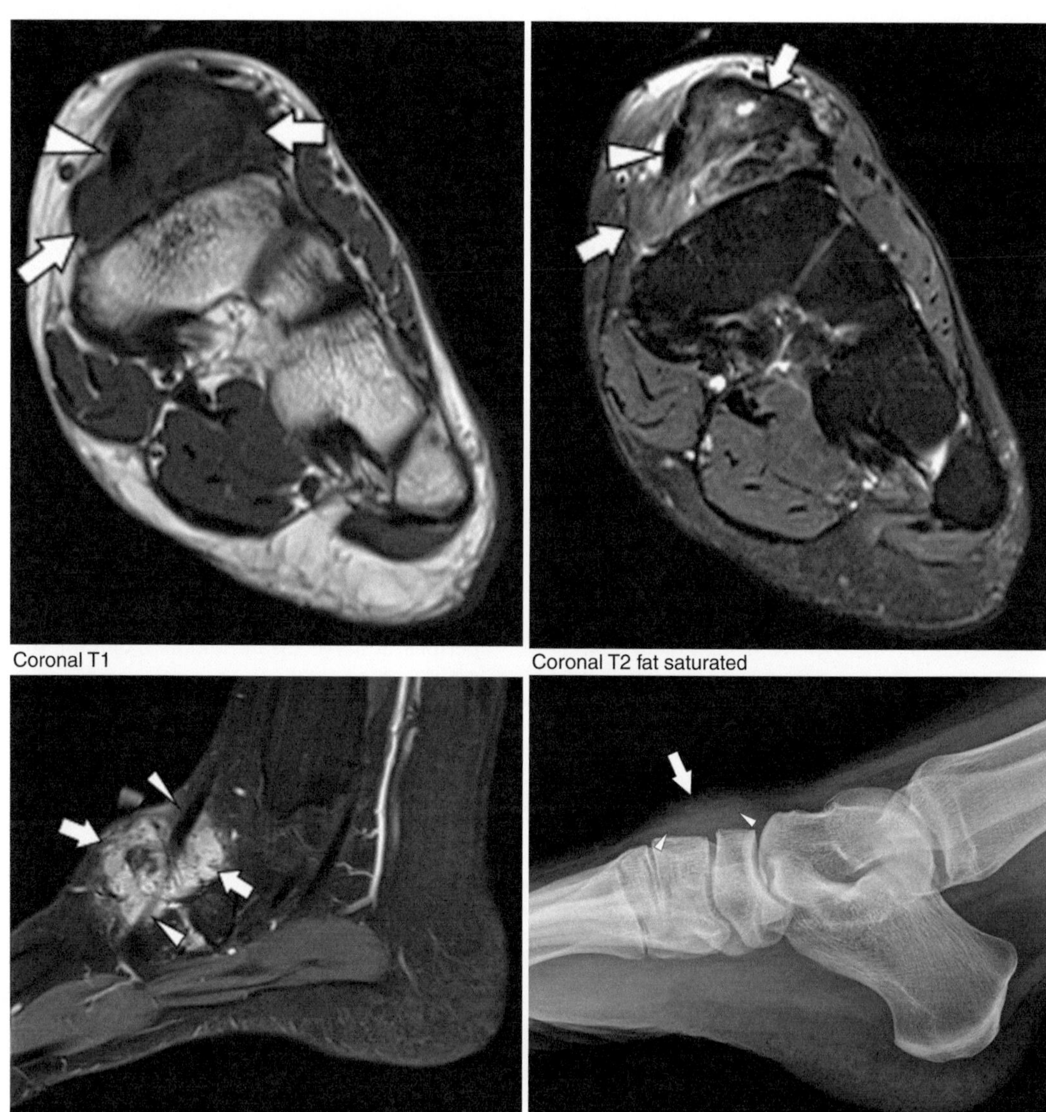

Findings

There is a 3.6 × 3.8 cm soft tissue mass (arrows) encasing the anterior tibialis tendon (arrowheads). The lesion is uniformly low signal on T1-weighted images and has heterogeneous, predominantly low signal on T2-weighted images.

There is avid internal enhancement after contrast administration. There is no remodeling of the adjacent bone, extension in the joint space or invasion of the adjacent muscles. There are foci of low signal on the post-contrast GRE T1 image (not shown) suggestive of hemosiderin deposit.

This lesion corresponds to the prior radiographs showing a soft tissue density mass encasing the anterior tibialis tendon. There are no calcifications on the radiographs.

Impression/Recommendation

Well-defined low signal intensity soft tissue mass encasing the anterior tibialis tendon, suggestive of tenosynovial giant cell tumor (TGCT) – focal type.

Discussion: Tenosynovial Giant Cell Tumor (TGCT) – Focal Type

Tenosynovial giant cell tumor (TGCT) is a benign tumor that arises from synovial tissue in joint, bursa, or tendons and is the preferred term over giant cell tumor of tendon sheath (GCT-TS) or pigmented villonodular synovitis (PVNS) which refers to the same entity. TGCT can have focal or diffuse types but are histologically the same tumor with mononuclear and inflammatory cells present. Focal TGCT occurs most commonly in the hands/wrist (85%) with the feet/ankle as the second most common site. The diffuse type is commonly seen in the knee. Patients usually present between 30 and 50 years of age and complain of a painless mass that enlarges over several years, ultimately becoming symptomatic. Large lesions can limit range of motion and making wearing footwear uncomfortable from mass effect on adjacent tissues. Intra-articular lesions can be especially problematic. TGCT is more common in women, more so with focal than the diffuse type. These lesions can be intra- or extra-articular depending on the anatomic structure involved.

TGCT have a characteristic appearance on MR imaging. Focal TGCT can be eccentrically located about the tendon or encase the tendon. These lesions are classically low signal on both T1- and T2-weighted images from the abundant collagen and hemosiderin. On gradient echo (GRE) sequences, "blooming" from hemorrhage can be present in the lesions as low signal foci. On post-contrast sequences, TGCT typi-cally have solid enhancement, but this can be variable. These MR imaging features can help distinguish TGCT from other common lesions about the hands and feet like ganglions, lipomas, and nerve sheath tumors. Moreover, the attachment of the tumor to a tendon is very helpful in diagnosis.

Treatment of TGCT is conservative for small stable lesions. However, large symptomatic or rapidly growing lesions are treated with en bloc resection. For focal types, recurrence after surgery is low but is higher for diffuse type or intra-articular lesions. TGCT have also been treated with imatinib, a tyrosine kinase inhibitor or radiation with variable results.

Report checklist
1. What is the size and location of the mass?
2. Is the mass attached to a tendon, within a bursa or intra-articular in location?
3. Is the mass low signal on T1 and T2 and has solid enhancement?
4. Is there "blooming" on gradient echo sequences?
5. Is there remodeling of the adjacent bone, extension in the joint space, or invasion of the adjacent muscles?
6. Are there multiple similar masses to suggest diffuse type of TGCT?

Suggested Reading

Gouin F, Noailles T. Localized and diffuse forms of tenosynovial giant cell tumor (formerly giant cell tumor of the tendon sheath and pigmented villonodular synovitis). Orthop Traumatol Surg Res. 2017;103:S91–7.

Mastboom MJL, Verspoor FGM, Hanff DF, Gademan MGJ, Dijkstra PDS, Schreuder HWB, Bloem JL, van der Wal RJP, van de Sande MAJ. Severity classification of Tenosynovial Giant Cell Tumours on MR imaging. Surg Oncol. 2018;27:544–50.

Wang C, Song RR, Kuang PD, Wang LH, Zhang MM. Giant cell tumor of the tendon sheath: Magnetic resonance imaging findings in 38 patients. Oncol Lett. 2017;13:4459–62.

Case 7.11

Indication   A 22-year-old male with palpable mass at the upper forearm and intermittent swelling. Prior radiographs show foci of calcifications, and ultrasound shows a vascular soft tissue mass.

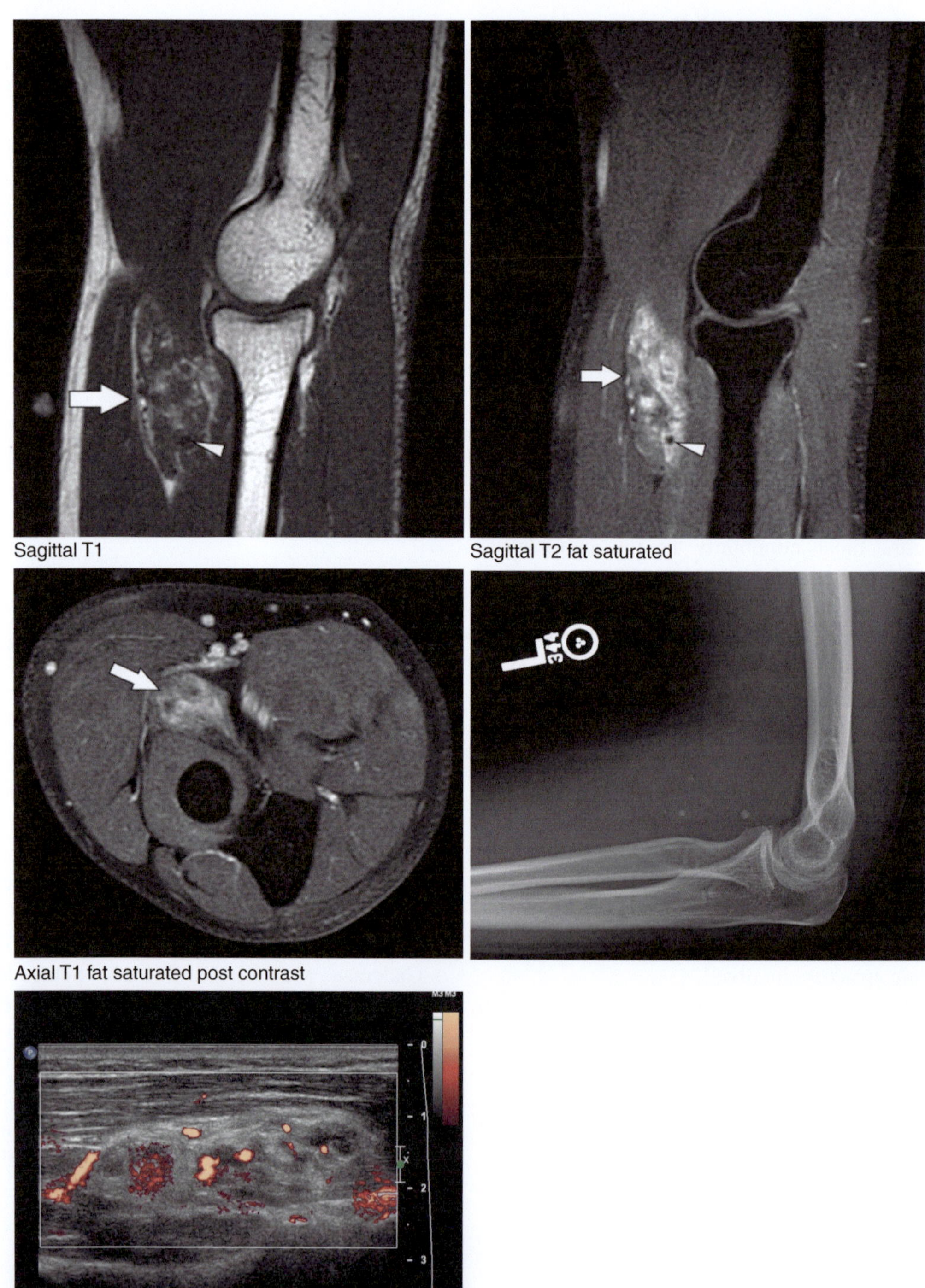

Sagittal T1

Sagittal T2 fat saturated

Axial T1 fat saturated post contrast

Color Doppler Ultrasound

Findings

There is a 3.1 × 1.9 × 2.5 cm lobulated soft tissue mass (arrows) in the anterolateral aspect of the elbow. On T1-weighted images, the lesion is heterogeneous and contains internal areas of high T1 signal that suppress with fat saturation consistent with fat. The lesion is hyperintense on T2-weighted images and has circular and tubular internal structures suggestive of vessels. There are small rounded foci (arrowheads) that are low signal on all sequences. These foci correspond to the calcifications seen on the radiographs and are consistent with phleboliths. There is avid internal enhancement after contrast administration corresponding to the vascularity seen on the prior ultrasound study. There are no feeding arteries to suggest a high-flow vascular lesion. The adjacent osseous structures are normal without bony remodeling or marrow edema.

Impression/Recommendation

Vascular malformation (low flow).

Discussion: Vascular Malformations

Vascular malformations are benign neoplasms that arise from dysplastic vascular channels and exhibit normal endothelial turnover. They can be subdivided into low-flow (venous, lymphatic, capillary, capillary-venous, and capillary-lymphatic-venous) or high-flow malformations (arteriovenous malformations or arteriovenous fistulas). Any lesion with a feeding artery should be considered a high-flow vascular malformation. For these soft tissue lesions, the terms "vascular malformation" and "hemangioma" have been used interchangeably in the medical literature leading to confusion. Hemangiomas are benign vascular tumors that typically occur shortly after birth, grow rapidly from cellular hyperplasia, and then involute. Vascular malformations are present at birth and have normal cellular growth but can increase as the patient grows. Thus most vascular lesions in adults are vascular malformations and are typically low-flow venous vascular malformations. Both hemangiomas and vascular malformations can be grouped under the term "vascular anomaly." Clinically, vascular malformations can manifest with bluish skin discoloration and have a history of size fluctuation depending on the amount of blood in the lesion from hormonal changes or trauma. Occasionally, pain may occur following exercise owing to shunting of blood flow away from the surrounding tissues into the lesion.

On MRI, vascular malformations appear as lobulated lesions with poorly defined margins and contain varying amounts of hyperintense T1 signal owing to either reactive fat overgrowth or hemorrhage. Areas of slow flow typically have high T2 signal intensity, while rapid flow can demonstrate a signal void on images obtained with a non-flow-sensitive sequence. Vascular malformations can contain serpentine vessels, fat, smooth muscle, hemosiderin, and phleboliths. Phleboliths are focal dystrophic calcifications in the vessel wall and appear as foci of low signal on all MRI sequences and corroboration on radiographs, or CT images can be helpful. Occasionally osseous changes can be seen such as periosteal reaction, bony remodeling, and marrow edema. It is important to search for feeding arterial vessels that can indicate the presence of a high-flow vascular lesion (*see supplementary images*), and pretreatment biopsy should be avoided. Lymphatic vascular malformation can contain fluid-fluid levels and often only have rim/septal enhancement (*see supplementary images*).

Hemangiomas often regress spontaneously making treatment unnecessary. Vascular malformations, on the other hand, do not regress. However, small or asymptomatic vascular malformations can be left alone. Symptomatic lesions are treated based on the whether they are low-flow (90%) or high-flow (10%) lesions. Low-flow lesions are treated with sclerotherapy (often requiring several treatments) whereas high-flow lesions are treated with embolization. These interventional procedures are preferred over surgery.

Supplementary Images

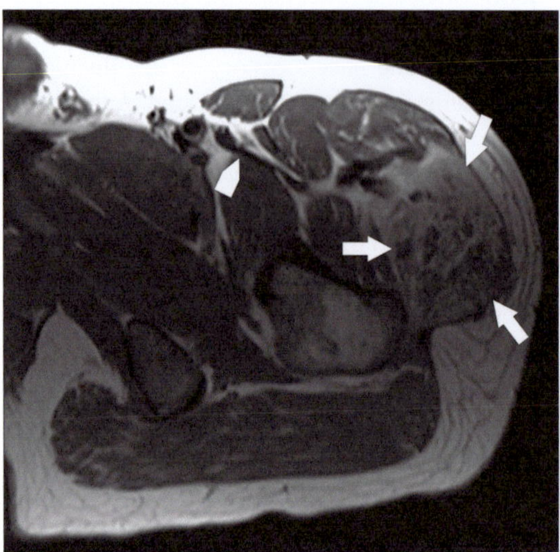

Axial T1

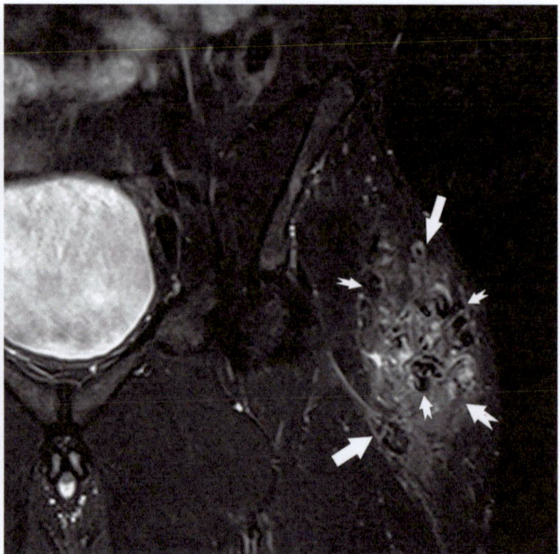

Coronal T2 fat saturated

High-flow arteriovenous malformation (AVM). There is a large 15 cm mass (arrows) in the lateral left hip which is heterogeneously hyperintense on T1- and T2-weighted *images. The lesion contains internal fatty signal. There are signal voids (notched arrows) in the lesion and a large feeding artery from the common femoral artery (block arrow)*

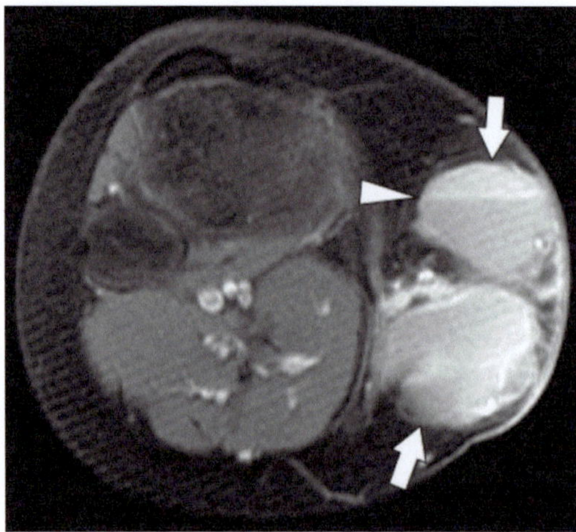

Axial T2 fat saturated

Lymphatic malformation (arrows) with fluid-fluid level (arrowhead).

Report checklist
1. What is the size and exact location of the mass?
2. Does the lesion have fatty areas, internal vessels, and ill-defined margins?
3. Are there phleboliths? Check prior radiographs and CT studies for soft tissue calcifications
4. Is there internal enhancement?
5. Are there feeding or draining vessels? Are any associated vessels arterial to suggest a high-flow lesion?
6. Are there fluid-fluid levels with rim enhancement to indicate a lymphatic malformation?
7. Are there adjacent bony changes (periosteal reaction, remodeling, marrow edema)?

Suggested Reading

Flors L, Leiva-Salinas C, Maged IM, Norton PT, Matsumoto AH, Angle JF, Hugo Bonatti M, Park AW, Ahmad EA, Bozlar U, Housseini AM, Huerta TE, Hagspiel KD. MR imaging of soft-tissue vascular malformations: diagnosis, classification, and therapy follow-up. Radiographics. 2011;31:1321–40.

Flors L, Leiva-Salinas C, Norton PT, Park AW, Ogur T, Hagspiel KD. Ten frequently asked questions about MRI evaluation of soft-tissue vascular anomalies. AJR Am J Roentgenol. 2013;201:W554–62.

Case 7.12

Indication A 48-year-old male with palpable swelling at the plantar aspect of the foot. Rule out soft tissue mass.

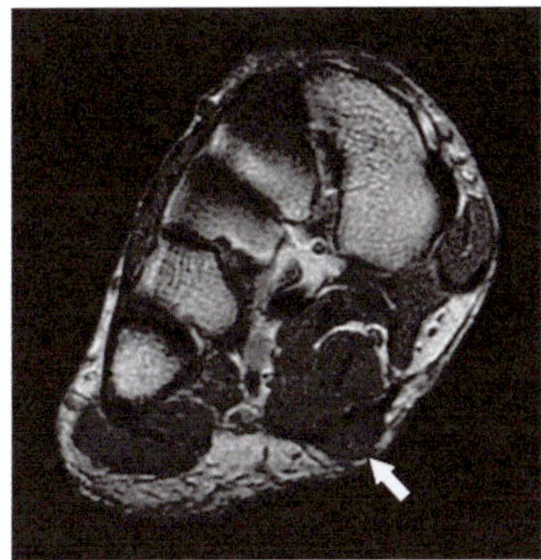

Coronal T1

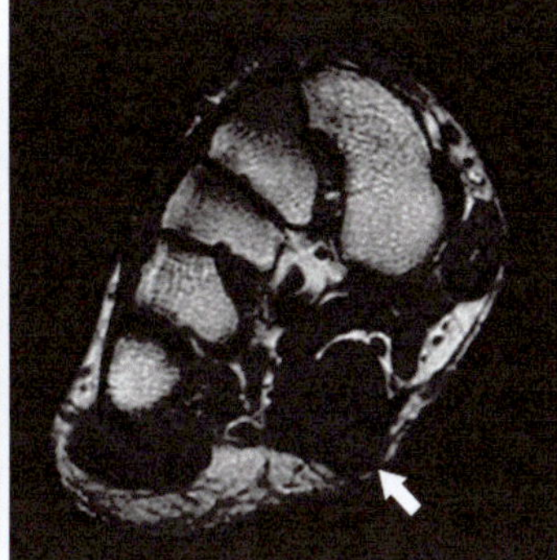

Coronal T2

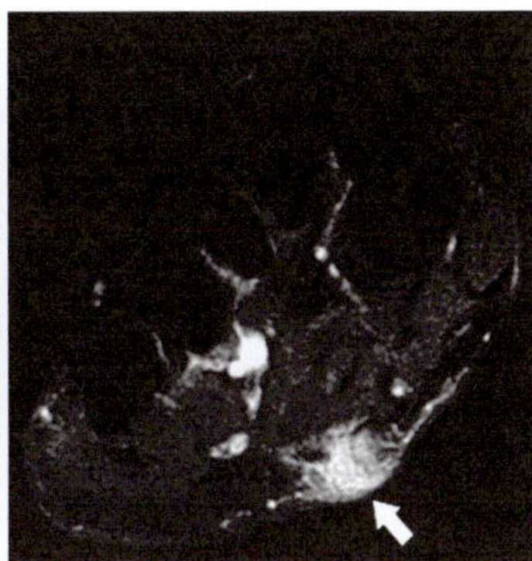

Coronal T1 fat saturated post contrast

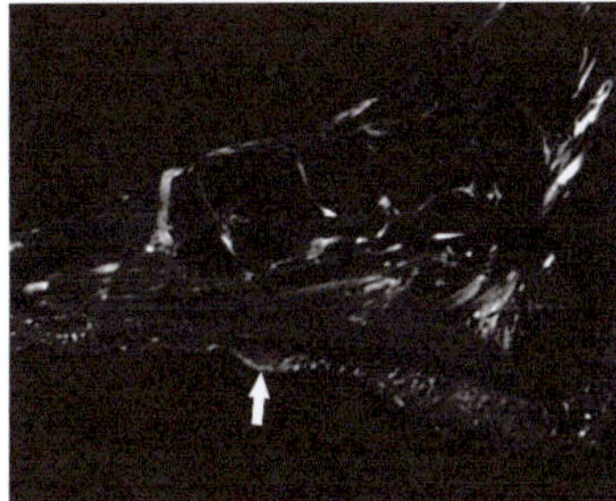

Sagittal STIR

Findings

There is a 1.5 cm soft tissue mass (arrows) arising from the central cord of the plantar fascia. The lesion is uniformly low signal on T1- and T2-weighted images and demonstrates solid internal enhancement. There are linear foci of enhancement/edema (arrowheads) along the fascia arising from the mass consistent with the "fascial tail sign."

Impression/Recommendation

Plantar fibroma.

Discussion: Plantar Fibroma

Plantar fibromas (Ledderhose disease) are the most common solid soft tissue tumor in the foot and ankle. It is composed of spindle cells, contains dense collagen, and typically arises along the plantar aponeurosis of the foot. Plantar fibromas are similar to palmar fibromas (Dupuytren disease) but are less likely to produce contractures which are common in the hand. Plantar fibromas are twice as common in men versus women and are typically seen over the age of 30 and very rare in children. The cause is unclear and believed to be a combination of trauma and genetics. Patients typically complain of a palpable mass along the plantar aspect of the foot and may experience mild pain after standing or walking for long periods. Lesions may be bilateral in 20–50% of patients.

On MR imaging, plantar fibromas are nodular masses adherent to the plantar aponeurosis, typically medial more than lateral. They can be hard to distinguish from the adjacent plantar musculature. Due to their high collagen content, plantar fibromas are uniformly low signal on T1- and T2-weighted images. However, more cellular lesions can have variable high signal on T2 sequences. Plantar fibromas typically have internal enhancement and can have a fascial tail sign where linear foci of enhancement extend from the lesion along the aponeurosis.

Treatment for small lesions is conservative with shoe inserts and orthotics. Steroid injections can also be helpful. However, very symptomatic or large lesions may require surgery. Unfortunately, plantar fibromas can have a relatively high recurrence rate of 20–40%.

Report checklist
1. What is the size and location of the mass?
2. Is the mass attached to the plantar aponeurosis?
3. Is the lesion low signal on T1- and T2-weighted images?
4. Is there solid enhancement or a fascial tail sign?
5. Are there multiple lesions?

Suggested Reading

Draghi F, Gitto S, Bortolotto C, Draghi AG, Ori Belometti G. Imaging of plantar fascia disorders: findings on plain radiography, ultrasound and magnetic resonance imaging. Insights Imaging. 2017;8:69–78.

Omor Y, Dhaene B, Grijseels S, Alard S. Ledderhose Disease: Clinical, Radiological (Ultrasound and MRI), and Anatomopathological Findings. Case Rep Orthop. 2015;2015:741461.

Robbin MR, Murphey MD, Temple HT, Kransdorf MJ, Choi JJ. Imaging of musculoskeletal fibromatosis. Radiographics. 2001; 21:585–600.

Arthropathy

Case 8.1

Indication A 69-year-old woman with worsening chronic hip pain.

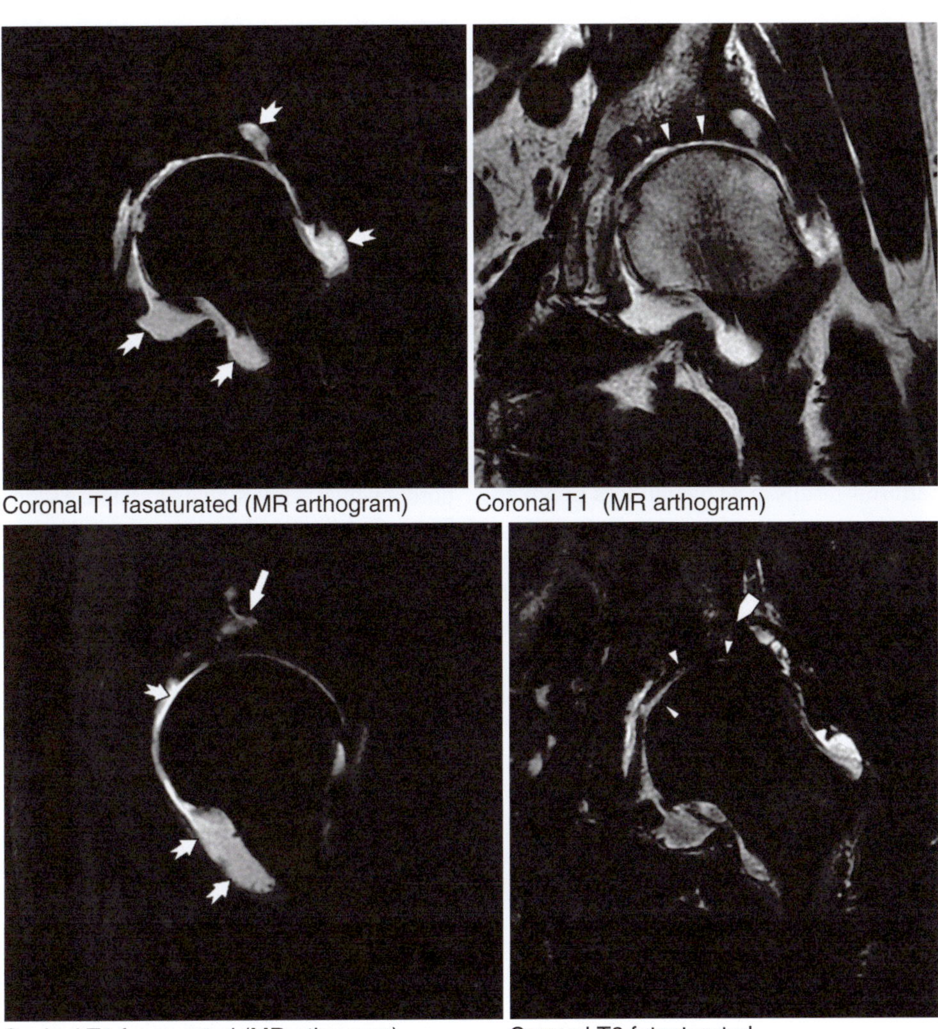

Coronal T1 fasaturated (MR arthogram)

Coronal T1 (MR arthogram)

Sagittal T1 fasaturated (MRarthogram)

Coronal T2 fatsaturated

© Springer Nature Switzerland AG 2020
T. M. Hegazi, J. S. Wu, *Musculoskeletal MRI*, https://doi.org/10.1007/978-3-030-26777-3_8

Findings

There is good distension of the hip joint with dilute gadolinium contrast (notched arrows). There are extensive full-thickness articular cartilage defects (arrowheads) at the weight-bearing portion of the superior femoral head and associated acetabulum. There are prominent subchondral cysts that fill with gadolinium contrast (arrow), best seen on the sagittal T1 fat saturated images. There is mild subchondral marrow edema along the lateral acetabulum (block arrow). There is a complex tear involving the anterior and superior labrum (not shown). There are no MRI signs for stress fracture, osteonecrosis, or marrow replacing lesions.

Impression/Recommendation

Severe osteoarthritis of the left hip with extensive full-thickness cartilage defects, subchondral cysts, and marrow edema along the acetabulum.

Discussion: Osteoarthritis

Osteoarthritis or degenerative joint disease is extremely common. It affects roughly 10% of men and 18% of women over the age of 60 worldwide. Osteoarthritis initially affects hyaline cartilage. Hyaline cartilage possesses a delicate balance of water which is determined by the amount of collagen fibers and proteoglycans. Osteoarthritis results in an overall loss of proteoglycans which increases the water content due to decrease "osmotic pull." This can weaken the collagen fibers and lead to inflammation of the synovial tissue. Eventually the amount of cartilage can decrease in thickness or breakoff as focal defects. This can lead to a cascade of injury to the adjacent bone and fibrocartilage such as the hip labrum or meniscus in the knee. Surrounding tendons and ligament can become thickened and fibrotic to compensate for joint instability and pain. Osteoarthritis can result from many causes including excessive weight, prior trauma, repetitive stresses, prior infection, osteonecrosis, or genetic factors. Patients commonly complain of joint pain and have limited range of motion and joint swelling.

Osteoarthritis can be diagnosed on radiographs as joint space narrowing, osteophytes, subchondral sclerosis, and subchondral cysts. However, MR imaging provides a more complete assessment. MRI is best at delineating the discrete cartilage defects, marrow edema, joint effusions, and injury to supporting structures such as fibrocartilage, tendons, and ligaments. Proton density images are ideal for showing the discrete cartilage defects. Hyaline cartilage defects that extend down to subchondral bone are described as full-thickness defects, whereas those that do not are called partial-thickness defects. Cartilage fissures extend perpendicular to the articular surface, and cartilage flaps are defects that extend oblique or parallel to the articular surface but exit the articular surface *(see supplementary images).* If focal areas of hyaline cartilage loss are present, one should search for loose bodies in the joint space. Subchondral cysts occur after the overlying hyaline cartilage is absent. Joint fluid or synovial tissue can enter the subchondral bone forming the cysts. The cysts often have a thin sclerotic border which is low signal on all pulse sequences. They can fill variably with contrast/fluid depending on the amount of fibrous or synovial tissue within them. Subchondral marrow edema is best seen on T2-weighted or STIR sequences and often overlie areas of full-thickness cartilage loss. If subchondral marrow edema is discovered, it is good practice to take extra time to evaluate the adjacent hyaline cartilage for focal defects.

Treatment for early/mild osteoarthritis is with physical therapy and alterations in activities that cause symptoms. NSAIDS and other pain medications can be helpful. Eventually the patient may require steroid injections to reduce pain long term. Various cartilage surgeries exist. In microfracture surgery, at the area of cartilage loss, the subchondral bone is drilled/pierced. This stimulates the filling in of blood clot and eventually with fibrous tissue. In osteochondral autograft transplantation (OATS), plugs of normal cartilage along with the subchondral bone are removed from non-weight-bearing portions and placed into areas of cartilage loss. In autologous chondrocyte implantation (ACI), healthy cartilage is removed and grown in tissue culture for 6–8 weeks. In a second surgery, the grown cartilage cells are placed over the cartilage defect with a collagen patch and allowed to fill the defect. Stem cells and platelet-rich plasma (PRP) are other treatment options. Patients with diffuse cartilage loss and persistent pain will ultimately require joint arthroplasty.

Supplementary images

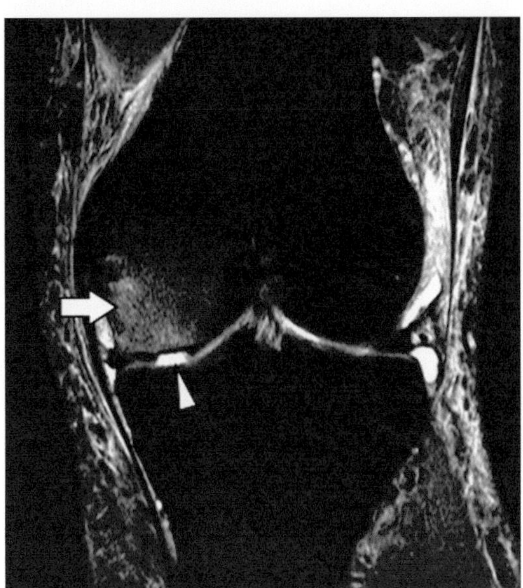

Coronal T1 fat saturated

There is an 11-mm full-thickness hyaline cartilage defect (arrowhead) in the medial femoral condyle with adjacent subchondral marrow edema (arrow)

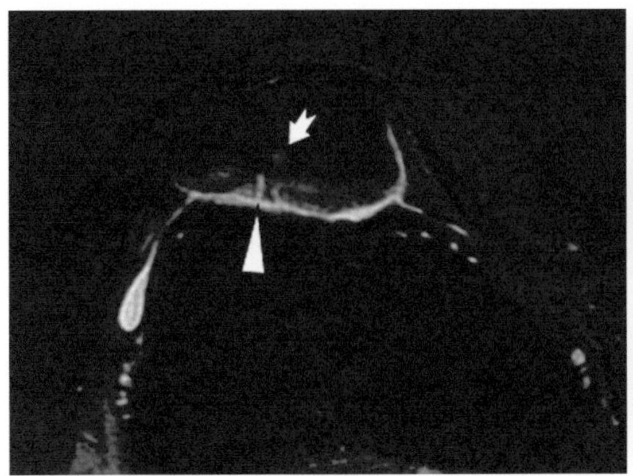

Axial T2 fat saturated

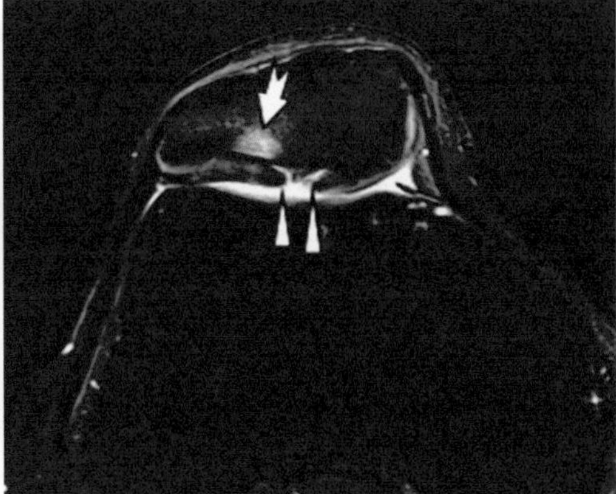

Axial T2 fat saturated

In the first image, there is a full-thickness cartilage fissure (arrowhead) that extends perpendicularly to the lateral patellar facet with associated subchondral marrow edema (notched arrow). In the second image (different patient), deep cartilage flaps (arrowheads) are seen extending obliquely to the lateral patellar facet bony surface, also with subchondral marrow edema (notched arrow)

Report checklist.
1. Where is the cartilage loss? Is it on both sides of the joint?
2. Are the hyaline cartilage defects full thickness, partial thickness, fissures, or flaps?
3. Are there any loose bodies?
4. Are there subchondral cysts?
5. Is there subchondral marrow edema? If yes, double-check for hyaline cartilage defects.
6. How are the supporting structures (menisci, labrum, tendons, ligaments)?

Suggested Reading

Hill CL. et al. Synovitis detected on magnetic resonance imaging and its relation to pain and cartilage loss in knee osteoarthritis. Ann Rheum Dis 2007;66:1599–603.

Loeuille D. et al. Macroscopic and microscopic features of synovial membrane inflammation in the osteoarthritic knee: correlating magnetic resonance imaging findings with disease severity. Arthritis Rheum. 2005;52:3492–501.

Menashe L. et al. The diagnostic performance of MRI in osteoarthritis: a systematic review and meta-analysis. Osteoarthritis Cartilage. 2012;20:13–21.

Case 8.2

Indication A 46-year-old woman with pain in the MCPs joints and normal radiographs

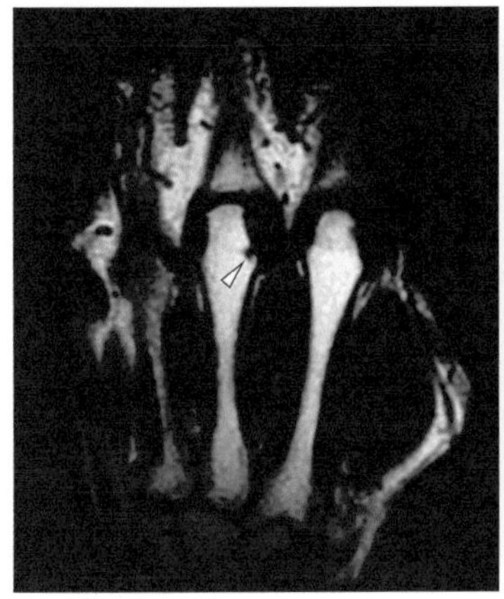

Coronal T1

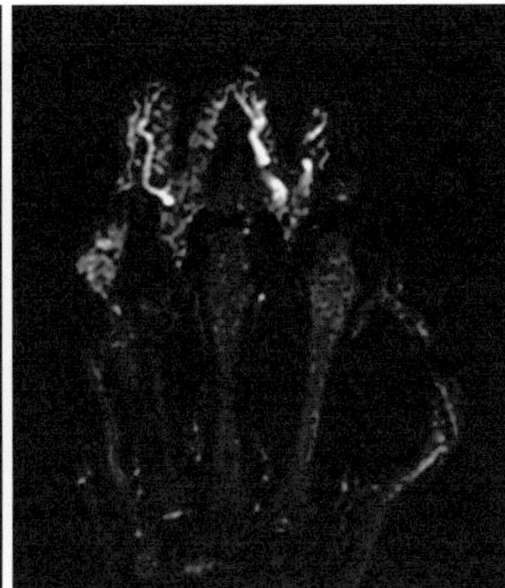

Coronal T2 fat saturated

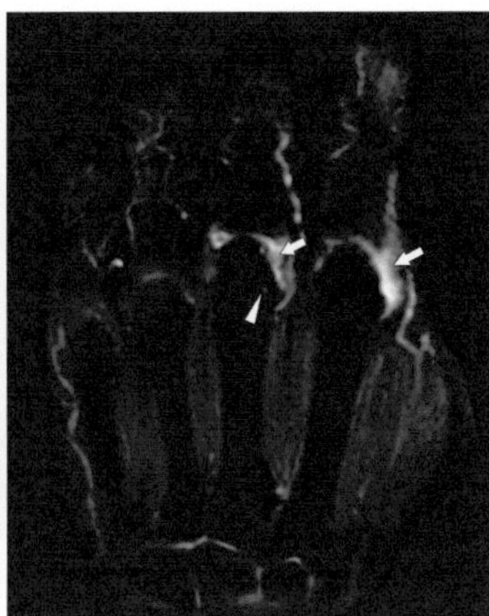

Coronal T1 fat saturated post contrast

Findings

There is prominent synovial enhancement of the index and long finger MCP joints (arrows). There is small margin erosion along the radial aspect of the longer finger metacarpal head (arrowheads). The radial aspects of the metacarpal heads also have subchondral irregularity and enhancement consistent with osteitis. There is no joint effusion, marrow edema, significant joint space narrowing, or abnormalities of the adjacent tendons.

Impression/Recommendation

Synovial enhancement of the index and long finger metacarpophalangeal MCP joints and marginal erosion of the longer finger metacarpal head consistent with an inflammatory arthropathy such as rheumatoid arthritis.

Discussion: Inflammatory Arthritis – Rheumatoid Arthritis

An inflammatory arthritis is characterized by inflammation of the joints and adjacent tissues (tendons, cartilage, bursa). The most common diseases in this group are rheumatoid arthritis, psoriatic arthritis, reactive arthritis, ankylosing spondylitis (AS), and systemic lupus erythematosus (SLE). Each of these arthritidies can affect characteristic joints, often in a specific pattern. For instance, rheumatoid arthritis classically affects the wrist and MCP joints. Psoriasis typically involves the hands, while reactive arthritis affects the feet. AS most commonly affects the spine, SI joints, and hips. These diseases are often autoimmune in origin, generally more common in women (except AS), but many have a multifactorial etiology. Symptoms depend on the joints involved, and early diagnosis with the initiation of anti-inflammatory medications (nonsteroidal anti-inflammatory drugs (NSAIDs) and disease-modifying antirheumatic drugs (DMARDs)) is the mainstay of treatment. The goal is to prevent joint destruction and delay surgical intervention.

MR imaging can be very helpful in establishing the early diagnosis of an inflammatory arthritis as findings on radiographs are typically only apparent in the later stages of the disease. The three main findings of an inflammatory arthritis on MRI are (1) synovitis, (2) osteitis, and (3) erosions. Synovitis, or synovial proliferation, is indicative of active disease and will appear as high signal on T2-weighted images and have enhancement on post-contrast images. It is important to distinguish synovial proliferation from joint fluid as the later will be high signal on T2 but will not have enhancement. Osteitis is the presence of bone marrow edema in a subarticular location and seen in the early stage of the disease process. Osteitis can coexist with the third main MRI findings, erosions, which represents the cumulative effect of the inflammatory pannus upon the bone and inflammation within the bone. They appear as focal defects in the bone, and most erosions in inflammatory arthritidies are in a marginal location. This is the anatomic location at the periphery of the bone and joint capsule where there is absence of articular cartilage. MRI has been shown to be seven times more sensitive than radiographs for detecting erosions. Other important MRI findings are the presence of tenosynovitis or bursitis as these structures can contain synovial tissue. Fluid can be seen in these structures and can be confused with tenosynovitis or septic bursitis. If in doubt, aspiration may be required to assess for an infection. In later-stage disease, the articular cartilage can be damaged and lead to focal defects and should be described in the report.

Report checklist
1. Is there synovitis?
2. Are there erosions?
3. Is there bone marrow edema (osteitis)?
4. Is there a joint effusion?
5. How is the articular cartilage?
6. Is there tenosynovitis?
7. What is the distribution of disease (single or multiple joints, which joints)?

Suggested Reading

Boesen M, Østergaard M, Cimmino MA, Kubassova O, Jensen KE, Bliddal H. MRI quantification of rheumatoid arthritis: current knowledge and future perspectives. Eur J Radiol. 2009;71:189–96.

Chang EY. Adult inflammatory arthritides: what the radiologist should know Radiographics. 2016;36:1849–70.

Narváez JA, Narváez J, De Lama E, De Albert M. MR imaging of early rheumatoid arthritis. Radiographics. 2010;30:143–63.

Case 8.3

Indication A 44-year-old woman with hand pain, skin lesions, and swelling of the metacarpophalangeal (MCP) joints of the index and small fingers.

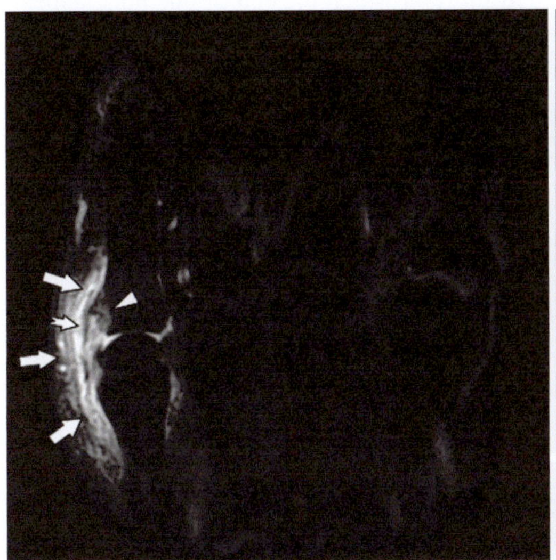

Coronal T1 fat saturated post contrast

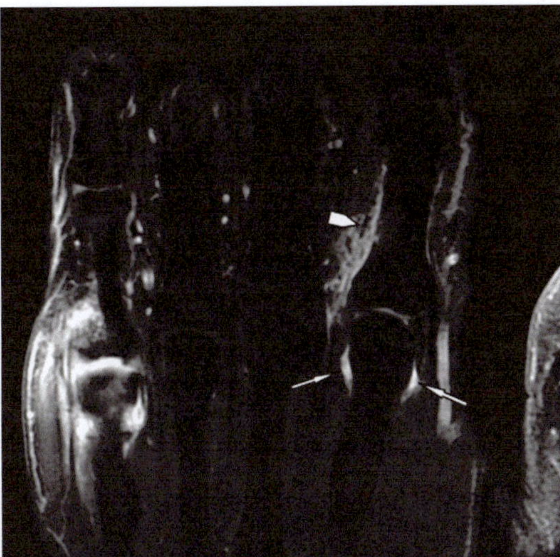

Coronal T1 fat saturated post contrast

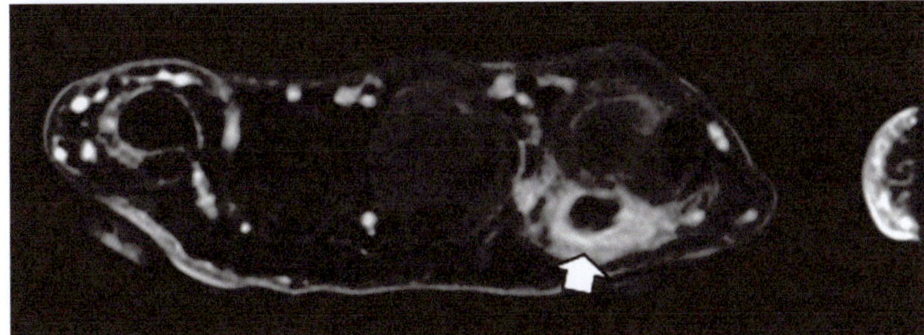

Axial T1 fat saturated post contrast

Findings

In the small finger MCP joint, there is enhancing proliferative synovitis with a small erosion (arrowhead) and marrow edema at the ulnar margin of the base of the proximal phalanx, not visible on the recent radiograph. There is also extensive soft tissue edema (arrows) surrounding the base of the proximal phalanx and the head of the metacarpal. There is thickening and edema of the ulnar collateral ligament (notched arrow). In the index finger, there is mild enhancing synovitis (thin arrows) about the metacarpal head and prominent marrow edema along the shaft of the proximal phalanx (block arrow) consistent with periostitis, greater on the ulnar side. There is extensive tenosynovitis (thick arrow) of the index finger flexor tendon, best seen on the axial images centered at the level of the MCP joint. There is no tendon tear.

Impression/Recommendation

1. Small erosion and extensive synovitis in the small finger MCP.
2. Tenosynovitis of the index finger flexor tendon without tear.
3. Moderate synovitis of the index finger MCP joint with periostitis about the proximal phalanx shaft.
4. Overall findings are compatible with an inflammatory arthropathy, likely psoriatic arthritis.

Discussion: Psoriatic arthritis

Psoriatic arthritis is an inflammatory arthropathy seen in patients with psoriasis, a chronic autoimmune disorder characterized by itchy plaque-like skin lesions. Psoriatic arthritis is also a seronegative spondyloarthropathy as it can affect the sacroiliac joints and less than half of patients are positive for HLA-B27. Patients typically develop painful swelling of the fingers and toes resulting in a sausage digit appearance, also called dactylitis. There can be associated pitting changes in the nail beds. The disorder is seen in 30% of patients with psoriasis and affects men and women equally. Patients typically have known psoriasis when joint issues occur, but in 10–20% of patients, the joint problems can precede skin changes. Early diagnosis is important in order to initiate prompt therapy and slow the progression of joint destruction.

On imaging, psoriatic arthritis is characterized by enthesitis, marginal erosions, synovitis, periostitis, and joint subluxations. For psoriatic arthritis, enthesitis occurs first and is then followed by synovitis. This is different than rheumatoid arthritis where synovitis is the main problem *(please refer to Case 8.2 for further discussion on rheumatoid arthritis)*. Enthesitis refers to inflammation at tendon, ligament, or joint capsule insertions, and therefore, abnormalities can occur outside the joint. Enthesitis is considered to be the primary site of joint inflammation in psoriatic arthritis and other spondyloarthropathies. Entheses can be classified as fibrous or fibrocartilaginous, and findings in psoriatic arthritis occur in the fibrocartilaginous type, such as the distal Achilles tendon or small muscles of the hands. An example of a fibrous enthesis would be the deltoid tendon insertion on the humeral shaft. On MRI, enthesitis will appear as edema and enhancement at these sites. Similar to other inflammatory arthropathies, synovitis is seen in psoriatic arthritis. This will appear as high signal on edema-sensitive sequences (T2 and STIR) and will enhance due to the hypervascularity of the synovium. Erosions can appear in a marginal location due to synovial proliferation.

Tenosynovitis can also be seen and typically affects the flexor tendons more than the extensors, similar to the case presented here. In late-stage disease, there can be a pencil-in-cup deformity in which the end of one bone appears like a pencil entering a cup. One should also look for changes (irregularity and edema) at the nail bed which is typical of psoriatic arthritis and can help differentiate it from rheumatoid arthritis. Lastly, MRI will identify changes of psoriatic arthritis much earlier than other imaging modalities such as radiographs, which can help with early diagnosis and prompt treatment.

Similar to other inflammatory arthropathies, treatment for psoriatic arthritis is with NSAIDs, disease-modifying antirheumatic drugs (DMARDS), and TNF inhibitors. Recently, phosphodiesterase-4 inhibitors, such as apremilast, have shown efficacy. These agents break down cyclic adenosine monophosphate, cAMP, resulting in the downregulation of various inflammatory factors and upregulation of some anti-inflammatory factors. Corticosteroid injections and joint replacement can be performed in later stages of the disease.

Report checklist

1. Is there enthesitis (i.e., edema and enhancement at capsular and tendinous attachments)?
2. Is there synovitis or erosions?
3. Are there signs of inflammation in other synovial tissues such as tenosynovitis?
4. Which joints are involved?
5. Are there nailbed findings?
6. Does the patient have a history of psoriasis?

Suggested Reading

Burge AJ. Imaging of inflammatory arthritis in adults status and perspectives on the use of radiographs, ultrasound, and MRI. Rheum Dis Clin N Am. 2016; 42:561–85.

Spadaro A, Lubrano E. Psoriatic arthritis: imaging techniques. Reumatismo. 2012; 64: 99–106.

Watad A, Eshed I, McGonagle D. Lessons learned from imaging on enthesitis in psoriatic arthritis. Isr Med Assoc J. 2017;19:708–11.

Case 8.4

Indication A 57-year-old man with swelling and pain of great toe.

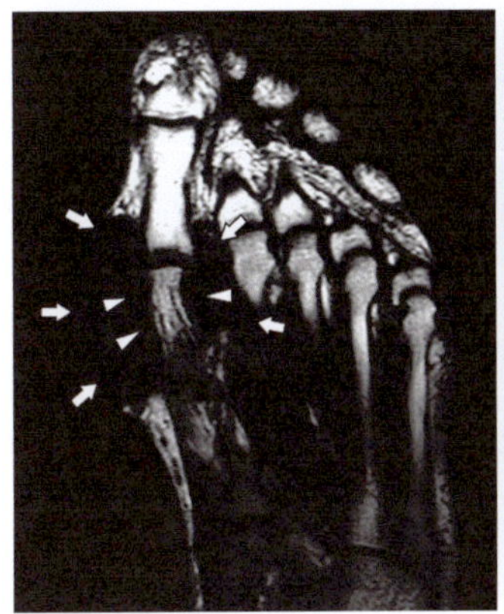

Axial T1

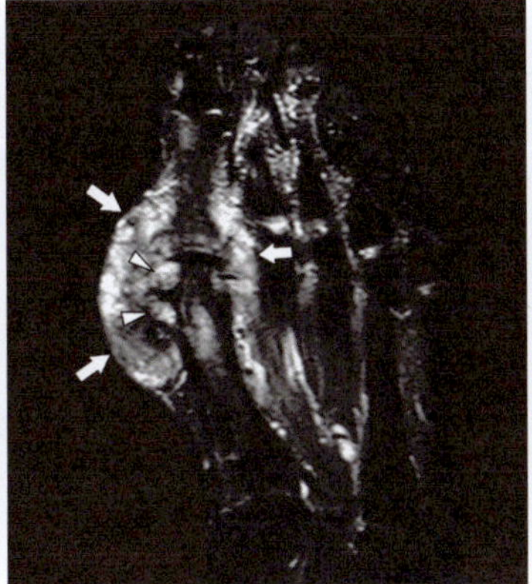

Axial T1 fat saturated post contrast

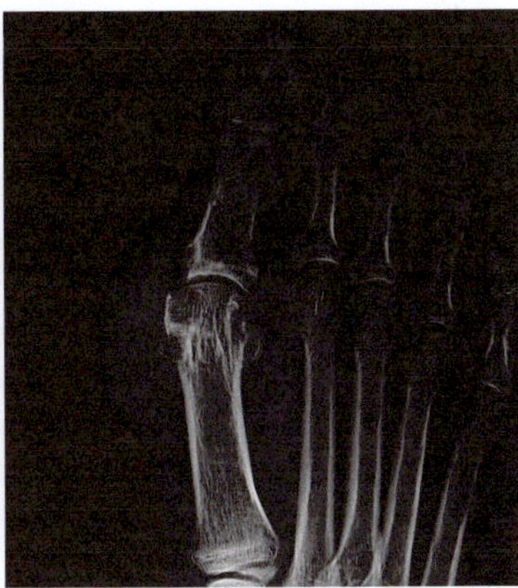

Findings

There are marginal and periarticular erosions (arrowheads) at the first MTP joint due to large soft tissue masses (arrows) that are low signal on T1-weighted images and heterogeneous on T2-weighted images (not shown). The masses are compatible with tophi as seen on the radiographs and have heterogeneous enhancement on the post-contrast images. There is moderate marrow edema and enhancement in the distal first metatarsal head and first proximal phalanx without replacement of the normal T1 marrow signal. There are no significant joint effusions.

Impression/Recommendation

Prominent erosions and soft tissue tophi at the first MTP joint compatible with tophaceous gout.

Discussion: Tophaceous Gout

Gout is an inflammatory arthritis due to high serum levels of uric acid and affects 1–2% of the US population. Most cases of gout, 90%, are due to the underexcretion of uric acid by the kidneys as opposed to overproduction. Gout can occur from a combination of genetics, diet (excess consumption of meat, beer, and seafood), certain medical conditions (obesity, metabolic syndrome, kidney disease, insulin resistance), and medications (diuretics). Symptoms occur from the crystallization of uric acid in and around joint tissue.

The great toe at the 1st MTP is the most classic location for gout (as in this case); however, any joint can be affected. Soft tissue deposits of uric acid, or tophi, can develop and appear as white or yellowish-white, chalky nodules. Their presence is pathognomonic for gout and occurs on average 10 years after the onset of the disease. Although gout is best known for its effects upon joints, untreated gout can lead to cardiovascular and renal complications.

The diagnosis of gout is made by identifying monosodium urate crystals in the joint fluid. The crystals will be negatively birefringent under polarized microscopy; however, identification of the crystals in joint fluid or synovial tissue can be hard, even during an acute flare. Imaging can be very helpful in these cases. Radiographs can demonstrate the characteristic peri- or juxta-articular erosions which occur outside the joint capsule. The slow formation of the erosions can give an overhanging edge appearance. Early in the disease process, the joint space is spared; however, during later stages of the diseases, the erosions can be in the joint space and are often marginal in location. Dual-energy CT can be especially helpful for the diagnosis for gout. Using two energy sources at different kVp values, tissue containing uric acid can be distinguished from tissue containing calcium. This allows for the earlier diagnosis of gout with higher sensitivity than other imaging modalities. MRI is best used for the evaluation of the soft tissue structures affected by gout and for marrow edema. This includes the presence of tophi and synovitis but is also helpful for early erosions appearing as discrete foci of high T2 signal. Tophi are classically uniformly low signal on T1-weighted images but are heterogeneously high signal on T2 and heterogeneously enhancing on post-contrast images. Bone marrow edema can be present, but is typically less severe than would be seen with osteomyelitis.

Similar to other arthropathies, early diagnosis and initiation of treatment is of high importance in order to prevent joint destruction. Treatment can begin with diet and lifestyle changes, such as limiting beer and meat intake and initiating an exercise program. Nonsteroidal anti-inflammatory drugs (NSAIDs), steroids, or colchicine can improve acute symptoms. During the preventive phase of gout, allopurinol or probenecid (uric acid lowering agents) can help prevent recurrent gout attacks.

Report checklist

1. What joints are involved?
2. Are there erosions and are they juxta-articular (outside the joint space)?
3. Is there soft tissue tophi or synovitis?
4. Is there bone marrow edema (presence of marrow edema is more common in infection versus gout)?
5. Is there a joint effusion? If present, the location should be described to aid with potential joint aspiration.

Suggested Reading

Chowalloor PV, Siew TK, Keen HI. 143 imaging in gout: a review of the recent developments. Ther Adv Musculoskel Dis. 2014;6:131.

Teh J, McQueen F, Eshed I, Plagou A, Klauser A. Advanced imaging in the diagnosis of gout and other crystal arthropathies. Semin Musculoskelet Radiol. 2018;22:225–36.

Terra MP, Maas M, Buckens CF. Computed tomography and MR imaging in crystalline-induced arthropathies. Radiol Clin N Am. 2017;52:1023–34.

Case 8.5

Indication A 51-year-old man with history of IV drug abuse and severe right hip pain, fever, and elevated white count.

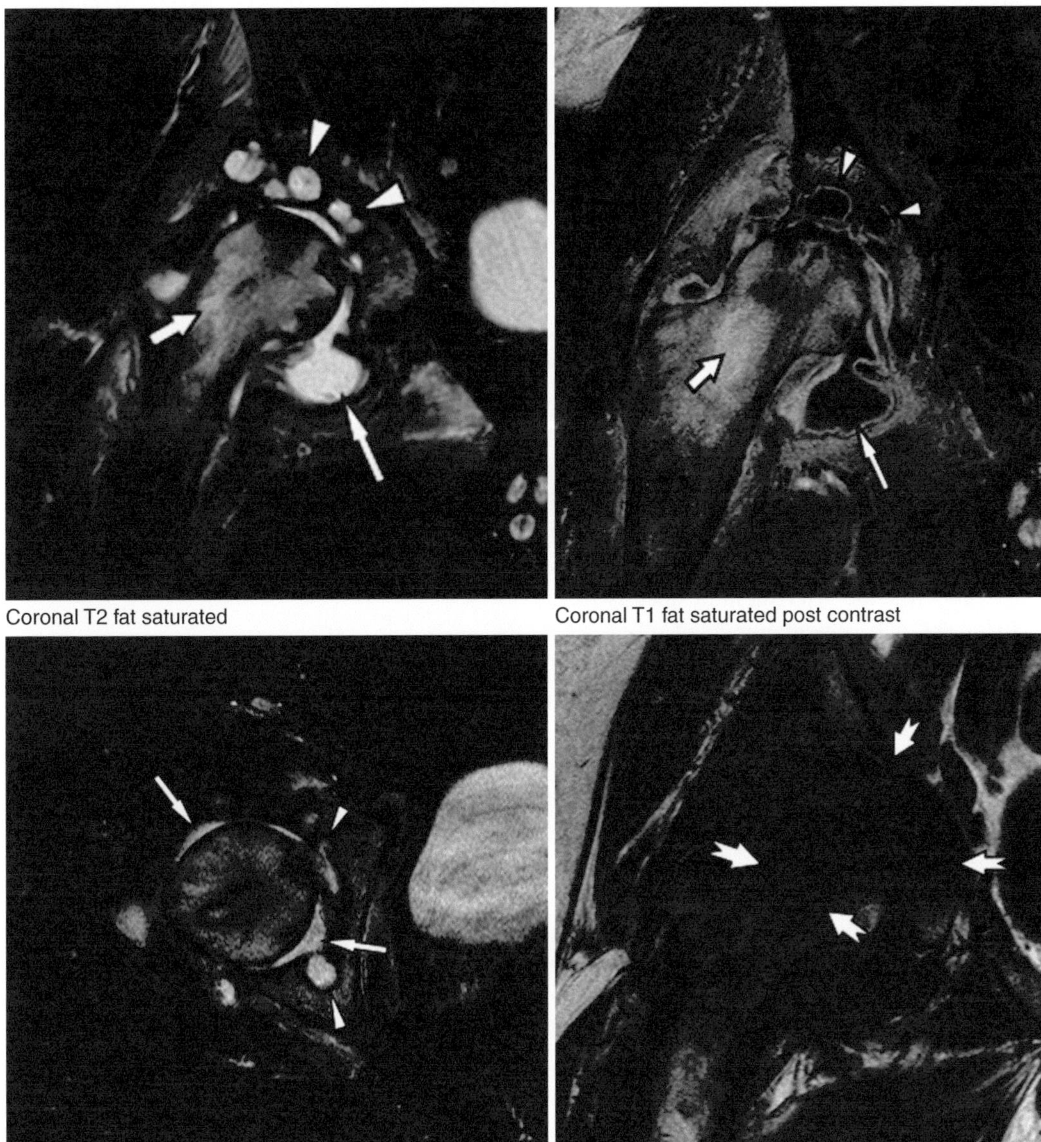

Coronal T2 fat saturated

Coronal T1 fat saturated post contrast

Axial T2 fat saturated

Cortonal T1

Findings

There is a large right hip joint effusion (thin arrows) with enhancement of the synovium and perisynovial edema. There are large erosions in the acetabulum (arrowheads) and smaller erosions along the femoral head. There is abnormal enhancement and marrow edema (arrows) in the proximal femur and the acetabulum. The marrow signal is hypointense to skeletal muscle (notched arrows) on the T1-weighted sequences, suspicious for osteomyelitis. There is prominent reactive edema in the surrounding muscles of the hip without rim-enhancing fluid collections.

Impression/Recommendation

Findings are highly suspicious for right septic hip arthritis with osteomyelitis of the proximal femur and acetabulum. Diagnostic arthrocentesis of the hip joint is recommended.

Discussion: Septic arthritis

Infection of the joint space is termed septic arthritis and has an incidence of 1 in 10,000 people in the USA. However, the rate is seven times higher in patients with a joint prosthesis or rheumatoid arthritis. Patients with IV drug abuse, diabetes, and who are immunocompromised are also at increased risk. The knee followed by the hip and then shoulder are the most commonly infected joints, although any joint can be infected. Most cases are the result of hematogenous spread. This is likely due to the fact that bacterial organisms can easily enter the synovial fluid since synovial tissue lacks a basement membrane. The most common causative organisms are *Staphylococcus aureus*. Patients typically present with joint pain, limited range of motion, fever, elevated white count, and elevated ESR. It is important to make the diagnosis quickly as delay in treatment can lead to joint destruction, secondary osteoarthritis, osteonecrosis, and sepsis.

MR imaging can be especially helpful in supporting the diagnosis of septic arthritis and is abnormal as early as 24 hours from the onset of infection. Synovial enhancement (98%), perisynovial edema (84%), and joint effusions (70%) are the most common MRI findings associated with septic arthritis. The lack of these findings can be helpful in excluding septic arthritis eliminating the need for arthrocentesis. Larger joints are more likely to have a joint effusion. Septic arthritis can be associated with osteomyelitis in which the bone marrow will have T1 signal that is

hypointense to skeletal muscle and can have erosions in the bare areas.

Treatment for septic arthritis should be initiated as early as possible. Although imaging and clinical features can be suggestive of septic arthritis, arthrocentesis with a positive culture of an infectious agent is the gold standard. Imaging can help with preprocedure targeting of the joint for attaining joint fluid. Joint fluid should be sent for microbiologic culture, gram stain, and cell count/differential in virtually all cases. A cell count of >50,000/μL with predominance of neutrophils is suggestive of infection. Crystal analysis, AFB, and fungal cultures can also be considered. Polymerase chain reaction (PCR) of synovial fluid and alpha-defensin assays of bacterial microbicidal peptides have become more popular and can identify the causative organism with a few hours of testing. The treatment of a septic joint is with joint lavage and systemic antibiotics tailored to the responsible organism.

Report checklist

1. Is there a joint effusion?
2. Is there synovial enhancement or perisynovial edema?
3. Are there associated changes in the bone to suggest osteomyelitis (low T1 marrow signal, marrow edema, erosions)?
4. Is there an associated soft tissue abscess or reactive edema in the surrounding soft tissues?
5. Does the patient have risk factors for septic arthritis (hardware, rheumatoid arthritis, HIV, diabetic, IVDA, fever, high WBC, or ESR)?

Suggested Reading

Bierry G, Huang AJ, Chang CY, Torriani M, Bredella MA. MRI findings of treated bacterial septic arthritis. Skeletal Radiol. 2012;41:1509–16.

Karchevsky M, Schweitzer ME, Morrison WB, Parellada JA. MRI findings of septic arthritis and associated osteomyelitis in adults. AJR Am J Roentgenol. 2004;182:119–22.

Case 8.6

Indication A 31-year-old woman with bilateral, right worse than left, lower back pain.

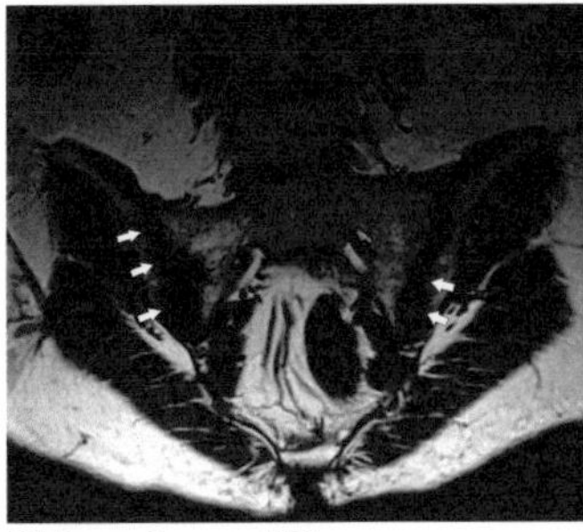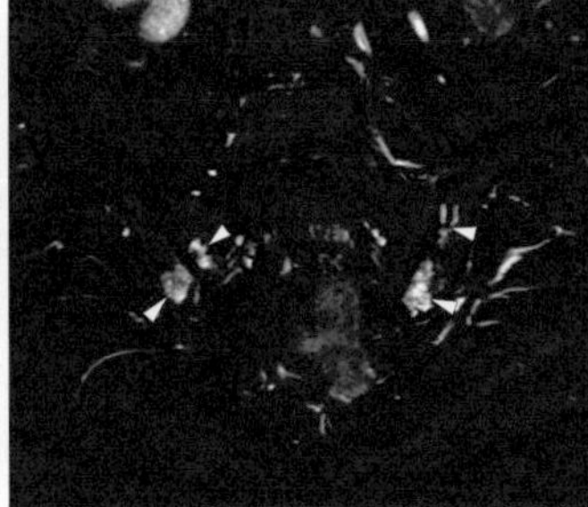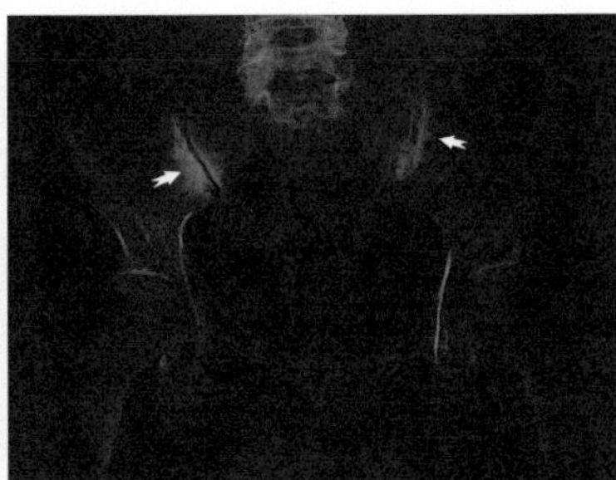

Oblique Coronal T1   Oblique Coronal T2 fat saturated

Findings

There are erosions at the inferior aspects of bilateral sacroiliac joints, right worse than left and more prominent on the iliac versus the sacral side. The erosions (arrows) are hypointense on T1-weighted images, and there is associated marrow edema (arrowheads). Findings correspond to areas of sclerosis (notched arrows) on the prior radiographs. There is no fluid in the SI joint on either side (case courtesy of Dr. Jennifer Ni Mhuircheartaigh).

Impression/Recommendation

There is bilateral sacroiliitis, worse on the right side. Findings are suggestive of an inflammatory spondyloarthropathy (SpA). Infection is felt to be less likely given the lack of SI joint fluid and bilateral involvement.

Discussion: Sacroiliitis

Sacroiliitis is inflammation of the SI joint and is a key finding in SpA, including ankylosing spondylitis, psoriatic arthritis, reactive arthritis, and arthritis of inflammatory bowel disease. These conditions are typically bilateral but can be symmetric or asymmetric. Features favoring SpA include a positive family history for SpA, HLA-B27 positivity, elevated C-reactive protein, and improvement with anti-inflammatory medications. Patients complain of lower back pain and can have other systemic symptoms depending on their underlying disease. Trauma, pregnancy, and infection can also affect the SI joint. Infection of the SI joint is typically unilateral; however, some SpAs can be unilateral during their early stages.

MR imaging is important in the evaluation of SpA. The criteria given by the Assessment of SpondyloArthritis International Society (ASAS), established in 2009, use four MRI findings for the imaging diagnosis of active sacroiliitis. These are osteitis (bone marrow edema), enthesitis, capsulitis, and synovitis. Osteitis or bone marrow edema is the most important criteria and appears as high signal on fluid-sensitive sequences. Enthesitis, capsulitis, and synovitis are best diagnosed as edema and enhancement at those sites. Erosions or fluid in the SI joint are additional supporting findings of sacroiliitis. At times, it can be difficult to distinguish a SpA from a septic SI joint (*see supplementary images*). Features favoring an infection include thick capsulitis, extracapsular fluid collection, and periarticular muscle edema. Abscess formation can extend from the SI joint in the psoas muscles. It is important to remember that the SI joint is unique in that it has both fibrous and synovial components. The posterosuperior portion if the joint is fibrous and the anteroinferior portion is synovial and the site affected in SpA. In addition, the cartilage on the sacral side is thicker than the iliac side and therefore more protective. Thus, findings of erosions, bone marrow edema, and subchondral sclerosis are typically more prominent on the iliac side versus the sacral side in SpA. If abnormalities are localized to the sacral side, an alternate diagnosis maybe present, such as a stress fracture. An oblique coronal plane depicting the entire SI joint should be included in dedicated SI joint MR protocols.

Treatment for sacroiliitis depends on the baseline disease process. Medical therapy with NSAIDs, TNF inhibitors, and DMARDS can be effective. Corticosteroid injections directly into the SI joint under fluoroscopic or CT guidance are also effective.

Supplementary images

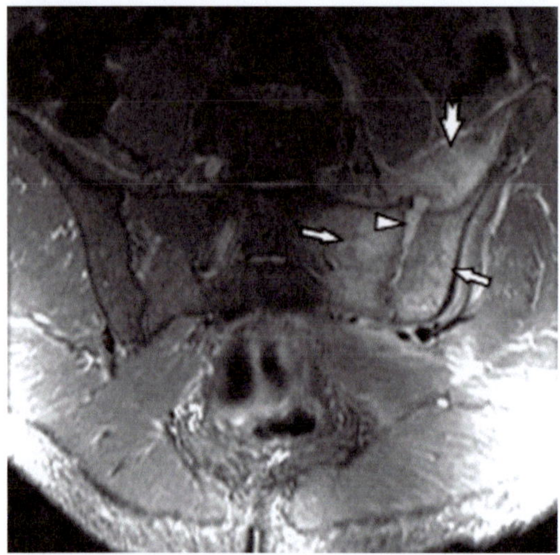

Oblique Coronal T2 fat saturated

A 35-year-old man with severe left lower back pain and history of IV drug use. There is marrow edema (arrows) in the sacrum and iliac bone with widening of this the SI joint (arrowhead). There is also abnormal edema in the left iliacus muscle (notched arrow). The right SI joint is normal. Unilateral sacroiliitis should be considered infectious until proven otherwise

Report checklist

1. Is there marrow edema about the SI joint? Is it more prominent on the iliac or sacral side?
2. Are there edema and enhancement in or at the periphery of the joint capsule to indicate synovitis and/or capsulitis
3. Are there bone erosions in the SI joint?
4. Is there fluid in the SI joint, extracapsular fluid collections, or muscle edema suggesting a septic SI joint?
5. Is the process unilateral or bilateral?

Suggested Reading

Ayd U, Ngöz A. Critical overview of the imaging arm of the ASAS criteria for diagnosing axial spondyloarthritis: what the radiologist should know. Diagn Interv Radiol. 2012; 18:555–65.

Chang EY. Adult inflammatory arthritides: what the radiologist should know. Radiographics 2016;36:1849–70.

Kang Y, Hong SH, Kim JY, Yoo HJ, Choi JY, Yi M, Kang HS. Unilateral sacroiliitis: differential diagnosis between infectious sacroiliitis and spondyloarthritis based on MRI findings. AJR Am J Roentgenol. 2015;205:1048–55.

Case 8.7

Indication A 57-year-old man with type 2 diabetes and chronic foot deformities. Now with pain, swelling, and deep plantar foot ulcer. Evaluate for osteomyelitis.

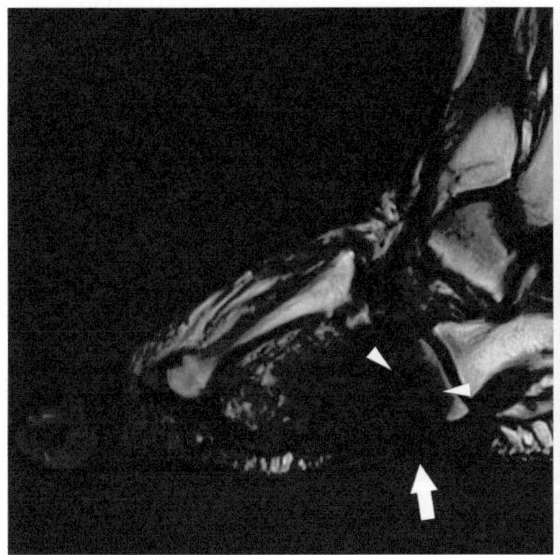

Sagittal T1

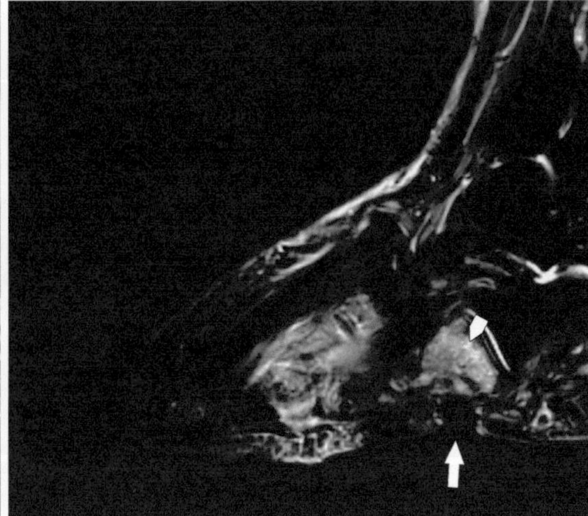

Sagittal T2 fat saturated

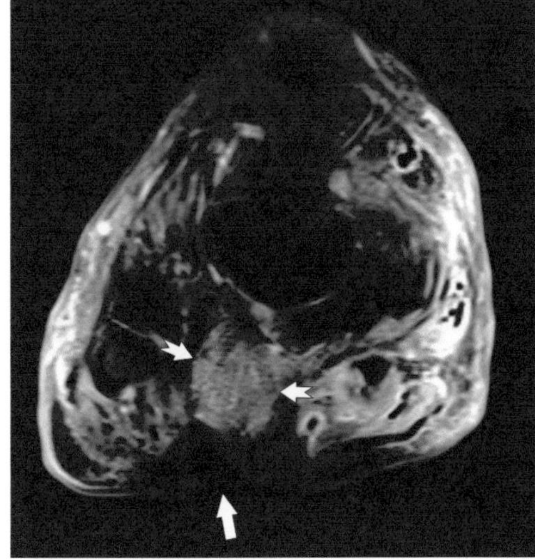

Coronal T1 fat saturated post contrast

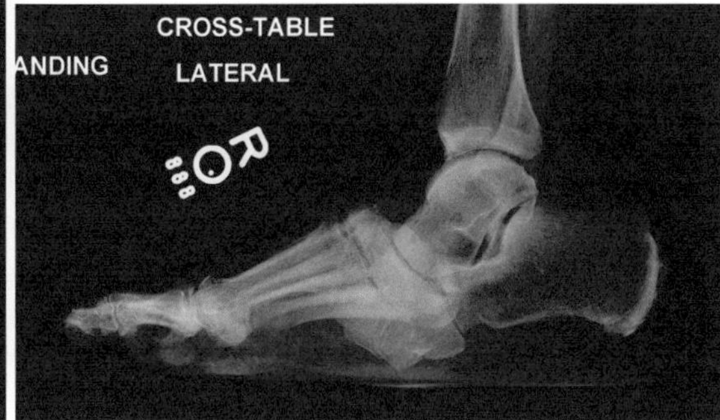

Findings

There are deformity of the midfoot with osseous fragmentation and inferior dislocation of the cuneiforms and navicular in relationship to the metatarsal bases, compatible with Charcot neuropathic arthropathy (CN), similar to the prior radiographs. There is a deep plantar soft tissue ulcer (arrows) that extends to the cuboid. On the T1-weighted image, the margins of the cuboid (arrowheads) are indistinct and replaced by low signal marrow signal which is isointense to skeletal muscle. There is abnormal marrow edema (block arrow) and enhancement (notched arrow) within the medullary portion of the cuboid on the T2 fat saturated and post-contrast T1-weighted images, respectively. These findings are consistent with osteomyelitis. There are no rim-enhancing abscess collections, tenosynovitis, or septic arthritis. The large veins are patent.

Impression/Recommendation

Osteomyelitis of the cuboid arising from a deep plantar soft tissue ulcer with background Charcot neuropathic arthropathy.

Discussion: Charcot neuropathic arthropathy

Charcot neuropathic arthropathy (CN) is a progressive disease that often affects the joints and soft tissue of the foot and ankle, typically in patients with diabetes. It occurs in 13% of patients with high-risk diabetic patients and up to 30% of patients with diabetic peripheral neuropathy. CN can also occur with other disorders besides diabetes such as trauma, rheumatoid arthritis, multiple sclerosis, alcoholism, syringomyelia, and leprosy. The prevailing theory for the pathogenesis of CN is that minor trauma or infection in a patient with peripheral neuropathy leads to a cascade of inflammatory changes that causes bone destruction. This injury induces the release of proinflammatory cytokines which causes the expression of receptor activator of nuclear factor kappa-B ligand (RANKL). Increase in RANKL results in osteoclast maturation and activation which leads to osteolysis. This osteolysis leads to bone injury which is not recognized by the patient due to the peripheral neuropathy and results in a vicious cycle. CN has two clinic phases. In the acute phase, the foot/ankle is warm, swollen, and red and should be without skin and soft tissue ulcers. C-reactive protein or erythrocyte sedimentation rate can be slightly elevated. Skin temperature is typically 2–6 °C higher than the contralateral foot. The patient may not have any pain due to their peripheral neuropathy. In the chronic phase, the warmth and redness have resolved, but swelling remains. Skin temperature differences are typically much improved. However, osseous deformities occur in this stage. Often a rocker-bottom deformity occurs in the midfoot due to fragmentation of the midfoot bones. Soft tissue ulcers can develop, leading to osteomyelitis.

CN can be well evaluated with radiographs; however, if there is suspicion for osteomyelitis in a patient with CN, then MRI is the best modality. On radiographs, CN can be characterized by the Eichenholtz classification. Stage 1 (bone dissolution) is the damaging acute phase and characterized by osteopenia, joint laxity, and a swollen and erythematous foot. In stage 2 (coalescence or repair phase), there are bone debris with osseous fusion or osteosclerosis and reduction in redness and warmth of the foot. In stage 3 (remodeling, chronic, or healed phase), there are bony remodeling, fragmentation, collapse of the foot, and rocker-bottom deformity without inflammation. The latter stages are characterized by the five or six "D"s of CN – distended (joint effusion), disorganized, dislocated, debris (intra-articular bodies and fracture fragments), increased density (sclerosis), and destruction. Disorganization and dislocation are combined if using five "D"s. There is also a stage 0 where clinical symptoms are present; however, radiographs are normal. MRI can be helpful in diagnosing CN, and findings can appear earlier than on radiographs. In the acute phase, edema-sensitive sequences (STIR or T2 fat saturated) can identify bone marrow edema, soft tissue edema, and joint effusion. The marrow edema is typically in the subchondral region and can be low signal on T1-weighted images. Marrow and soft tissue enhancement will be present. There can be associated injury of the ligamentous structures, such as the Lisfranc ligament complex. In the chronic phase, there can be low signal on both T1 and edema-sensitive sequences due to osteosclerosis. Subchondral cysts can be present, and there is decrease in the marrow edema when compared to the acute phase. There is typically extensive bone injury and abnormal alignment.

A major diagnostic problem with Charcot arthropathy is whether osteomyelitis is also present. This is a common dilemma for physicians treating patients with diabetes as clinical and imaging findings can be confusing. MRI is likely the best imaging modality in these cases. The presence of soft tissue ulcers extending to bone or rim-enhancing fluid collections are highly concerning for osteomyelitis. Disappearance of previously seen subchondral cysts or bone fragments are also concerning. Although edema in the bone is present with CN, the degree of edema can be increased with osteomyelitis and extend to the medullary cavity instead of only involving the subchondral bone. T1 marrow signal will be isointense or hypointense to skeletal muscle in osteomyelitis. Diffusion-weighted imaging or dynamic contrast enhancement may help distinguish CN from CN with osteomyelitis.

Treatment of CN begins with offloading the foot to decrease pressure to the foot and ankle with orthotics, removable walkers, half shoes, and total contact cast (TCC). TCCs are especially helpful in improving clinical symptoms and in preventing disease progression. Bisphosphonates can be used to treat CN because the pathogenesis is partially due to increased osteoclastic activity. TNF-α antagonists (infliximab, etanercept) and RANK-L antagonists (denosumab) can also be used, but their efficacy is still to be determined. Surgery with debridement and/or hardware fixation can be helpful in the chronic phase of CN but should be avoided in the acute phase.

Report checklist

1. Is there joint distension, disorganization, dislocation, debris (intra-articular bodies and fracture fragments), increased density (sclerosis), and osseous destruction to suggest CN?
2. On MRI, is there bone marrow edema (subchondral), soft tissue edema, or joint effusion in the midfoot?
3. Is there a soft tissue ulcer? And does it extend to bone?
4. Is there intramedullary bone marrow edema or enhancement to support osteomyelitis?
5. Is there replacement of the T1 marrow edema (isointense or hypointense to muscle) to support diagnosis of osteomyelitis?
6. Is there an associated soft tissue abscess or reactive edema in the surrounding soft tissues?

Suggested Reading

Ergen FB, Sanverdi DE, Oznur A. Charcot foot in diabetes and an update on imaging. Diabet Foot Ankle. 2013;4:21884.

Mautone M, Naidoo P. What the radiologist needs to know about Charcot foot. J Med Imaging Radiat Oncol. 2015;59:395–402.

Leone A, Cassar-Pullicino VN, Semprini A, Tonetti L, Magarelli N, Colosimo C. Neuropathic osteoarthropathy with and without superimposed osteomyelitis in patients with a diabetic foot. Skeletal Radiol. 2016;45:735–54.

Case 8.8

Indication A 27-year-old woman with severe left knee pain, swelling, and limited range of motion.

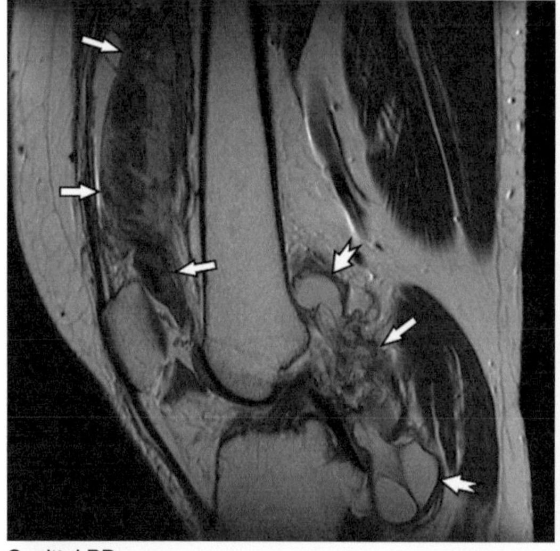

Sagittal PD

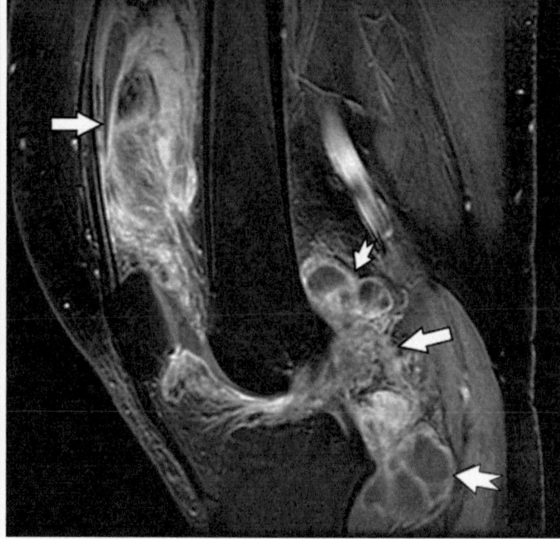

Sagittal T2 fat saturated

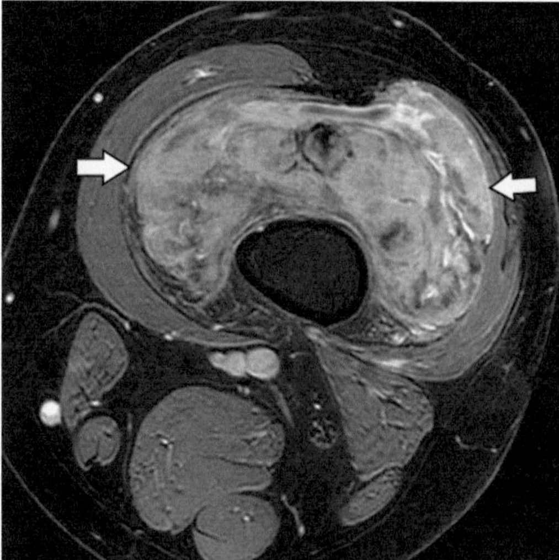

Axial T1 fat saturated post contrast

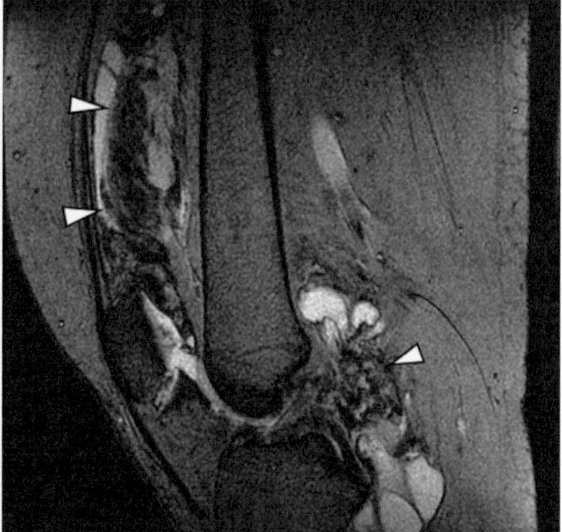

Sagittal T2 weighted Gradient Echo (GRE)

Findings

There are several intra-articular masses (arrows) throughout the joint space anteriorly and posteriorly, most prominent within the suprapatellar recess and posteriorly at the midline. These masses are predominantly low signal on proton density and T1-weighted images and heterogeneously hyperintense on T2-weighted images. Moreover, they demonstrate solid internal enhancement. These masses have blooming artifact (arrowheads) on the gradient echo sequences consistent with hemorrhage. The suprapatellar component measures 10 × 10 × 3 cm. There is similar material in the posterior aspect of the joint space adjacent to the posterior cruciate ligament measuring 3.5 cm in craniocaudal dimension, best seen on series 11, image 19. The more inferior aspect of the posterior masses are cystic (notched arrows) in nature. There is no significant joint effusion. The bones are intact without bony erosions or marrow edema.

Impression/Recommendation

Several large enhancing intra-articular masses anteriorly and posteriorly in the knee, most consistent with tenosynovial giant cell tumor, diffuse type.

Discussion: Tenosynovial Giant Cell Tumor (TGCT) – diffuse type

Tenosynovial giant cell tumor (TGCT) is a benign tumor that arises from synovial tissue in a joint, bursa, or tendon and is the preferred term over giant cell tumor of tendon sheath (GCTTS) or pigmented villonodular synovitis (PVNS) which refer to the same entity. TGCT can have focal or diffuse types but are histologically the same tumor *(please refer to Case 7.10 for further discussion on the focal type)*. The diffuse type, as seen in this case, can mimic an arthropathy, so we have chosen to place it in this section. The diffuse type most commonly occurs in the knee and then the ankle, but can affect any joint. Patients usually present in the third or fourth decade of life, and symptoms are typically from the hypervascular synovial tissue that is prone to bleed. This can cause pain and limit range of joint motion.

Diffuse-type TGCT typically appears as several intra-articular masses and can have variable MRI signal characteristics depending on the amount of hemorrhagic components. Diffuse-type lesions are often low signal on T1 and heterogeneously hyperintense on T2-weighted images. On gradient echo (GRE) sequences, "blooming" from hemorrhage can be present in the lesions and are seen as low signal foci. Diffuse type is more likely to have blooming than the focal type of TGCT due to the hemorrhagic synovium. It is important to perform a gradient echo sequence in suspected cases of TGCT when protocolling these cases. The masses should enhance after contrast administration. There can be an associated joint effusion and osseous erosions *(see supplementary images)*, which can mimic an inflammatory arthropathy.

Treatment of TGCT is dependent on symptoms. For mild symptoms, conservative management can suffice. This can include NSAIDS and imatinib, a tyrosine kinase inhibitor. For high disease burden, treatment is with surgery. It is important to comment in the MR report on the exact distribution of disease as this can have implications for surgery. For instance, lesions in the suprapatellar recess of the anterior knee can be removed arthroscopically; however, posterior lesions require open surgery for removal. The recurrence rate for diffuse-type TGCT is 28% versus 7% for the focal type. Recurrence rates are higher if only a partial versus full synovectomy is performed. However, a full synovectomy can lead to increased risk for joint stiffness and accelerated osteoarthritis.

Supplementary images

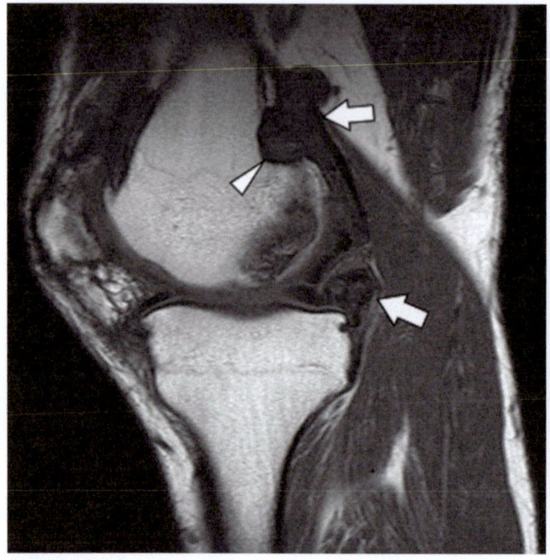

Sagittal T2 fat saturated

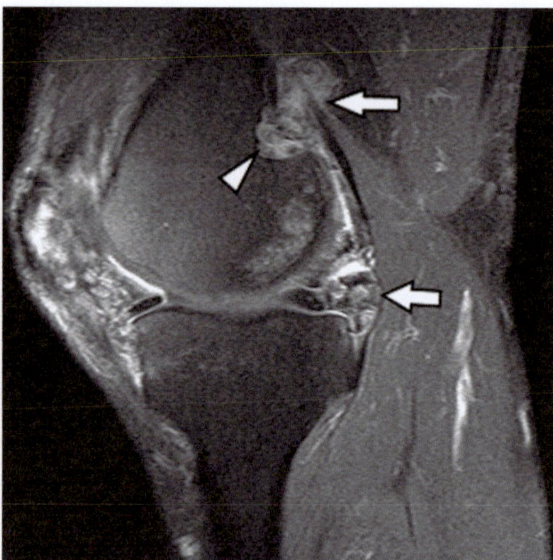

Sagittal T1

A 34-year-old man with diffuse-type TGCT. There are low signal intra-articular masses(arrows) in the posterior aspect of the joint and a large erosion (arrowheads) along the posteromedial aspect of the distal femur

Report checklist
1. What are the size and location of the masses?
2. Are the masses intra-articular?
3. Do the masses enhance?
4. Is there "blooming" artifact on the gradient echo sequences?
5. Is there remodeling of the adjacent bone or bone marrow edema? Are there bone erosions?
6. Is there a joint effusion?

Suggested Reading

Gouin F, Noailles T. Localized and diffuse forms of tenosynovial giant cell tumor (formerly giant cell tumor of the tendon sheath and pigmented villonodular synovitis). Orthop Traumatol Surg Res. 2017;103:S91–7.

Noailles T, Brulefert K, Briand S, Longis PM, Andrieu K, Chalopin A, Gouin F. Giant cell tumor of tendon sheath: Open surgery or arthroscopic synovectomy? A systematic review of the literature. Orthop Traumatol Surg Res. 2017;103:809–14.

Case 8.9

Indication A 64-year-old woman with left shoulder pain and limited range of motion.

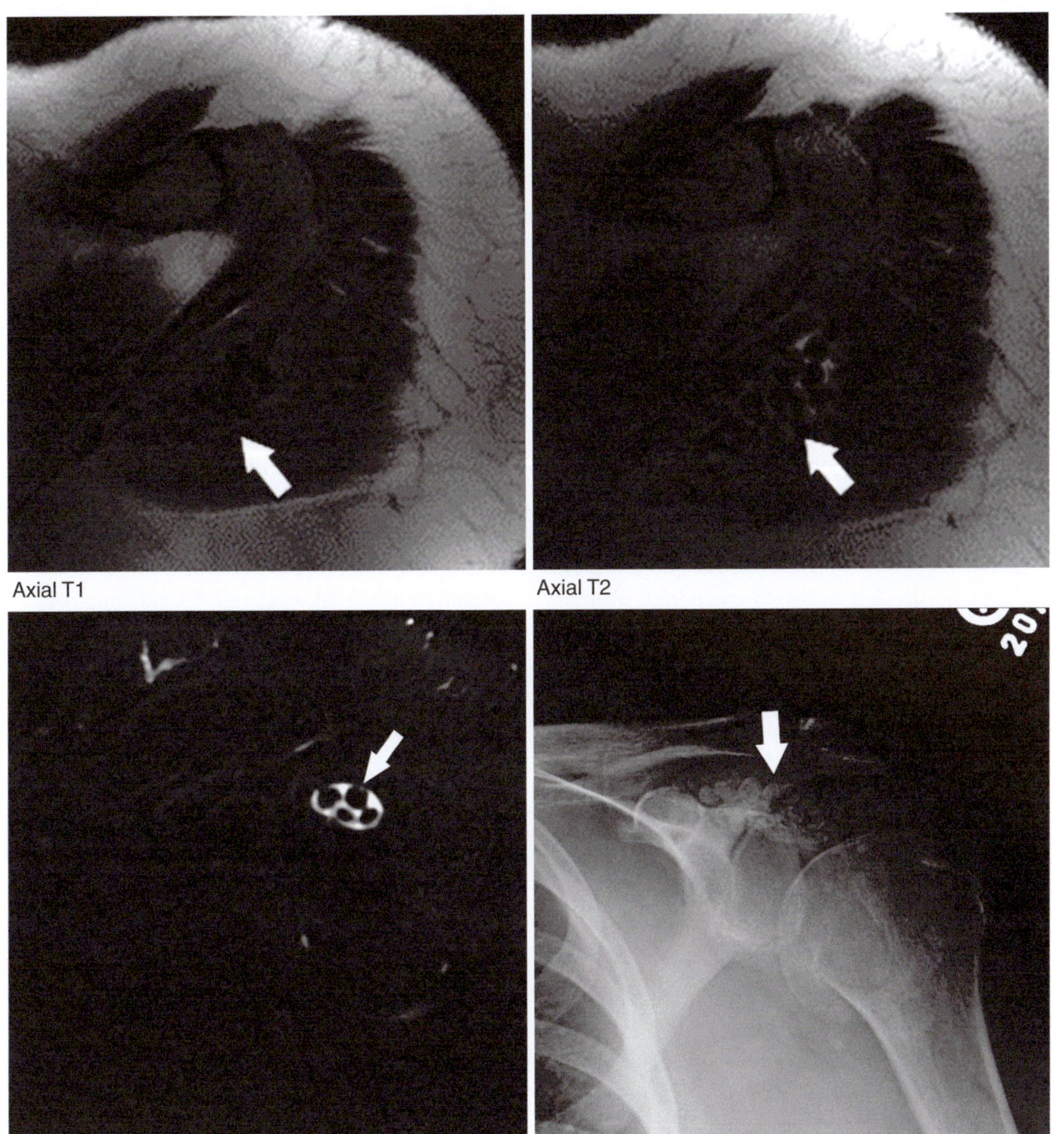

Axial T1

Axial T2

Sagittal T2 fat saturated

Findings

There are numerous small subcentimeter ossified foci (arrows) in the subdeltoid bursa posterior to the infraspinatus muscle. The foci are similar in size measuring roughly 0.5 cm each. They are low signal on all pulse sequences and correspond to ossified loose bodies on the prior radiographs. There is a small amount of fluid in the subdeltoid bursa. There is no edema in the adjacent muscles or bone marrow. There are degenerative changes of the glenohumeral joint (not shown); however, the loose bodies are separate from the joint space.

Impression/Recommendation

Numerous ossified loose bodies in the posterior subdeltoid bursa consistent with synovial osteochondromatosis.

Discussion: Synovial chondromatosis/ osteochondromatosis

Synovial chondromatosis/osteochondromatosis is a benign process where there is nodular metaplasia of synovial tissue within the joint, tendon sheath, or bursa. The nodules can detach and become loose and grow. This disorder is typically a mono-articular process, is more common in men, and presents in the third to fifth decade of life. The most common sites affected are the knee followed by the hip, elbow, and shoulder. However, it can affect any synovial structure and is not uncommonly seen in the temporomandibular joint. The loose bodies are often similar in size and can become ossified. The ossified form (as in this case) is called synovial osteochondromatosis. The disorder can be divided into two categories. Primary synovial chondromatosis occurs in a normal joint, whereas secondary synovial chondromatosis occurs in joints with severe osteoarthritis, can be bilateral, and occurs in older patients. Patients complain of limited range of motion, swelling, and pain; however, it can also be asymptomatic. The loose bodies can damage adjacent structures such as the rotator cuff tendons. There are three phases to the primary form: (1) initial, formation of syno-vial metaplastic cartilaginous nodules; (2) transitional, nodules detach; (3) inactive, synovial proliferation resolves, and nodules remain.

On MR imaging, synovial chondromatosis/osteochondromatosis has a characteristic appearance. There are several loose bodies, similar in size, within the joint, tendon sheath, or bursa. The loose bodies are typically low signal on T1-weighted images but can have variable signal intensity on T2-weighted images depending on the degree of ossification and calcification. If the bodies are predominantly cartilaginous, they will be high signal on T2; however, calcified or ossified lesions will be low signal on T2. There is typically no enhancement of the bodies; however, there can be enhancement of the adjacent synovium. Occasionally the nodules can cause mass effect upon the adjacent structures, so it is important to assess and comment upon the status of the tendons, muscles, and bones. Furthermore, the presence or absence of osteoarthritis in the adjacent joint should be commented upon, as primary synovial (osteo)chondromatosis can be confused with osteoarthritis with multiple loose bodies. Diffuse tenosynovial giant cell tumor (TGCT) can also be confused with this process. However, in TGCT, the lesions are adherent to the synovial tissue, can have hemorrhage, and typically have a larger joint effusion.

Symptomatic synovial chondromatosis is treated with synovectomy and removal of the loose bodies. The recurrence rate is 3–23% and is higher for patients who undergo only loose body removal without synovectomy. Synovectomy should be considered in patients in the initial active phase of the disorder as opposed to the inactive phase where the synovium is normal. There have been rare reports of malignant transformation (5%) of synovial chondromatosis to chondrosarcoma, which is characterized by an enlarging mass with cortical destruction and bone marrow invasion. This is more common in patients with multiple recurrences.

Report checklist

1. Are there several loose bodies of similar size in a joint, tendon sheath, or bursa?
2. Are the loose bodies calcified?
3. Is there osteoarthritis of the joint?
4. Are the loose bodies causing mass effect and injuring the adjacent structures (tendons, muscles, bone)?
5. Is this is a recurrence process, and are there signs of malignant transformation (cortical destruction with bone marrow invasion)?
6. Could this be PVNS or osteoarthritis with loose bodies?

Suggested Reading

Murphey MD, Vidal JA, Fanburg-Smith JC et-al. Imaging of synovial chondromatosis with radiologic-pathologic correlation. Radiographics. 2007;27:1465–88.

Ryan RS, Harris AC, O'Connell JX, Munk PL. Synovial osteochondromatosis: the spectrum of imaging findings. Australas Radiol. 2005;49:95–100.

Case 9.1

Indication A 29-year-old female for evaluation of incidental bone marrow abnormalities partially seen on recent MRI of the knee.

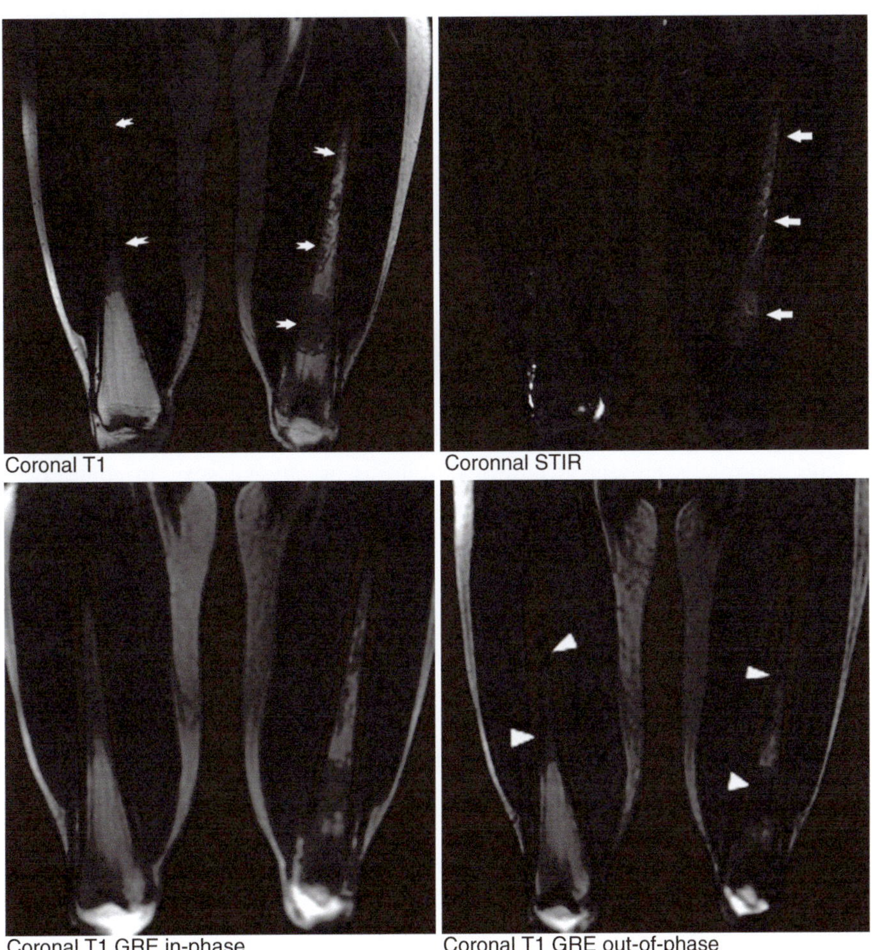

© Springer Nature Switzerland AG 2020
T. M. Hegazi, J. S. Wu, *Musculoskeletal MRI*, https://doi.org/10.1007/978-3-030-26777-3_9

Findings

There are bilateral patchy areas of bone marrow signal abnormalities within the femurs, most prominent in the left distal femur. The lesions are low signal intensity on the T1-weighted images (notched arrows); however, they are hyperintense relative to the adjacent skeletal muscle. They are hyperintense on the STIR sequence (arrows). There is also diffuse drop in signal (arrowheads) on the out-of-phase images when compared to the in-phase images indicating the internal presence of fat. There is no cortical destruction.

Impression/Recommendation

Normal red marrow. No further workup required.

Discussion: Normal versus abnormal bone marrow

The increasing use of MRI has resulted in the increased detection of incidental findings in the bone marrow on routine imaging. Radiologists are often presented with the dilemma of what to do with these incidentally detected signal alterations and whether a biopsy or other diagnostic test should be recommended. As many hematologic neoplasms are often asymptomatic early in the disease process, these findings could be the initial signs of an underlying malignancy, and hence, these findings should not be taken lightly.

Normal bone marrow is composed of variable proportions of hematopoietic cells and fat. Red (hematopoietic) marrow is present at birth and contains 40% fat cells, 40% hematopoietic cells, and 10% structural elements. Red marrow then transitions to yellow (fatty) marrow as one ages. Yellow (fatty) marrow contains 80% fat cells, 10% hematopoietic cells, and 10% structural elements. The conversion of red to yellow marrow occurs in a predictable, orderly, and symmetrical pattern occurring first in the appendicular skeleton followed by the axial skeleton. The process starts in the hands and feet and works centrally, distal first, then proximal. In the long bones, the epiphysis and diaphysis undergo conversion first, then the distal metaphysis and lastly the proximal metaphysis *(see supplementary images)*. The process is usually completed by 25 years of age. In an adult, the red marrow is mainly located in the appendicular skeleton in the metaphysis and near the vertebral endplates.

On MRI, yellow marrow has hyperintense signal intensity on T1- and T2-weighted sequences, with drop of signal on the fat-suppressed sequences, while red marrow has relative hypointense signal compared to fat on T1 (but higher signal intensity than muscle) and intermediate to slightly hyperintense signal relative to fat on fluid-sensitive sequences, due to its high cellular content.

When there is a demand for increased hematopoiesis, marrow reconversion occurs. This pattern follows an orderly sequence that is the reverse order as the pattern observed in marrow conversion with aging. In the long bones, it begins in the proximal metaphysis, followed by distal metaphysis and finally the diaphysis. Marrow reconversion can occur due to multiple reasons, including obesity, smokers, living in high altitude, marathon runners, anemia patients, or patients treated with marrow-stimulating medications (e.g., GCSF therapy). However, hematologic malignancies can also cause marrow reconversion. A few useful discriminators favoring benign marrow hyperplasia over neoplasm include having bilateral symmetric involvement, having the signal intensity of red marrow isointense or slightly hyperintense to muscle on T1-weighted sequences, and having a nonconfluent patchy pattern and the lack of aggressive features such as cortical destruction. Also, red marrow should not extend past the physis or physeal scar. In contrast, pathologic marrow infiltration tends to have signal intensity that is lower than muscle on T1-weighted images *(see supplementary images)*, and hence the T1-weighted sequences are key. It is important to note that although marrow reconversion can be seen on MRI, the exact etiology is difficult to determine on imaging alone, and correlation with patient's clinical history and laboratory values is recommended. A pitfall is that multiple myeloma can have signal intensity that is slightly hyperintense to muscle, suggesting red marrow.

Sometimes it can be difficult to determine whether the abnormal signal is truly isointense or hyperintense to skeletal muscle. In these situations, chemical shift imaging (in- and out-of-phase) can be useful to determine whether a signal abnormality is due to red marrow or a neoplastic process. Red marrow contains microscopic fat and hence would demonstrate greater than 20% loss of signal on the out-of-phase images as compared to the in-phase images *(see supplementary images)*. Neoplastic lesions replacing bone marrow will not have signal dropout *(see supplementary images)*. According to a recent study, using a relative signal intensity ratio of 0.81, chemical shift imaging has a sensitivity and specificity of 95% for the detection of bone marrow neoplasm. It is important to emphasize that chemical shift imaging does not differentiate between benign and malignant lesions but between bone marrow replacing and non-bone marrow replacing lesions. Additional MRI techniques as diffusion-weighted imaging (DWI), dynamic contrast enhancement, and MR spectroscopy can be performed. Lastly, in equivocal cases, short-term follow-up with MRI and bone marrow biopsy are reasonable recommendations.

Bone marrow disorders can be classified into marrow proliferative disorders, marrow replacement disorders, marrow depletion, and lastly marrow edema. Marrow proliferative disorders are related to the overproduction of, typically normal, bone marrow elements with examples including myelofibrosis *(see supplementary images)*, polycythemia vera, leukemia, and mul-

tiple myeloma. They demonstrate diffuse low signal intensity on T1- and variable signal on T2-weighted sequences. Marrow replacement disorders are related to infiltration of cells that do not belong in the bone marrow. They are typically focal or multifocal, but not diffuse *(see supplementary images)*. Examples include metastases, bone tumors, osteomyelitis, and lymphoma. Marrow depletion is related to ablation or failure of red marrow elements. On MRI, this appears as hyperintense signal on both T1- and T2-weighted images, similar to fat. The distribution may be diffuse or regional depending on the underlying cause with examples including aplastic anemia, radiation therapy *(see supplementary images)*, or chemotherapy.

When presented with a case of bone marrow abnormality, assessing the distribution of the disease helps to narrow the differential diagnosis. If the process is diffuse and symmetric bilaterally, then think of marrow reconversion or marrow proliferative diseases such as multiple myeloma, leukemia, polycythemia vera, and myelofibrosis. If the abnormality is focal, then the differential could be a red marrow island, tumor, trauma, infection, degenerative, or postradiation. If the lesions are multifocal, then it could be related to metastases or myeloma.

Supplementary Images

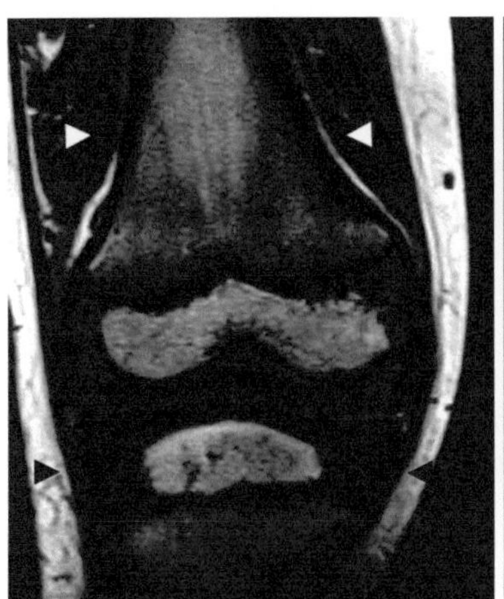

Coronal T1

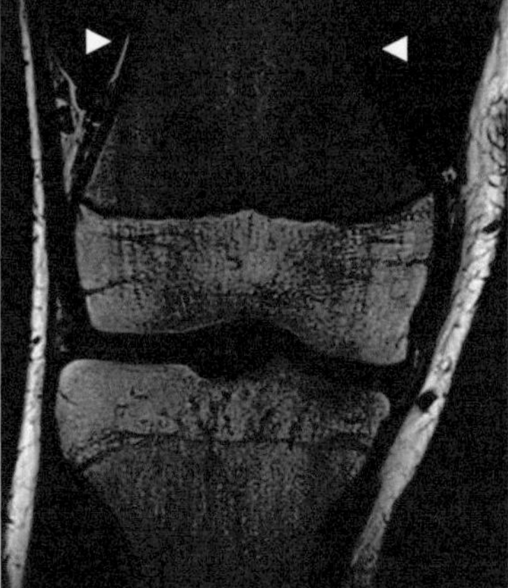

Coronal T1

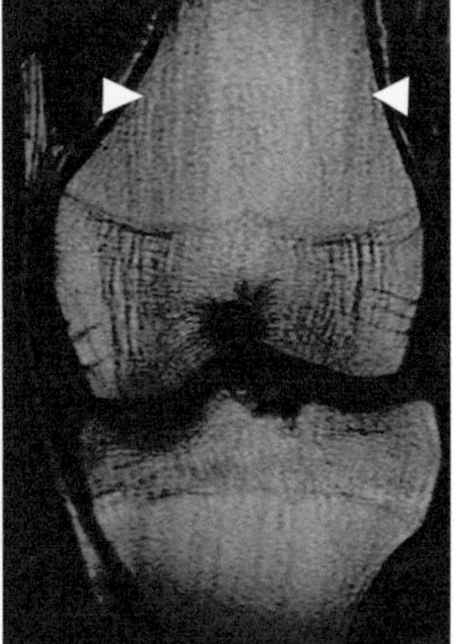

Coronal T1

Normal bone marrow conversion appearance on MRI. T1-weighted images of different patients from left to right at 2 years old, 14 years old, and 42 years old. Notice how the normal marrow conversion from red to yellow with advancing age. The signal intensity in the distal femur (arrowheads) is slightly hyperintense to the surrounding skeletal muscle. (Images courtesy of Mary Hochman)

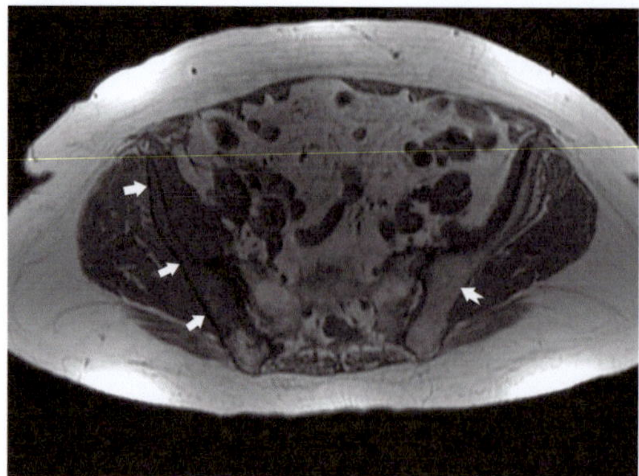

Axial T1

Axial STIR

Marrow replacing disorder on MRI. There is diffuse low T1 signal (arrows) in the right iliac bone that is iso−/ hypointense to the adjacent skeletal muscle, suspicious for a marrow replacement disorder. The contralateral left iliac bone (notched arrow) has red marrow which is *mildly hypointense on T1, but hyperintense relative to skeletal muscle. There are soft tissue mass and muscle edema arising from the right iliac bone (arrowheads) that are hyperintense on the T2-weighted images. Biopsy revealed B cell lymphoma*

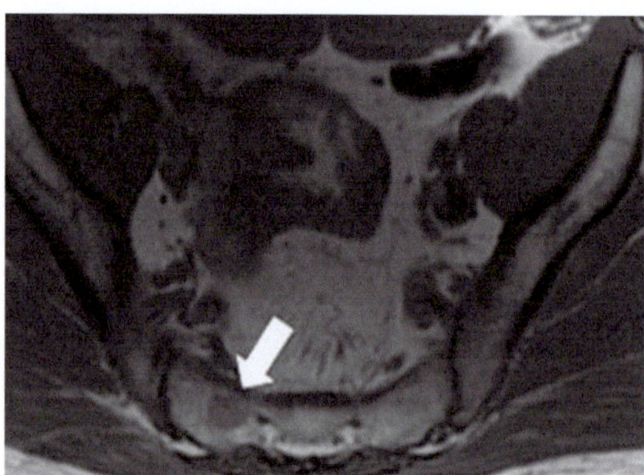

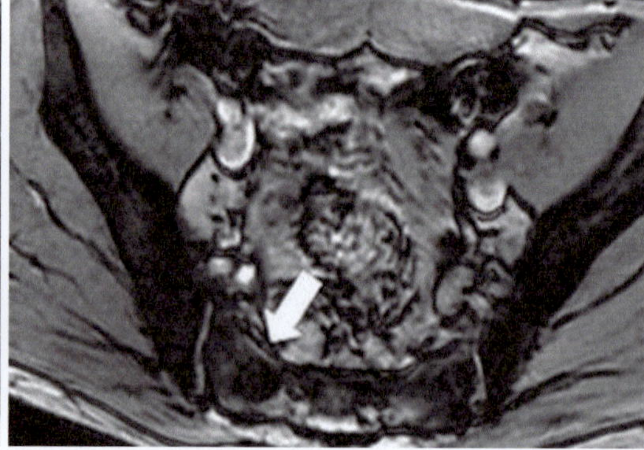

Axial T1 GRE in-phase

Axial T1 GRE out-of-phase

Red marrow island. There is a 1.3 cm lesion (arrows) in the right sacral ala that is isointense to adjacent skeletal muscle and demonstrates diffuse drop in sig- *nal on the out-of-phase image compatible with a normal island of red marrow*

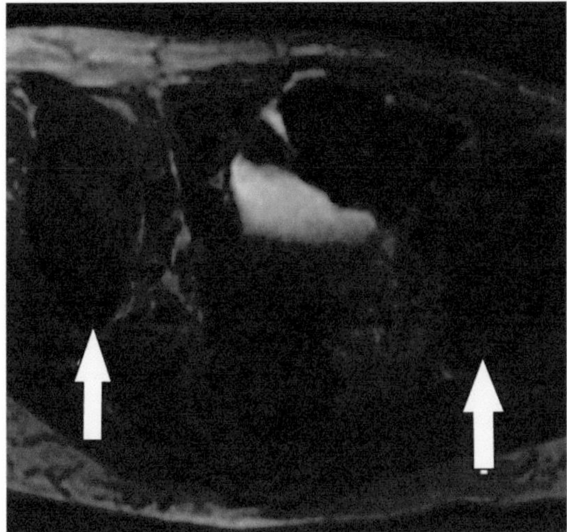

Axial T1 GRE in-phase

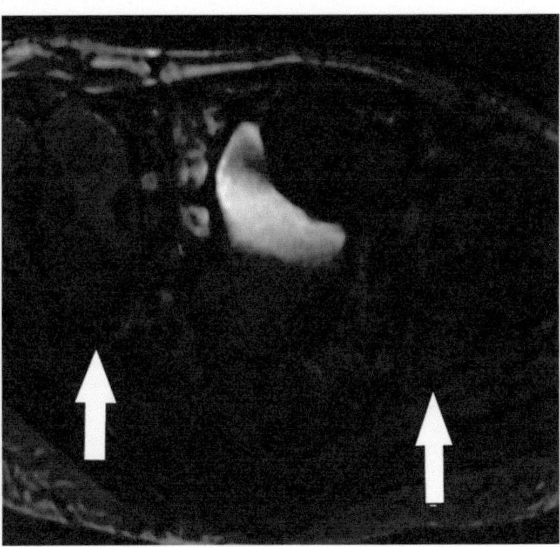

Axial T1 GRE out-of-phase

In- and out-of-phase chemical shift imaging. There is diffuse low signal intensity of the pelvic bones bilaterally that is hypointense to surrounding skeletal muscle and does not drop in signal on the out-of-phase images. This suggests a diffuse bone marrow replacing process. (Lymphoma in this case)

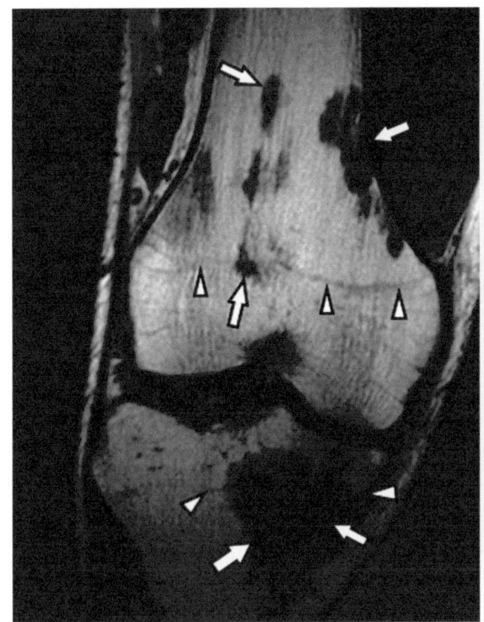

Coronal T1

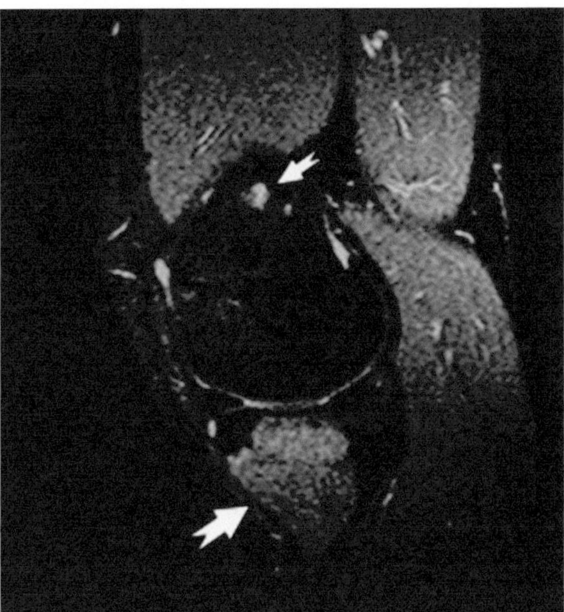

Sagittal T2 fat saturated

There are multiple focal TI hypointense lesions (arrows) in the proximal tibia and distal femur that are hypointense to surrounding skeletal muscle and hyperintense (notched arrows) on T2-weighted images. The lesions cross the physeal scar (arrowheads) which should not occur with red marrow. Findings suggest an abnormal marrow replacing lesion. (Breast cancer metastases in this case)

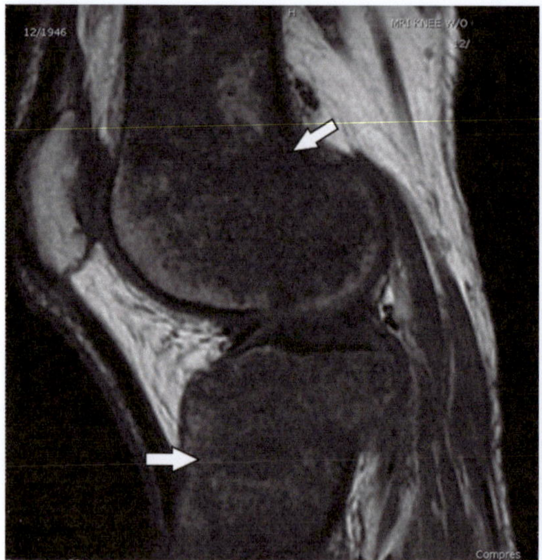

Sagittal T1

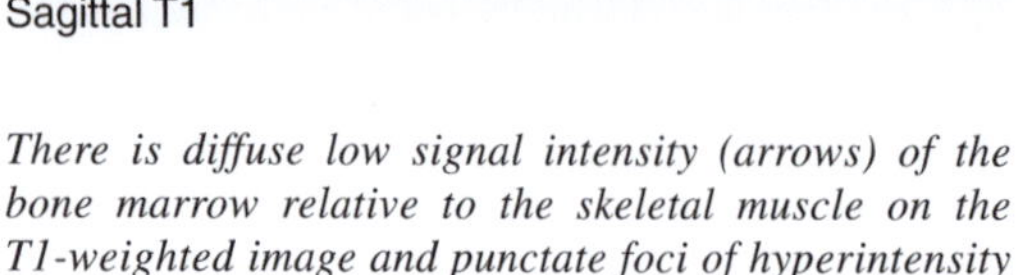

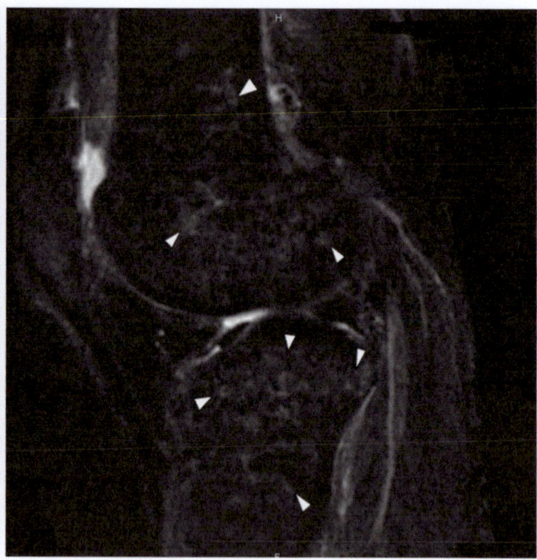

Sagittal T2 fat saturated

There is diffuse low signal intensity (arrows) of the bone marrow relative to the skeletal muscle on the T1-weighted image and punctate foci of hyperintensity *(arrowheads) on the T2-weighted image. Findings suggest a diffuse marrow proliferative disorder. (Myelofibrosis in this case)*

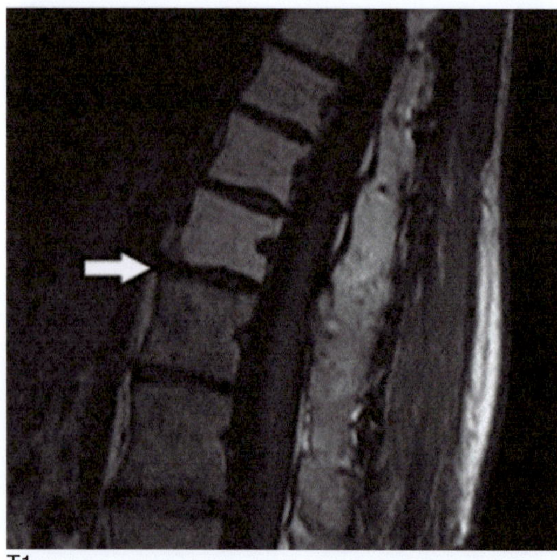

T1

Postradiation bone marrow changes. There is diffuse high signal intensity in the upper thoracic vertebral bodies when compared to the lower lumbar vertebral bodies on this T1-weighted image compatible with marrow depletion and fatty marrow related to radiation treatment for breast cancer. The arrow denotes the inferior edge of the radiation treatment field (arrow)

Report checklist
1. What is the distribution of the bone marrow signal abnormalities (diffuse, focal, or multifocal)?
2. How is the signal on the T1-weighted images (hyperintense, isointense, or hypointense relative to the adjacent skeletal muscle)? If difficult to tell, consider doing in- and out-of-phase images to tell if it is red marrow or a marrow replacing lesion.
3. Do the lesions cross the physis?
4. Are there aggressive features as cortical destruction or periosteal reaction?

Suggested Reading

Grønningsæter IS, Ahmed AB, Vetti N, Johansen S, Bruserud Ø, Reikvam H. Bone marrow abnormalities detected by magnetic resonance imaging as initial sign of hematologic malignancies. Clin Pract. 2018;8:1061.

Kung JW, Yablon CM, Eisenberg RL. Bone marrow signal alteration in the extremities. AJR Am J Roentgenol. 2011;196:W492–510.

Case 9.2

Indication A 28-year-old soccer player with sudden onset of left anterior thigh pain and swelling.

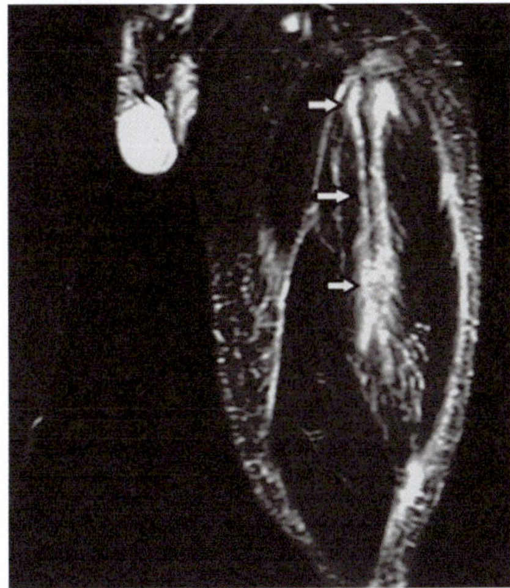

Coronal STIR

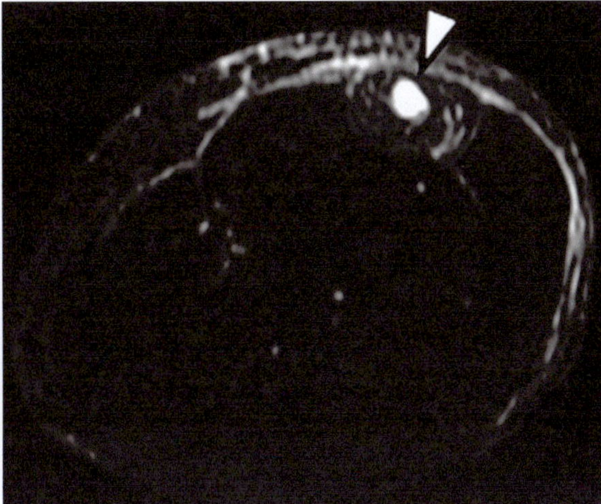

Axial T2 fat saturated

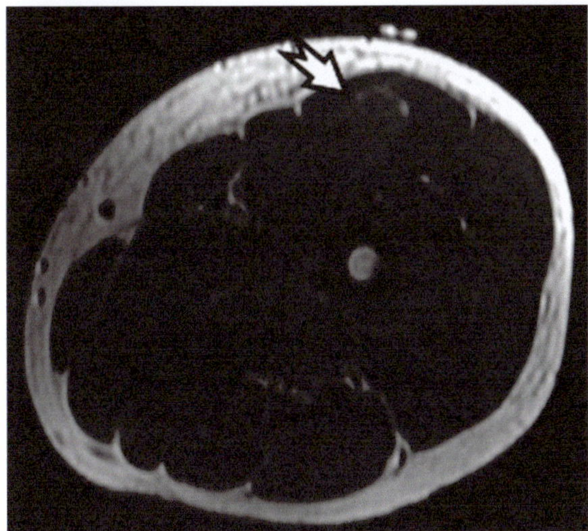

Axial T1

Findings

There is partial tear at the proximal myotendinous junction of the left rectus femoris muscle with surrounding intramuscular edema (arrows). The tear involves approximately 20% of the cross-sectional area of the muscle. This injury is associated with a 2.5 cm intramuscular hematoma with T2 (arrowhead) and T1 (notched arrow) hyperintensity making this a grade 2 injury. There is no muscle rupture or muscle retraction. There is no fatty atrophy of the muscle.

Impression/Recommendation

Partial tear of the left rectus femoris muscle (grade 2 strain) with small subacute intramuscular hematoma.

Discussion: Muscle injuries/tear

Muscle injuries are common, often occurring during sports-related activities and can be especially debilitating for professional athletes lengthening the time for return to play. Although most muscle injuries are diagnosed clinically, imaging plays a crucial role to confirm and assess the extent of injury, which can guide appropriate management and gauge the time needed for return to play. Muscle injuries are classified depending on the mechanism of injury into muscle strains related to an indirect stretching injury, a muscle contusion related to a direct blow, or muscle laceration from penetrating trauma.

The most common type of muscle injury is muscle strain. This typically occurs as an indirect injury during eccentric muscle contraction, with the majority occurring at the myotendinous junction. During eccentric contraction, the muscles lengthen despite contraction, often due to a strong external force. Moreover, muscles that contain "fast twitch" fibers and muscles that cross two joints (rectus femoris, gastrocnemius, biceps) are particularly affected. The most commonly affected muscles in the extremities include the hamstrings, the adductors and flexors of the hip, the rectus femoris, and the medial head of the gastrocnemius. Patients typically present with sudden onset of acute pain in the affected muscle group at the time of activity. The degree of muscle strain on imaging has been graded along a spectrum from grade 1–3 injury/strain. This grading system is commonly used to facilitate communication between referring physicians; however, this system does not adequately represent the extent of an injury and lacks diagnostic accuracy since it does not properly cover the full spectrum of muscle injury features. It is important to provide a full assessment of the muscle injury.

A grade 1 strain is a mild injury without identifiable muscle disruption. On MRI, this appears as feathery edema within the muscle at the myotendinous junction *(see supplementary images)*. The presence of visible muscle fiber discontinuity with distortion of muscle architecture and hematoma formation around the myotendinous junction signifies a grade 2 strain. Try to give an approximate percentage of muscle disruption with respect to the entire cross section of the muscle as this is crucial information to the referring clinician. A grade 3 strain on MRI is represented by complete disruption and retraction of the myotendinous junction with a hematoma filling the gap created by the tear. The degree of muscle retraction should be indicated in the report. After a complete tear and immobilization, muscle atrophy may ensue, which is characterized on MRI by reduction in the size of the muscle and usually starts within 10 days of immobilization; however, this is reversible. With continued immobilization, fatty degeneration of the muscle occurs and starts at approximately 4 months and is irreversible *(see supplementary images)*.

Muscle contusion occurs following a direct blow to the muscle resulting in injury to the deep layers of the muscle from compression of the muscle between the object and underlying bone. On MRI, they present as diffuse intramuscular edema that has an indistinct feathery appearance. Edema within the overlying subcutaneous soft tissues may indicate the direct trauma mechanism. This can be accompanied by the development of an intramuscular hematoma in more severe cases. The MRI appearance of an intramuscular hematoma depends on the age of the lesion. Acute hematomas appear isointense to muscle on the T1-weighted images and hypointense on T2-weighted images. Subacute hematomas have high signal on both T1- and T2-weighted sequences. Chronic hematoma would have low signal on both T1- and T2-weighted sequences due to hemosiderin deposition.

Muscle contusions usually heal quickly with rest and immobilization with expected return to play in 1–2 weeks. Grade 1 and 2 strains are generally treated conservatively with rest and immobilization first and then with physiotherapy, and recovery may take up to 6 months. Complete full-thickness tears require surgical repair to prevent fatty atrophy of the involved muscle.

Supplementary Images

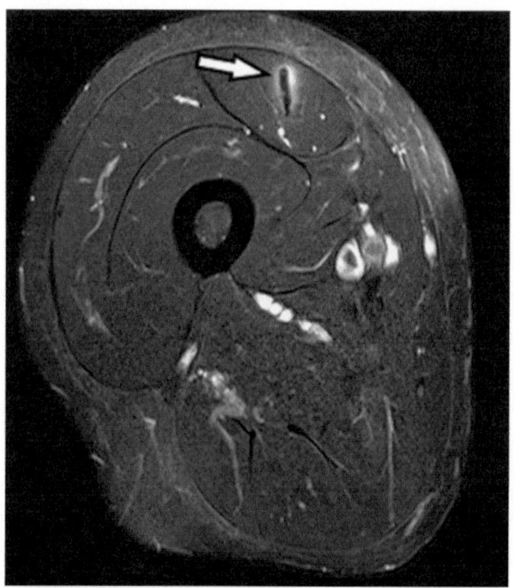

Axial T2 fat saturated

There is mild intramuscular edema at the proximal myotendinous junction (arrow) of the rectus femoris muscle without visible muscle fiber discontinuation or architectural distortion, compatible with a grade 1 strain

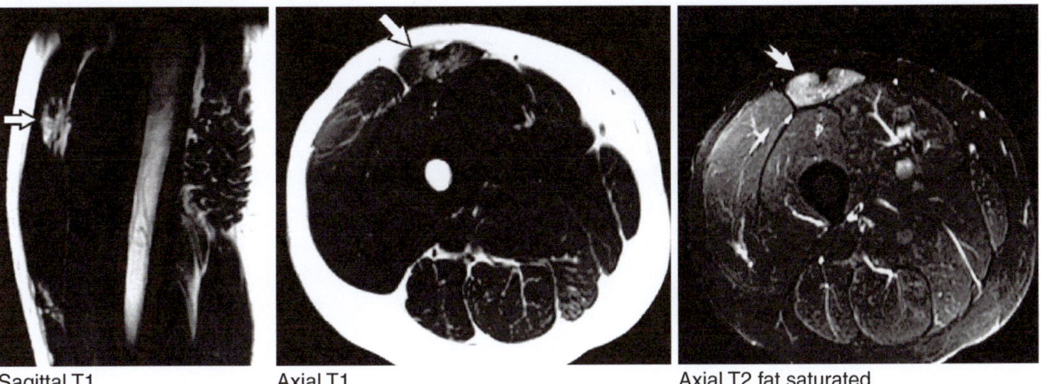

Sagittal T1   Axial T1   Axial T2 fat saturated

There is a chronic tear at the proximal myotendinous junction (arrow) of the rectus femoris muscle with associated decreased muscle bulk and mild fatty atrophy best *seen on the T1 images. There is mild muscle edema (notched arrow) on the T2-weighted image*

Report checklist

1. Is there a muscle tear? Which muscle is involved? Where is the precise location of the tear (tendon/bone interface, tendon, proximal myotendinous junction, or muscle belly)?
2. What is the extent of the tear (grade 1, 2, or 3 strain)? Hematomas indicate at least a grade 2 injury.
3. If it is a partial tear, then how much of the cross-sectional area of the muscle belly is involved?
4. If a complete tear, is there retraction of the muscle belly?
5. Is there muscle fatty atrophy to suggest a chronic injury?

Suggested Reading

Flores DV, Mejía Gómez C, Estrada-Castrillón M, Smitaman E, Pathria MN. MR imaging of muscle trauma: anatomy, biomechanics, pathophysiology, and imaging appearance. Radiographics. 2018;38:124–48.

Guermazi A, Roemer FW, Robinson P, Tol JL, Regatte RR1, Crema MD. Imaging of muscle injuries in sports medicine: sports imaging series. Radiology. 2017;282:646–63.

Case 9.3

Indication A 57-year-old woman with difficulty in walking, rising from a chair, raising her arms above her head, and combing her hair for the past month. Patient has elevated CPK serum values.

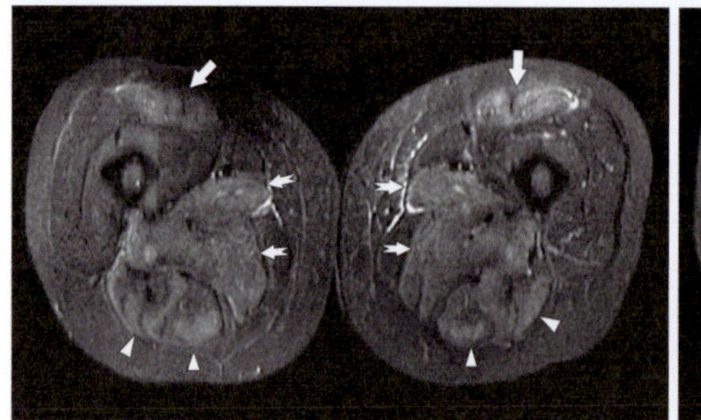
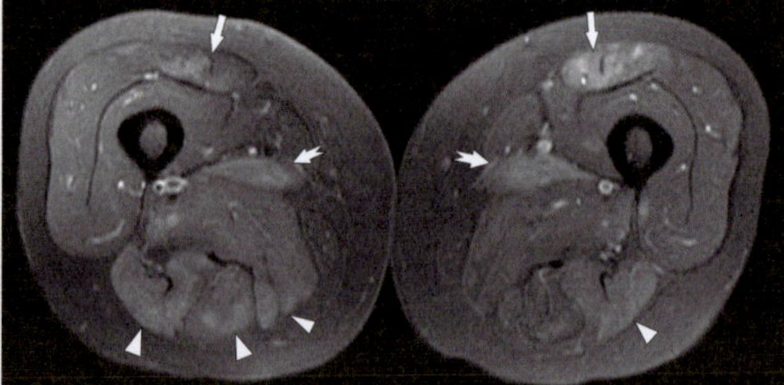

Axial STIR   Axial T1 fat saturated post contrast

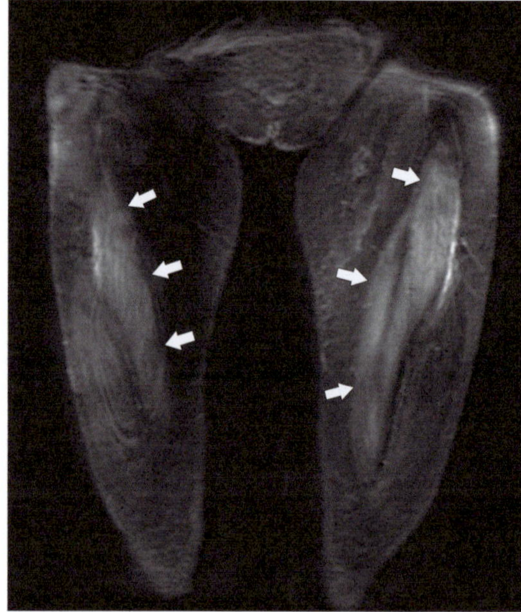
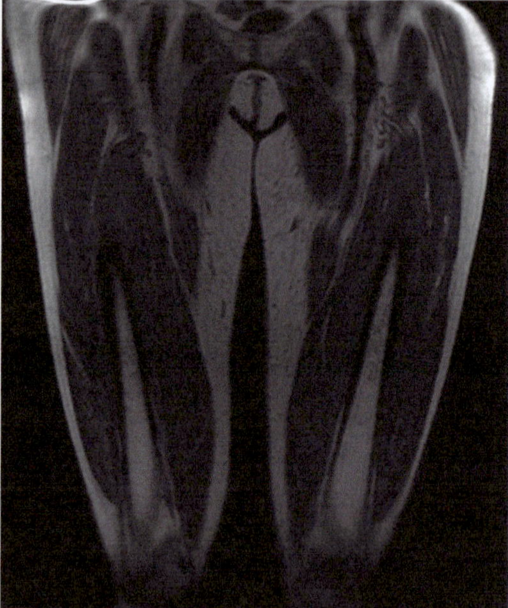

Coronal STIR   Coronal T1

Findings

There is prominent muscle edema in the rectus femoris (arrows), adductors (notched arrows), and hamstrings (arrowheads) muscles bilaterally on the STIR images. After contrast administration, the areas of highest enhancement are in left rectus femoris, left adductor longus, and the right biceps femoris muscles. There is no fatty muscle atrophy or rim-enhancing fluid collections to suggest abscess or muscle necrosis. The subcutaneous soft tissues and bony structures are normal.

Impression/Recommendation

Bilateral patchy areas of muscle edema in both thighs which is nonspecific but can be seen with an inflammatory myopathy such as polymyositis or dermatomyositis. Other conditions to consider would be drug-induced myopathy such as with statin medications or trauma. There are focal areas of enhancement in the left rectus femoris, left adductor longus, and the right biceps femoris muscles. If muscle biopsy is being considered, these muscles will likely have the highest diagnostic yield.

Discussion: Muscle edema

Muscle edema is nonspecific and can have a wide variety of causes. The major causative categories are trauma, infection, denervation, disuse, myopathy, ischemia/necrosis, and iatrogenic/drug-related causes. In order to arise at the correct diagnosis, clinical history and laboratory values are very important. In a patient who just ran 10 miles after a long period of inactivity, delayed-onset muscle soreness would be the most suspected cause. In the patient with bilateral calf pain and recent initiation of medication for high cholesterol, statin-induced drug-related myopathy would be a possible cause. Patients with inflammatory myopathies (polymyositis, dermatomyositis, inclusion body) can have slow but progressive muscle weakness beginning in the proximal muscles. Classically, dermatomyositis has a skin rash that precedes or accompanies the muscle symptoms. In the later stages, there can be muscle calcifications and wasting. Patients with diffuse muscle edema can have elevated serum creatine kinase (CK) which can be a marker of muscle damage. Patients with severe muscle damage can have CK levels 10X normal (typically >1000 U/L) and are considered to have rhabdomyolysis, a life-threatening condition with rapid muscle breakdown. Patients can have muscle pain, vomiting, confusion, tea-colored urine, and renal failure due to accumulation of protein myoglobin.

Muscle edema represents an increase in free water and is best depicted by MRI. Fluid-sensitive sequences are particularly good at detecting muscle edema, either T2-weighted images with chemically selective fat suppression or STIR sequences. T2-weighted sequences have the advantage of higher signal-to-noise ratio (SNR) and specific fat suppression, but they are more susceptible to inhomogeneous fat suppression. Conversely, STIR has homogeneous fat suppression but relatively low SNR; moreover, the signal suppression is not specific for fat but rather for substances with a particular T1 value. On both of these sequences, muscle edema appears as increased signal intensity within the substance of the muscle. Edematous muscle can also increase in size as a result of increased fluid content. Depending on the underlying abnormality, focal fluid collections can also be seen indicating muscle necrosis or abscess, and their detection can be aided by post-contrast images. T1-weighted images are also useful in depicting intramuscular fat in muscle atrophy, the end stage of many of the disease processes that produce muscle edema. In the setting of muscle atrophy, T1-weighted images may show a loss of muscle volume, which is usually replaced by fat that has signal intensity identical to subcutaneous fat (high signal intensity on T1-weighted images). In many muscle disorders, the degree of muscle edema parallels disease activity, and MRI can highlight areas for direct muscle biopsy for histopathologic diagnosis. It is important to describe the muscles that have the most edema and enhancement in the report to aid with surgical biopsy. In general, the muscle samples obtained with percutaneous core needle biopsies are too small for diagnosis for many of these muscle disorders, and an open surgical biopsy is needed. However, you should check with the pathologists at your own institution.

Due to the vast array of diseases that can cause muscle edema, treatment depends on the exact cause. Most disorders are self-limiting and resolve with rest or cessation of the inciting agent, such as in delayed-onset muscle soreness or drug-related myopathy, respectively. Polymyositis and dermatomyositis are treated with steroids and other anti-inflammatory agents.

Report checklist
1. Is there muscle edema?
2. Which muscles are involved? Is it bilateral? Symmetric?
3. Is there enhancement of the muscle?
4. Are there rim-enhancing fluid collections to suggest abscess or muscle necrosis?
5. Is there fatty atrophy and/or decrease in muscle size to suggest a chronic process?
6. What are the clinical and laboratory findings to help narrow the differential for muscle edema?

Suggested Reading

Kumar Y, Wadhwa V, Phillips L, Pezeshk P, Chhabra Avneesh. MR imaging of skeletal muscle signal alterations: systematic approach to evaluation. Eur J Radiol. 2019;85:922–35.

McMahon C, Wu JS, Eisenberg RE. Patterns in imaging: muscle edema. AJR. 2010;194(4): W284–92.

Case 9.4

Indication A 47-year-old woman with diabetes and great toe ulcer.

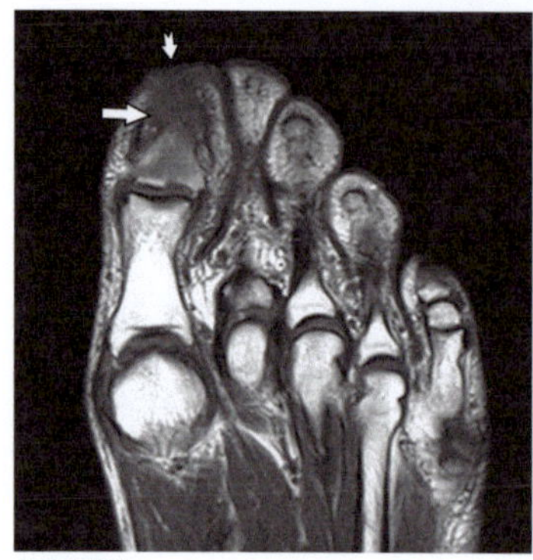

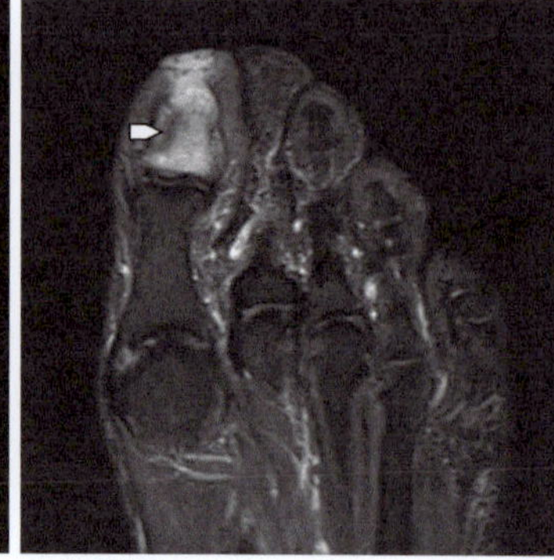

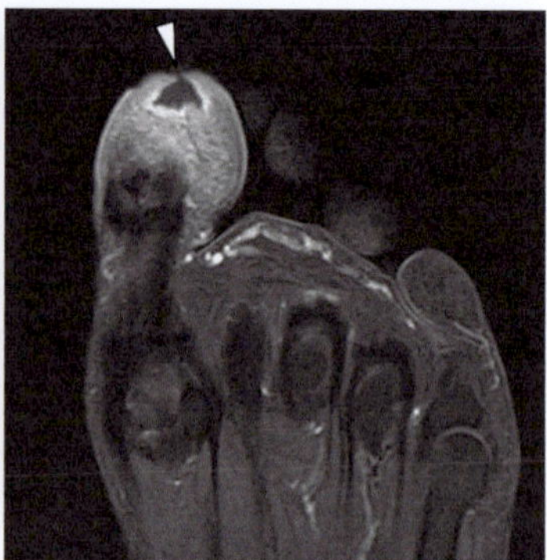

Axial T1   Axial T2 fat saturated   Axial T1 fat saturated post contrast

Findings

There is low signal replacing the normal T1 fatty marrow signal in the distal aspect of the first distal phalanx (arrow) adjacent to a soft tissue ulcer (notched arrow). There is also marrow edema (block arrow) throughout the entire first distal phalanx and adjacent soft tissues. In the plantar soft tissue of the distal first toe, there is a 9 × 6 mm rim-enhancing collection (arrowhead) extending to the ulcer. There is no joint effusion in the first IP joint to suggest septic arthritis or tenosynovitis.

Impression/Recommendation

Osteomyelitis of the distal aspect of the great toe with adjacent 9 mm soft tissue abscess.

Discussion: Diabetes related osteomyelitis and soft tissue abscess

Infections of the feet in patients with diabetes are a major cause of amputations and can lead to poor quality of life and high medical costs. Peripheral neuropathy can occur in patients with long-standing diabetes which results in poor sensation in the feet and low detection of this injury. This puts the patients at risk for developing soft tissue ulcers at points of contact with poor fitting shoes. The ulcers often occur at the tips of the toes, medial aspect of the 1st MTP joint, lateral aspect of the 5th MTP joint, and heel. The ulcers can become infected and lead to osteomyelitis and soft tissue abscess by direct extension. Approximately 50% of diabetic foot ulcers presenting at hospitalization

are infected, and 20% of those cases have concurrent osteomyelitis. Roughly 85% of these cases with osteomyelitis will require amputation or surgical debridement. Clinically, it can be difficult to determine if osteomyelitis is present. The patients may not elicit the same clinical symptoms or abnormal blood tests suggestive of infection as nondiabetic patients. If there is a positive probe to bone (PTB) test, the sensitivity and specificity of osteomyelitis is around 90% for both. In this test, a metallic probe is inserted into the ulcer in an attempt to touch bare bone. When the PTB test is negative, diagnosing osteomyelitis can be very challenging.

In equivocal cases of osteomyelitis, imaging, especially MRI, can be very helpful. Radiographs should be the initial tests, but the findings of osteomyelitis (soft tissue gas, bony destruction, loss of the cortical line) occur during the later stages of the infection. CT and nuclear medicine tests have their relative strengths and weaknesses, but MRI is likely the best overall test with sensitivity and specificity around 80–90%. The most important feature for diagnosing osteomyelitis on MRI is replacement of the normal fatty signal on T1-weighted sequences with low signal intensity. The signal intensity should be isointense or hypointense to skeletal muscle, at times making the bone disappear on T1 sequences as it is obscured by the adjacent soft tissue edema or muscle. The bone will then reappear on the post-contrast images or T2-weighted images, and this finding has been termed the "ghost sign" (*see sup-*

plementary images). Other MRI findings supportive of osteomyelitis are bone marrow edema, enhancement of the medullary bone, cortical destruction, sinus tracts, and an adjacent soft tissue ulcer. In our experience nearly all cases of diabetic foot ulcers are associated with an adjacent soft tissue ulcer. So it is important to carefully scrutinize the images and read the clinical notes to identify a soft tissue ulcer. Moreover, if there is exposure of bone to the air, that constitutes osteomyelitis, even if the MRI findings are not conclusive. Besides assessing for osteomyelitis, it is also important to assess for soft tissue abnormalities such as cellulitis and abscess. Invariably there will be soft tissue edema and enhancement to suggest cellulitis, but this should be apparent clinically. An abscess is diagnosed when there is a peripherally enhancing fluid collection. In the later stages, the wall of the abscess can be more rim-like and distinct as the abscess mature.

However, early on during abscess formation, there can simply be mass-like enhancement consistent with a phlegmon. It is important to comment on the presence or absence of an abscess as they often require drainage since antibiotic therapy can have difficulty entering through the thick wall of the abscess. One should also comment on fluid in the adjacent tendon sheath or joint space to exclude tenosynovitis or septic arthritis, respectively.

Minor cases of diabetic foot infections can be treated with antibiotics and carefully monitoring of their efficacy. However, most cases required surgical debridement. Percutaneous biopsy of suspected diabetic osteomyelitis should be avoided as the biopsy needle will traverse infected soft tissue before entering the bone for sampling. If no osteomyelitis is present initially, the act of biopsy may seed the previously normal bone, producing osteomyelitis.

Supplementary Images

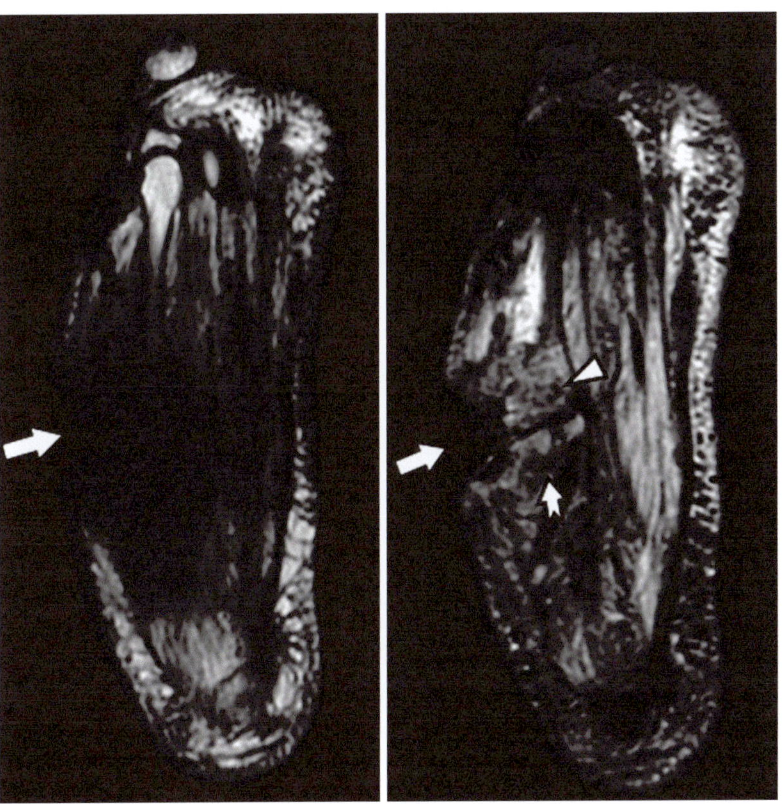

"Ghost sign" in osteomyelitis. There is soft tissue ulcer along the lateral midfoot. The base of the 4th metatarsal (arrowhead) and cuboid (notched arrows) are not well seen on the T1 image but reappear on the T2 fat saturated image

Report checklist

1. Is there a soft tissue ulcer and where is it located? Check patient or clinical notes if unsure.
2. Is there low T1 signal with poor visualization of the bone?
3. Are there marrow edema and enhancement?
4. Is there bony destruction, periostitis, and/or sinus tract formation?
5. How are the surrounding soft tissues? Is there an abscess, tenosynovitis, or joint effusion to suggest septic arthritis?

Suggested Reading

Fridman R, Bar-David T, Kamen S, Staron RB, Leung DK, Rasiej MJ. Imaging of diabetic foot infections. Clin Podiatr Med Surg. 31(2014):43–56.

Mandell JC, Khurana B, Smith JT, Czuczman GJ, Ghazikhanian V, Smith SE. Osteomyelitis of the lower extremity: pathophysiology, imaging, and classification, with an emphasis on diabetic foot infection. Emerg Radiol. 2018;25:175–88.

Case 9.5

Indication A 54-year-old man with lump along the volar aspect of the wrist 2 months after cardiac catheterization procedure.

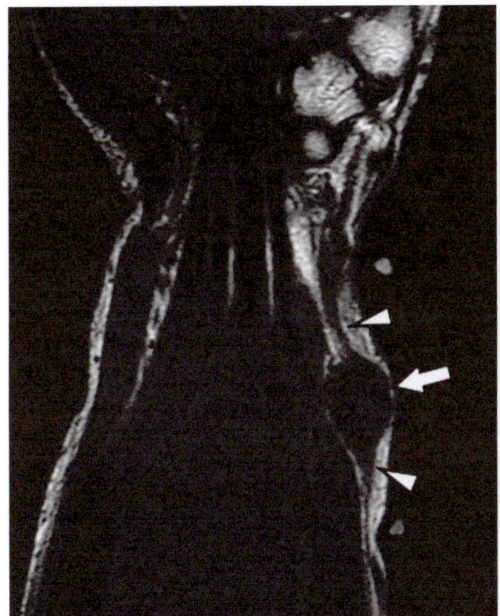

Coronal T1

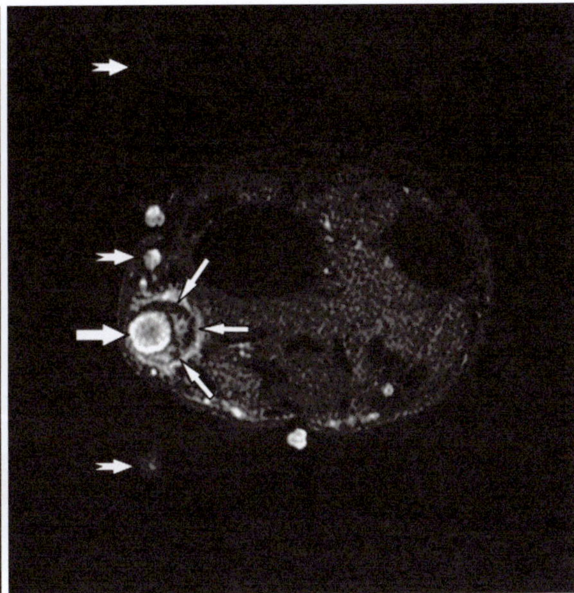

Axial T1 fat saturated post contrast

Findings

There is a 2.4 × 1.5 cm mass (arrow) along the volar aspect of the wrist, 6 cm proximal to the wrist joint. The mass appears to arise from the radial artery (arrowheads) and is at the expected entry site for vascular access from the prior cardiac procedure. The mass is low signal on T1-weighted images and slightly hyperintense on T2-weighted images. There is pulsation artifact (notched arrows) suggesting a vascular lesion. The lesion has heterogeneous central enhancement and peripheral C-shaped area (thin arrows) of nonenhancement suggestive of thrombus.

Impression/Recommendation

Radial artery pseudoaneurysm with pulsation artifact.

Discussion: Aneurysms

This case is being included as it highlights two important issues when interpreting MSK MRIs. The first point is the importance of knowing the complete clinical history. In the actual radiology report for this case, the lesion was misread as a peripheral nerve sheath tumor with a "target sign" appearance on the post-contrast images, and a percutaneous core needle biopsy was recommended. During preprocedural workup for biopsy planning, it was discovered that the patient had undergone cardiac catheterization 2 months prior to the MRI and the mass was then correctly diagnosed as a radial artery pseudoaneurysm and the biopsy was not performed. The initial radiologist failed to investigate the complete history for the patient, and a biopsy of the mass could have been disastrous. This case highlights the importance of reading the clinical history and investigating any prior surgeries or procedures at the site of interest.

The second important feature of this case is the pulsation artifact. Most of the time, we view artifacts on MRI as a negative, compromising the interpretability of the exam. However, at times, artifacts can be helpful. Pulsation or motion artifact occurs in the phase-encoded direction and results from tissue motion during the scan. This can occur from arterial pulsation, respiratory motion, peristalsis, or physical motion. Ghosting can occur, which is when tissue reappears throughout the image, in evenly spaced intervals. The spacing depends on the repetition time and frequency of the motion *(please refer to Case 9.7 for further discussion on MRI artifacts)*. In this case, the radial artery in cross section is repeated in an AP direction throughout the image. Had the initial radiologist realized that arterial pulsation artifact was present, he may not have mistaken the radial artery for a nerve. Another important use of MR artifact is using chemical shift artifact during "in- and out-of-phase" imaging. Bone lesions that contain macroscopic fat will have dropout on the "out-of-phase" T1 images when compared to the corresponding "in-phase" images. This technique is extremely helpful in distinguishing red marrow from a neoplasm.

Radial artery pseudoaneurysms are not uncommon and have been increasing due to the increase number of interventional radiology and cardiac procedures that require arterial access. They have also been described as an occupational injury in tailors and cheesemakers and from compression by the extensor pollicis longus tendon. Radial artery pseudoaneurysms are initially treated with compression. Thrombin injection and surgical closure may be needed in more severe cases.

Report checklist

1. Have you read the clinical history and do you understand the reason for the exam?
2. If the provided clinical history is sparse, have you looked at the medical records for additional information?
3. Have there been any surgeries or procedures in the area of concern?
4. Are there any MRI-related artifacts? Can you explain the cause of the artifact?
5. If there is pulsation artifact, is that structure a vessel?

Suggested Reading

Alabsi H, Goetz T, Murphy DT. Radial artery aneurysm secondary to dynamic entrapment by extensor pollicis longus tendon: a case of snapping thumb. Skelet Radiol. 2019;48:971–5.

Krupa K, Bekiesińska-Figatowska M. Artifacts in magnetic resonance imaging. Pol J Radiol. 2015;80:93–106.

Case 9.6

Indication A 34-year-old man with persistent foot pain and worsening soft tissue swelling 3 weeks after walking barefoot in his backyard.

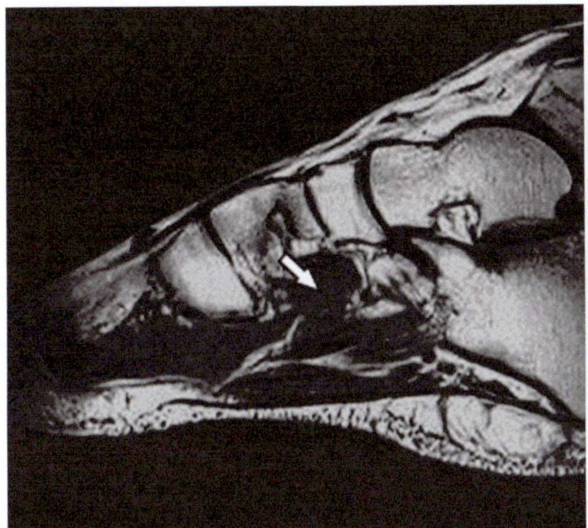

Sagittal T1

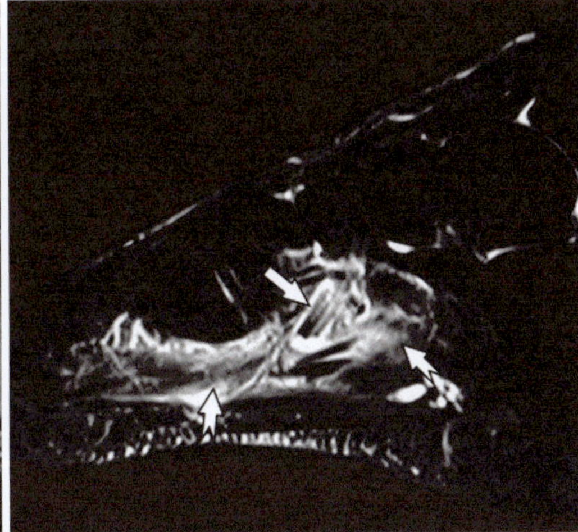

Sagittal T2 fat saturated

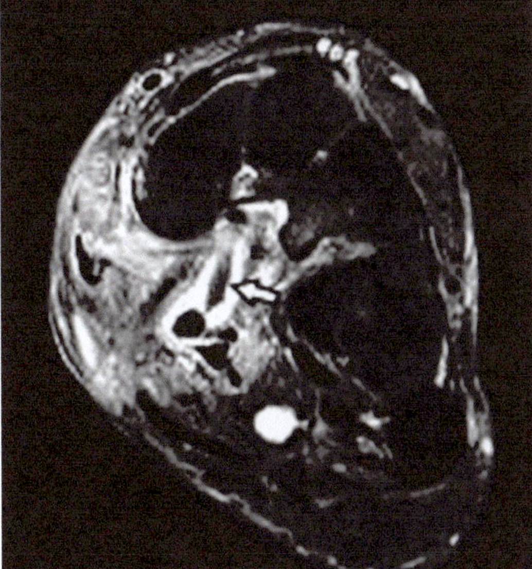

Coronal T2 fat saturated

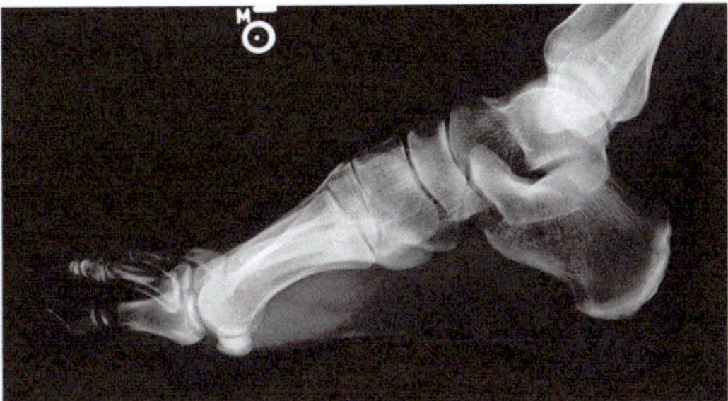

Findings

There is a 1.5-cm rectangular-striated low signal structure (arrows) in the plantar muscles, inferior to the medial and intermediate cuneiforms most consistent with a retained foreign body. There is fluid surrounding the structure and edema (notched arrows) in the surrounding plantar foot muscles. T1 marrow signal in the bones is preserved, and there are no MRI signs of osteomyelitis. There is no fluid in the adjacent tendon sheaths or joint spaces to indicate tenosynovitis or septic arthritis. No radiopaque material is seen on the prior radiographs.

Impression/Recommendation

Retained foreign body, likely wood splinter, in the plantar aspect of the midfoot with surrounding abscess and myositis.

Discussion: Retained foreign bodies

Puncture wounds to the feet are common and can lead to retained foreign bodies. These injuries are more common in the summer and fall months due to increase outdoor activity. Up to 10% of these injuries can have complications such as foreign body granuloma, abscess, osteomyelitis, and chronic pain. These complications are more likely to occur if the foreign body has been present for greater than 48 hours. At times, the patients may not recall any penetrating injury. This can be common for patients with diabetes with peripheral neuropathy. The main goal in the diagnosis and treatment of pedal puncture wounds is to identify the presence and location of the foreign body for quick removal before complications develop.

It is important to take a careful history as to what type of foreign body is suspected in order to select the best imaging test. In general radiographs are the initial imaging test, and they are excellent at detecting metallic objects such as nails and needles, but are poor for wood, rubber, hair, plastic, or clear glass. Tinted glass can have variable appearance on radiographs due to the presence of some metal that provides color to the glass. CT is excellent in the detection of soft tissue gas and has higher sensitivity than radiographs for detection of foreign bodies, but wood and other non-radiopaque material may still not be evident on CT. The USA is likely the best modality at identifying the location and presence of a foreign body since most substances, including wood, will be visible and cause posterior acoustic shadowing regardless of its composition *(see supplementary images)*. But ultrasound cannot assess many of the complications that can occur with pedal puncture wounds. MRI is likely the best modality at assessing these complications. It can detect the presence of osteomyelitis, cellulitis, abscess, and foreign body granuloma better than other imaging modalities. On MRI, most foreign bodies are low signal on both T1- and T2-weighted sequences. However, fresh wood can have high signal on T2-weighted images due to some water content. MRI is ideal for identifying the presence of osteomyelitis which classically appears as hypointense signal on T1-weighted sequences relative to skeletal muscle. The presence of fluid around the foreign body can suggest an abscess, and a sinus tract to the skin may be present. A foreign body granuloma will appear as an enhancing mass encasing the foreign body, often with surrounding soft tissue edema and enhancement. Lastly, the foreign body may fragment, and the various components may separate from each other and migrate away from the initial entry time over time. So it is important to perform a careful search for additional foreign bodies.

Treatment for a retained foreign body is with debridement and surgical removal of the foreign body followed by irrigation of the wound. The patient's tetanus status should be reviewed, and a booster dose can be given if the patient has equivocal or negative immune status.

Supplementary Images

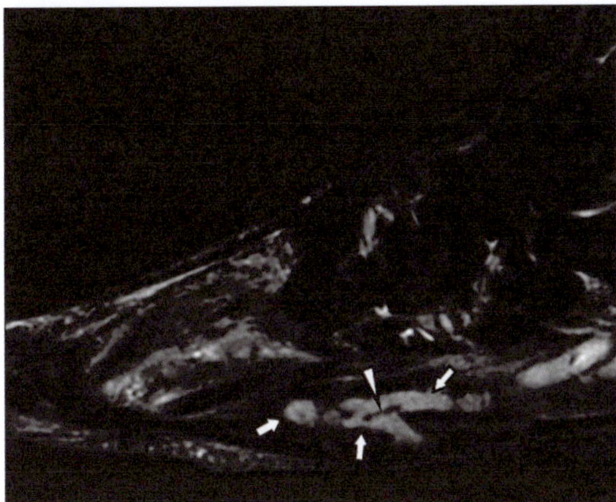

Sagittal STIR

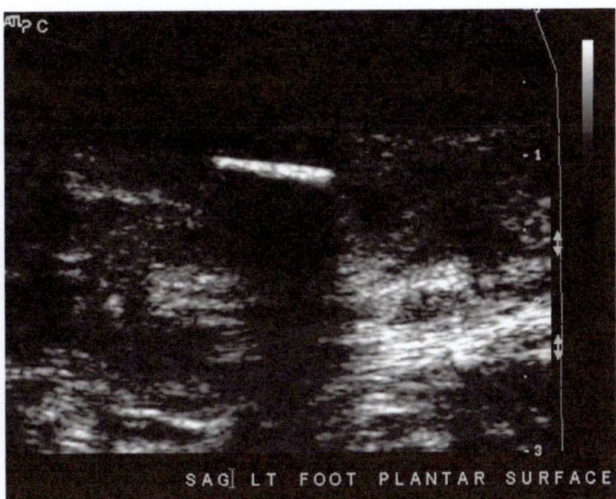

Longitudinal gray scale ultrasound image

Retained wood splinter in the foot. MR image shows a linear 1.3 cm low signal structure (arrowhead) in the lateral midfoot with surrounding fluid (arrows) consistent with abscess. The wood splinter is highly echogenic and has *posterior acoustic shadowing on the ultrasound image. Ultrasound is likely the best overall test at identifying a foreign body regardless of composition*

Report checklist

1. Is there a history of penetrating trauma? What is the composition of the suspected foreign body?
2. Is there a low signal structure near the puncture site? What is its exact location of the foreign body to aid in surgical removal?
3. Is there fluid surrounding the foreign body to suggest an abscess?
4. Are there signs of cellulitis or osteomyelitis?
5. Are there more than one foreign body?

Suggested Reading

Pattamapaspong N, Srisuwan T, Sivasomboon C, Nasuto M, Suwannahoy P, Settakorn J, Kraisarin J, Guglielmi G. Accuracy of radiography, computed tomography and magnetic resonance imaging in diagnosing foreign bodies in the foot. Radiol Med. 2013;118:303–10.

Peterson JJ, Bancroft LW, Kransdorf MJ. Wooden foreign bodies: imaging appearance. AJR. 2002;178:557–62.

Racz RS, Ramanujam CL, Zgonis T. Puncture wounds of the foot. Clin Podiatr Med Surg. 2010;27:523–34.

Case 9.7

Indication A 38-year-old female with palpable lump on the right arm. Assess for underlying mass.

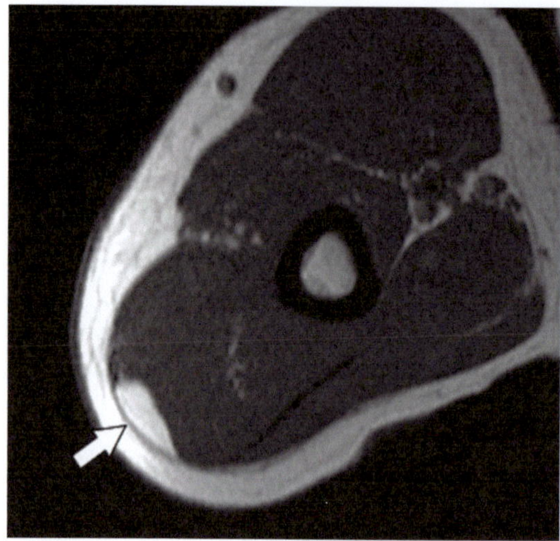

Axial T1

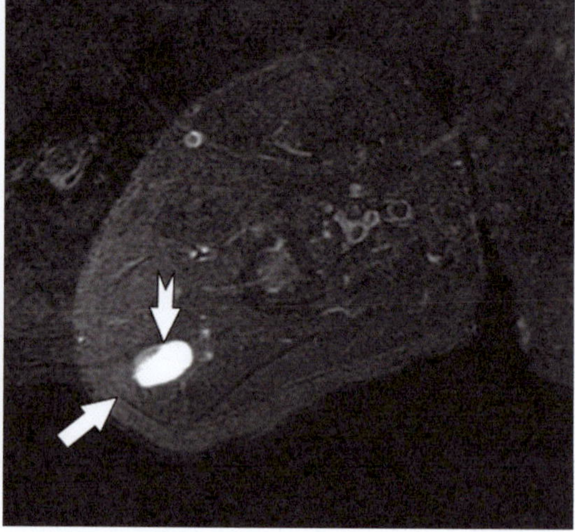

Axial T2 fat saturated

Findings

There is a 2.5 × 1.5 cm intramuscular fatty lesion (arrows) at the lateral aspect of the triceps muscle that is hyperintense on T1-weighted images and suppresses on fat saturated images. The imaging characteristics are compatible with a simple lipoma. On the T2 fat saturated images, there is 2 cm hyperintense lesion (notched arrow) projecting near the area of concern which corresponds to a sebaceous cyst at the patient's upper back. This is due to wraparound artifact.

Impression/Recommendation

1. Small intramuscular lipoma. No concerning features.
2. Wraparound artifact causes a 2 cm cyst to project over the area of concern in the arm and is likely a known sebaceous cyst in the patient's upper back.

Discussion: MRI artifacts in MSK imaging

MRI of the musculoskeletal (MSK) system is subject to a number of potential artifacts which may affect image quality or simulate pathologic conditions and hence can result in interpretation errors. Although a detailed review of MRI artifacts is beyond the scope of this discussion, we will discuss a few common artifacts we see in daily practice and how to overcome them.

Motion artifacts are probably one of the most common artifacts in MSK imaging. These artifacts can be divided into periodic and nonperiodic motion. Periodic motion results from various physiologic processes including cardiac motion, respiration, and vascular flow. Nonperiodic motion includes inadvertent patient motion and is more commonly seen in elderly and pediatric patients. Ghosting and smearing are common artifacts that occur with motion which results in the moving structure being reconstructed repeatedly "ghost" in the phase-encoding direction *(see supplementary images)*. This can be problematic as the ghosting artifact may extend through the area of anatomic interest. Patient motion can be reduced by reassuring the patient, immobilizing the limb within the coil by using soft pads or towels, using sequences with shorter acquisition times, or performing the study under sedation. Periodic motion can be compensated by increasing the number of acquired signals or switching the direction of the phase and frequency-encoding gradients to direct the ghosting artifact away from area of concern.

Wraparound artifact, also known as "aliasing" artifact, is also a commonly encountered artifact in MSK imaging and occurs when the field of view is too small to include the tissue being imaged. This results in folding or wraparound of the phase-encoded signal outside the field of view to the opposite side of the image and is always encountered in the phase-encoding direction like in this case. The artifact may be reduced by increasing the field of view, applying an oversampling technique or by applying saturation pulses on the undesired structures. Alternatively, switching the frequency and phase-encoding directions may help reduce these artifacts.

Susceptibility artifact occurs due to inhomogeneity of the local magnetic field producing spatial misregistration. These artifacts are more severe in areas with ferromagnetic material as joint prosthesis, metallic implants, surgical implants or metallic foreign bodies *(see supplementary images)*. If the artifact is caused by an external metallic object, then simply removing it corrects the artifact. *There are various ways of reducing metal artifacts that is discussed in more detail in Case 4.10.*

Fat saturated sequences are one of the main sequences used in MSK imaging to highlight areas of pathology; however, occasionally with these sequences, there may be areas of heterogeneous signal with parts of the image showing lit-tle or no fat suppression. This is usually related to inhomogeneity in the magnetic field and is more commonly seen in images performed with a large field of view. They are also commonly seen when imaging the post-peripheral extremities such as the foot and hand. This can be problematic as it may cause confusion if an area of high signal intensity is related to edema or from the artifact. One of the simplest ways of correcting this is using a STIR sequence rather than a standard fat-suppressed sequence *(see supplementary images)*. Alternatively, decreasing the field of view or repositioning the patient might help reducing this artifact.

Lastly, another commonly encountered artifact is what has been described as the "magic angle phenomenon." This artifact is seen in sequences with short echo time (TE) as T1 and PD sequences and occurs when the fibers being imaged are oriented at an angle of about 55° to the main magnetic field. Examples include the distal rotator cuff, ankle tendons, and the patellar tendon. This pitfall can be overcome by closely comparing the signal abnormalities with this on the T2-weighted images or repositioning the patient *(see supplementary images)*.

Supplementary Images

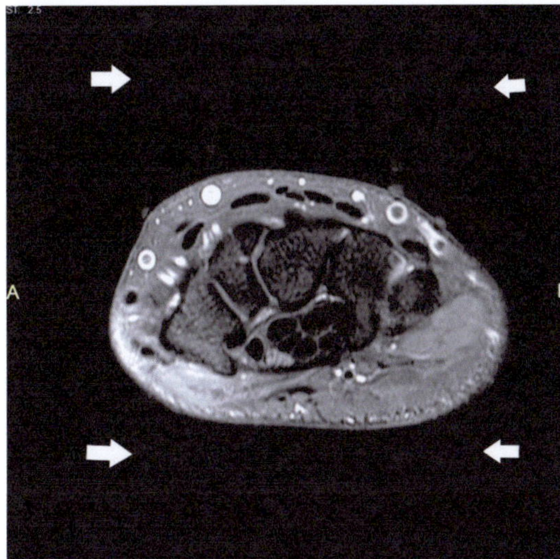

Axial T2 fat saturated

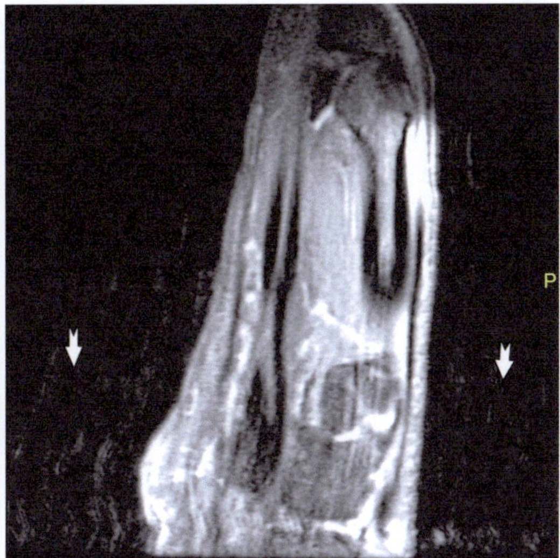

Sagittal T2 fat saturated

Motion artifacts. The first image demonstrates a pulsing ghost artifact (arrows) in the phase-encoded direction from the vascular structures of the wrist. The second *image demonstrates smearing of the image as well as ghosting artifact (notched arrows) related to patient motion in the foot*

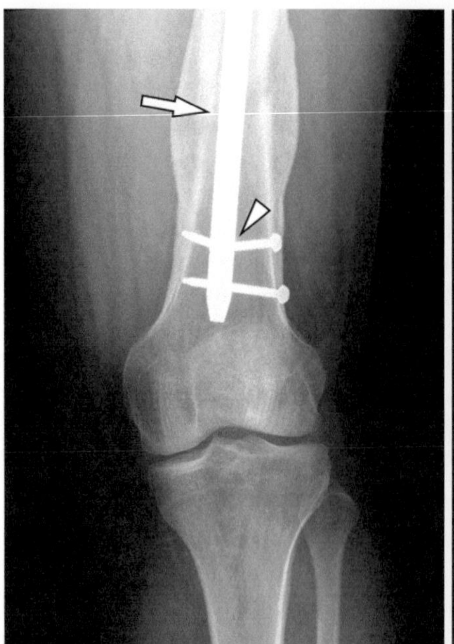

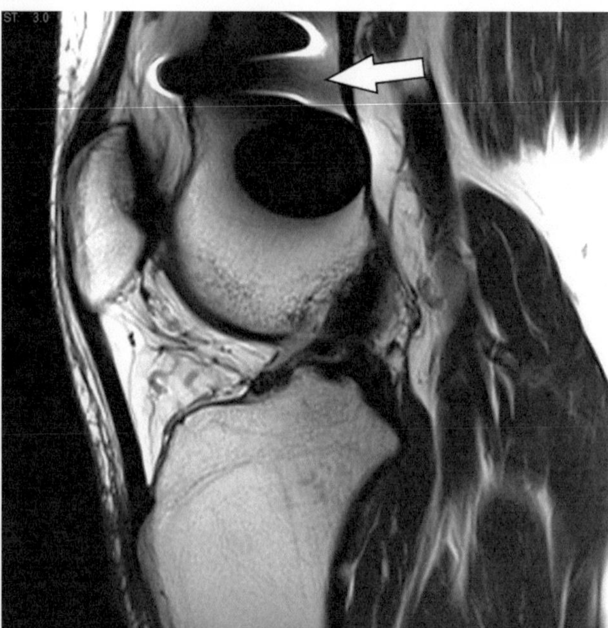

Sagittal PD

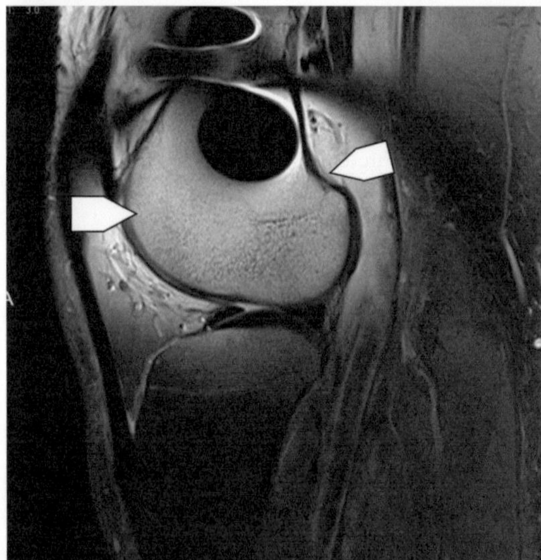

Sagittal T2 fat saturated

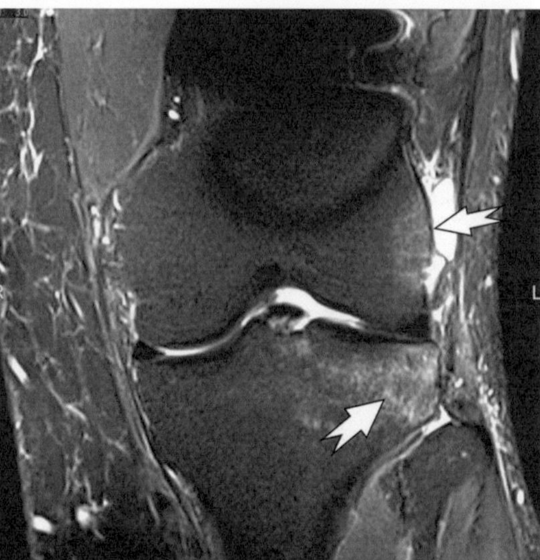

Coronal T2 STIR

Susceptibility artifact. There is an intramedullary rod (arrow) in the distal femur with broken screw (arrowhead) which causes significant distortion of the image related to magnetic field inhomogeneity. This causes issues with fat suppression. The distal femur is hyperintense (block arrows) on the T2 fat saturated image due to field inhomogeneity from the hardware. Note how using the STIR sequence improves that fat suppression and now the bone marrow edema (notched arrows) seen at the lateral femoral condyle and lateral tibial plateau is better visualized

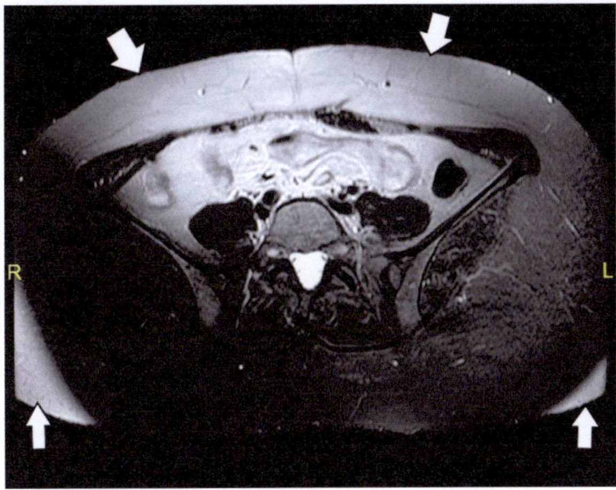

Axial T2 fat saturated

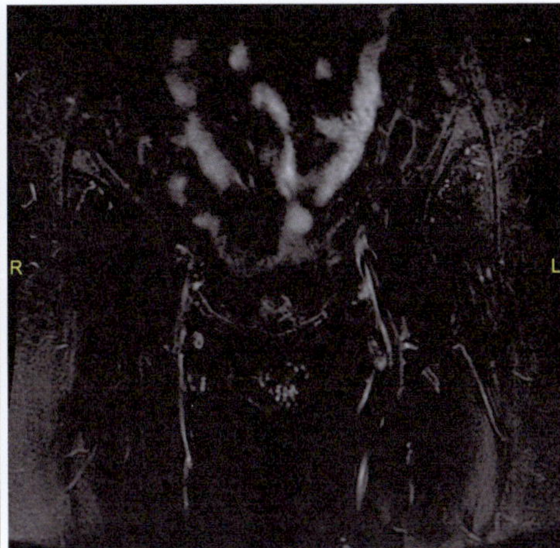

Coronal STIR

Incomplete fat suppression. Due to the large size of the patient and large field of view. The peripheral and anterior portions of the image (arrows) demonstrate little fat *suppression which is related to magnetic field inhomogeneity at the periphery. Note the improved fat suppression on the STIR sequence*

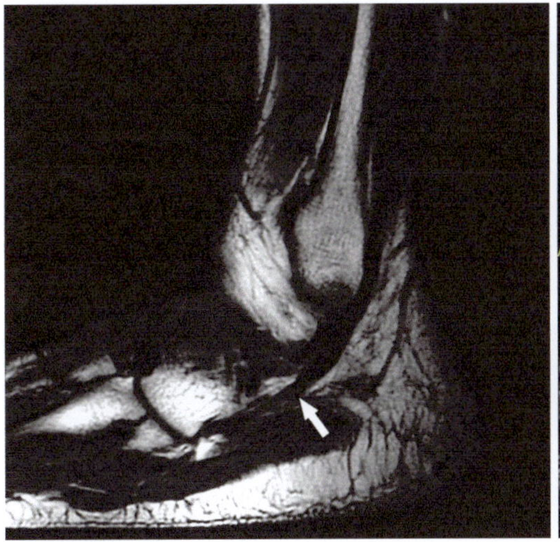

Sagittal T1

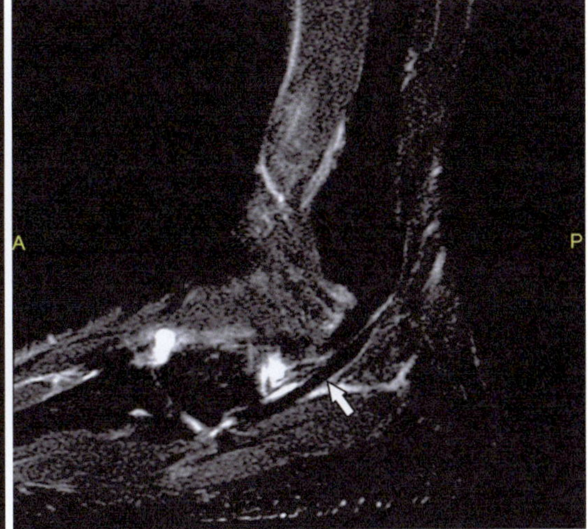

Sagittal T2 fat saturated

Magic angle phenomenon. There is artifactual high signal intensity on the T1-weighted images within the peroneal tendon (arrows) as it curves below the lateral malleolus *giving a false impression of pathology. Note how this is improved by closely scrutinizing the same area on the T2-weighted image*

Suggested Reading

Roth E, Hoff M, Richardson ML, Ha AS, Porrino J. Artifacts affecting musculoskeletal magnetic resonance imaging: their origins and solutions. Curr Probl Diagn Radiol. 2016;45:340–6.

Singh DR, Chin MS, Peh WC. Artifacts in musculoskeletal MR imaging. Semin Musculoskelet Radiol. 2014;18:12–22.

Sample MSK MRI Reports 10

SHOULDER

EXAMINATION:

[MRI SHOULDER]

INDICATION: [ ]

TECHNIQUE:
Multiplanar images of the shoulder were performed without the administration of intravenous or intra-articular contrast using a routine MRI shoulder protocol. Sequences include: (Axial PD FS, Coronal Oblique T2 FS, Sagittal Oblique T2 FS, Sagittal Oblique T1).

COMPARISON:

Compared to prior study from [ ].

FINDINGS:
Supraspinatus: [Normal. There is no focal tear or tendinosis.]
Infraspinatus: [Normal. There is no focal tear or tendinosis.]
Teres minor: [Normal. There is no focal tear or tendinosis.]
Subscapularis: [Normal. There is no focal tear or tendinosis.]
Rotator Cuff: [Normal. There is no fatty atrophy or decrease muscle bulk.]

Acromio-clavicular joint: [Normal. There are no significant degenerative changes.]

Biceps tendon: [The biceps tendon is well seated within the bicipital groove and attaches normally to the superior labrum.]

Glenoid labrum: [The labrum is intact without focal tear. There is no SLAP or labral Bankart injury.]

Glenohumeral joint: [There is no joint effusion.]

Hyaline cartilage: [Cartilage is preserved without focal defects or subchondral marrow edema.]

Bone marrow: [There is no abnormal marrow edema or marrow replacing lesions.]

Soft tissues: [There is no lymphadenopathy or abnormal masses. Neurovascular structures are within normal limits.]

IMPRESSION:

[Normal MRI examination of the shoulder.]

© Springer Nature Switzerland AG 2020

T. M. Hegazi, J. S. Wu, *Musculoskeletal MRI*, https://doi.org/10.1007/978-3-030-26777-3_10

SHOULDER ARTHROGRAM

EXAMINATION:

[MRI SHOULDER ARTHROGRAM]

INDICATION: [ ]

TECHNIQUE:

Multiplanar images of the shoulder were performed after the injection of intra-articular gadolinium contrast using a MRI shoulder arthrogram protocol. Sequences include: Axial T1 FS, Coronal Oblique T1 FS, Coronal Oblique T2 FS, Sagittal Oblique T1 FS, Coronal Oblique T1.

COMPARISON:

Compared to prior study from [ ].

FINDINGS:

There is good distention of the glenohumeral joint space with dilute gadolinium contrast. There is no extension of contrast into the subacromial/subdeltoid space to indicate a full-thickness rotator cuff tear.

Supraspinatus: [Normal. There is no focal tear or tendinosis.]
Infraspinatus: [Normal. There is no focal tear or tendinosis.]
Teres minor: [Normal. There is no focal tear or tendinosis.]
Subscapularis: [Normal. There is no focal tear or tendinosis.]
Rotator Cuff Muscles: [Normal. There is no fatty atrophy or decrease muscle bulk.]

Acromio-clavicular joint: [Normal. There are no significant degenerative changes.]

Biceps tendon: [The biceps tendon is well seated within the bicipital groove and attaches normally to the superior labrum.]

Glenoid labrum: [The labrum is intact without abnormal contrast extension to indicate a focal tear. There is no SLAP or labral Bankart injury.]

Glenohumeral joint: [The joint is distended with contrast.]

Hyaline cartilage: [Cartilage is preserved without focal defects or subchondral marrow edema.]

Bone marrow: [There is no abnormal marrow edema or marrow replacing lesions.]

Soft tissues: [There is no lymphadenopathy or abnormal masses. Neurovascular structures are within normal limits.]

IMPRESSION:

[Normal MRI arthrogram examination of the shoulder.]

PECTORALIS MAJOR

EXAMINATION:

MRI PECTORALIS MAJOR (CHEST WALL)

INDICATION: [ ]

TECHNIQUE:

Multiplanar images of the upper lateral chest wall at the humeral attachment of the pectoralis major were performed without the administration of intravenous contrast using a pectoralis major protocol. Sequences include: Axial T1, Axial STIR, Coronal Oblique T1, Coronal Oblique STIR, Sagittal Oblique STIR.

COMPARISON:

Compared to prior study from [ ].

FINDINGS:

[The common tendon of the pectoralis major muscle is normal in signal intensity without focal tear or tendinosis.] [The tendon has a normal attachment onto the bicipital groove of the proximal humerus.] [The pectoralis major muscle belly is normal without muscle edema, hematoma, or fatty atrophy.]

[There is normal marrow signal without edema or focal lesions.] [There is no glenohumeral joint effusion.] [The neurovascular structures are normal.]

IMPRESSION:

Normal examination of the pectoralis major without focal tear or muscle injury.

ELBOW

EXAMINATION:

MRI ELBOW

INDICATION: [ ]

TECHNIQUE:

Multiplanar images of the elbow were performed without the administration of intravenous or intra-articular contrast using a routine MRI elbow protocol. Sequences include: Axial T1, Axial T2 FS, Coronal T1, Coronal T2 FS, Coronal T2* GRE, Sagittal PD FS.

COMPARISON:

Compared to prior study from [ ].

FINDINGS:

Biceps tendon: [There is no focal tear or tendinosis. The tendon has a normal insertion on the radial tuberosity.]
Brachialis tendon: [There is no focal tear or tendinosis. The tendon has normal insertion onto the ulna.]
Triceps tendon: [There is no focal tear or tendinosis. There is a normal distal attachment at the olecranon.]

Radial collateral ligament: [Within normal limits.]
Ulnar collateral ligament: [Within normal limits.]
Lateral ulnar collateral ligament: [Within normal limits.]

Common extensor tendon: [Within normal limits.]
Common flexor tendon: [Within normal limits.]

Joint space: [There is no joint effusion or osteoarthritis.] [No osteochondral lesions are seen.]

Bone marrow signal: [There is no marrow edema or marrow replacing lesions.]

Muscles: [Muscle mass is preserved, without muscle edema or atrophy.]

Nerves: [No abnormal signal or lesions seen within the expected location of the median, ulnar, or radial nerves.]

Cubital tunnel: [Normal]

IMPRESSION:

Normal Elbow MRI examination.

ELBOW ARTHROGRAM

EXAMINATION:

MRI ELBOW ARTHROGRAM

INDICATION: [ ]

TECHNIQUE:

Multiplanar images of the elbow were performed after the injection of intra-articular gadolinium contrast using a MRI elbow arthrogram protocol. Sequences include: Axial T1, Axial T1 FS, Coronal T1 FS, Coronal T2 FS, Coronal T2* GRE, Sagittal T1 FS.

COMPARISON:

Compared to prior study from [ ].

FINDINGS:

There is good distention of the elbow joint space with dilute gadolinium contrast.

Biceps tendon: [There is no focal tear or tendinosis. The tendon has a normal insertion on the radial tuberosity.]
Brachialis tendon: [There is no focal tear or tendinosis. The tendon has normal insertion onto the ulna.]
Triceps tendon: [There is no focal tear or tendinosis. There is a normal distal attachment at the olecranon.]

Radial collateral ligament: [Within normal limits. There is no abnormal extension of contrast into the adjacent soft tissues.]
Ulnar collateral ligament: [Within normal limits. There is no abnormal extension of contrast into the adjacent soft tissues.]
Lateral ulnar collateral ligament: [Within normal limits.]

Common extensor tendon: [Within normal limits.]
Common flexor tendon: [Within normal limits.]

Joint space: [There is distension with dilute gadolinium contrast.] [Hyaline cartilage is preserved.] [No osteochondral lesions are seen.]

Bone marrow signal: [There is no marrow edema or marrow replacing lesions.]

Muscles: [Muscle mass is preserved, without muscle edema or atrophy.]

Nerves: [No abnormal signal or lesions seen within the expected location of the median, ulnar, or radial nerves.]

Cubital tunnel: [Normal]

IMPRESSION:

Normal Elbow MRI arthrogram examination.

WRIST

EXAMINATION:

[MRI WRIST]

INDICATION: [ ]

TECHNIQUE:
Multiplanar images of the wrist were performed without the administration of intravenous or intra-articular contrast using a routine MRI wrist protocol (Axial PD, Axial T2 FS, Coronal T1, Coronal T2 FS, Coronal 3D T2* GRE, Sagittal T2).

COMPARISON:

Compared to prior study from [ ].

FINDINGS:
Triangular fibrocartilage: [The central disc, radial and ulnar components are normal.]
Scapholunate ligament: [The dorsal, membranous, and volar components are normal.]
Lunotriquetral ligament: [The dorsal, membranous, and volar components are normal.]

Flexor tendons: [Normal. There is no tenosynovitis or focal tear.]

Extensor tendons: [Normal. There is no tenosynovitis or focal tear.]

Carpal tunnel: [There is no abnormal bowing. The median nerve is normal in signal and size.]
Guyon's canal: [Within normal limits.]

Bone marrow: [Within normal limits.] [No bone marrow edema or marrow replacing lesions.] [No erosions are seen.]

Joint effusion: [No joint effusion seen.] [No ganglia are seen.]

Muscles: [Muscles about the wrist within normal limits without edema or fatty atrophy.]
Masses: [There are no abnormal masses detected about the wrist.]

IMPRESSION:

Normal MRI of the wrist

WRIST ARTHROGRAM

EXAMINATION:

[MRI WRIST ARTHROGRAM]

INDICATION: [ ]

TECHNIQUE:
Multiplanar images of the wrist were performed after the injection of intra-articular gadolinium contrast using a MRI wrist arthrogram protocol. Sequences include: Axial T1 FS, Coronal T1 FS, Sagittal T1 FS, Coronal T2 FS, Coronal T1, Axial T2 FS.

COMPARISON:

Compared to prior study from [ ].

FINDINGS:
Triangular fibrocartilage: [The central disc, radial and ulnar components are normal.][There is no contrast in the distal radioulnar joint to indicate a full thickness tear.]
Scapholunate ligament: [The dorsal, membranous, and volar components are normal.] [There is no contrast in the midcarpal row to indicate a full thickness tear.]
Lunotriquetral ligament: [The dorsal, membranous, and volar components are normal.] [There is no contrast in the midcarpal row to indicate a full thickness tear.]

Flexor tendons: [Normal. There is no tenosynovitis or focal tear.]

Extensor tendons: [Normal. There is no tenosynovitis or focal tear.]

Carpal tunnel: [There is no abnormal bowing. The median nerve is normal in signal and size.]

Guyon's canal: [Within normal limits.]

Bone marrow: [Within normal limits.] [No bone marrow edema or marrow replacing lesions.] [No erosions are seen.]

Joint effusion: [The wrist joint is distended with dilute gadolinium contrast.] [No ganglia are seen.]

Muscles: [Muscles about the wrist within normal limits without edema or fatty atrophy.]
Masses: [There are no abnormal masses detected about the wrist.]

IMPRESSION:

Normal MRI of the wrist arthrogram.

HAND/FINGER/THUMB

EXAMINATION:

[MRI HAND FINGER]

INDICATION: [ ]

TECHNIQUE:

Multiplanar images of the hand/finger/thumb were performed without the administration of intravenous or intra-articular contrast using a routine MRI hand/finger/thumb protocol (Axial PD, Axial T2 FS, Sagittal T2, Coronal T1, Coronal T2* GRE).

COMPARISON:

Compared to prior study from [ ].

FINDINGS:

Bone marrow: [Normal.] [There is no bone marrow edema or marrow replacing lesions.] [No erosions are seen.]

Flexor tendons: [The tendons have normal signal without focal tear, tendinosis or tenosynovitis.] [There is no bowstringing of the tendon to suggest a pulley injury.]

Extensor tendons: [The tendons have normal signal without focal tear, tendinosis or tenosynovitis.]

Joint: [The collateral ligaments are intact without thickening or increase signal.] [No joint effusion seen.] [No ganglia are seen.]

Muscles: [Muscles about the hand and fingers are within normal limits without edema or fatty atrophy.]

Soft tissues: [There are no abnormal masses.]

IMPRESSION:

Normal MRI examination of the hand/finger/thumb.

PELVIS

EXAMINATION:

[MRI Pelvis]

INDICATION: [ ]

TECHNIQUE:

Multiplanar images of pelvis (top of the iliac crests through the lesser trochanters bilaterally) were performed
without the administration of intravenous or intra-articular contrast using a routine MR orthopedic pelvis protocol.
Sequences include: Axial T1, Axial T2 FS, Coronal T1, Coronal STIR.

COMPARISON:

Compared to prior study from [ ].

FINDINGS:

[There is normal marrow signal in the proximal femurs bilaterally.] [There are no signs for avascular necrosis or
stress fracture.] [The marrow signal throughout the rest of the pelvis is preserved.] [There is normal marrow signal
at the sacroiliac joints and in the lower lumbar spine.]

[There is no hip joint effusion on either side.] [No paralabral cysts are seen.] [There is no greater trochanteric
bursitis on either side.] [The hamstring insertions onto the ischial tuberosities are normal.] [There is normal muscle
bulk without fatty atrophy.]

[The visualized intra-abdominal contents are within normal limits.]

IMPRESSION:

Normal MRI of the bony pelvis.

UNILATERAL HIP

EXAMINATION:

MRI [right or left] HIP

INDICATION: [ ]

TECHNIQUE:

Multiplanar images of the [] hip were performed [without] the administration of intravenous contrast using a unilateral [] hip MR protocol. Sequences include: Coronal T1 (bilateral large FOV), Coronal STIR (bilateral large FOV), Axial Oblique PD FS (unilateral), Coronal PD FS (unilateral), Sagittal PD FS (unilateral).

COMPARISON:

Compared to prior study from [ ].

FINDINGS:

[There is normal marrow signal within the proximal femurs bilaterally.] [There are no signs for avascular necrosis or stress fracture.] [The marrow signal throughout the rest of the pelvis is preserved.] [There is normal signal at the sacroiliac joints and lower lumbar spine.]

[Focused imaging of the [right] hip demonstrates no significant joint effusion.] [The articular cartilage is relatively preserved.] [There are no displaced labral tears.] [There is no greater trochanteric bursitis. [The hamstring insertion onto the ischial tuberosity is normal.] [There is normal muscle bulk without fatty atrophy.]

[The visualized intra-abdominal contents are within normal limits.]

IMPRESSION:

[Normal exam of the [] hip.]

UNILATERAL HIP ARTHROGRAM

EXAMINATION:

MRI [right or left] HIP ARTHROGRAM

INDICATION: [ ]

TECHNIQUE:

Multiplanar images of the [] hip were performed after the injection of intra-articular dilute gadolinium contrast using a unilateral hip MR arthrogram protocol. Sequences include: Coronal T1 FS, Axial Oblique T1 FS, Sagittal T1 FS, Coronal T2 FS, Coronal T1.

COMPARISON:

Compared to prior study from [ ].

FINDINGS:

[There is good distention of the hip joint with dilute gadolinium contrast.] [The hip labrum is normal without displaced or intrasubstance tears. The transverse ligament and ligamentum teres are intact. The articular cartilage is preserved without focal defects. The femoral head and neck has a normal contour without signs of cam or pincer type femoral acetabular impingement. The alpha angle is normal at [ ] degrees.] There are no paralabral cysts.

[There is normal marrow signal in the proximal femur.] [There are no signs for avascular necrosis or stress fracture.] [The marrow signal throughout the rest of the pelvis is preserved.] [The hamstring insertion onto the ischial tuberosity is normal.] [There is normal muscle bulk without fatty atrophy.]

[The visualized intra-abdominal contents are within normal limits.]

IMPRESSION:

[Normal MR arthrogram of the [] hip.]

SACROILIAC JOINTS

EXAMINATION:

[MRI SACROILIAC JOINTS WITH INTRAVENOUS CONTRAST]

INDICATION: [ ]

TECHNIQUE:

Multiplanar images of bilateral sacroiliac joints were performed before and after the administration of intravenous or intra-articular contrast using a MR sacroiliac joint protocol. Sequences include: Sagittal T1, Coronal Oblique T1, Coronal Oblique STIR, Axial Oblique T1, Axial Oblique STIR, Axial 3D SPGR T1 Pre, Axial 3D SPGR T1 Post

COMPARISON:

Compared to prior study from [ ].

FINDINGS:

[There is no abnormal marrow edema or erosions of either sacroiliac joints to indicate sacroilitis.] [No fluid is seen in the sacroiliac joints.] [The iliacus, psoas, and iliopsoas muscles are normal bilaterally without atrophy or edema.] [After the administration of intravenous gadolinium contrast, there is no abnormal enhancement.]

[Limited evaluation of the lower lumbar spine is unremarkable without compression deformities or significant degenerative disc disease.] [The proximal femurs and rest of the marrow signal throughout the pelvis is normal.] [There is no hip joint effusion on either side.]

[The visualized intra-abdominal contents are within normal limits.]

IMPRESSION:

Normal MRI examination of the sacroiliac joints.

KNEE

EXAMINATION:

[MRI KNEE]

INDICATION: [ ]

TECHNIQUE:

Multiplanar images of the knee were performed without the administration of intravenous contrast using a routine MR knee protocol. Sequences include: Axial PD FS, Sagittal PD,Sagittal T2 FS, Coronal PD FS.

COMPARISON:

Compared to prior studies from [ ].

FINDINGS:

Medial meniscus: [There is normal morphology without focal tear.]
Lateral meniscus: [There is normal morphology without focal tear.]

Anterior cruciate ligament: [There is normal alignment without focal tear.]
Posterior cruciate ligament: [There is normal alignment without focal tear.]

Medial collateral ligament: [Normal]
Lateral collateral ligamentous complex: [The iliotibial band, fibular collateral ligament, biceps femoris tendon, and popliteus are normal.]

Extensor mechanism: [The quadriceps tendon and patellar tendon are normal. There is normal fatty signal in Hoffa's fat pad. There is no prepatellar bursitis.]

Baker's cyst: [None]

Joint effusion: [None]

Patellofemoral articular cartilage: [The cartilage is preserved without focal defects or subchondral marrow edema.]
Medial articular cartilage: [The cartilage is preserved without focal defects or subchondral marrow edema.]
Lateral compartment cartilage: [The cartilage is preserved without focal defects or subchondral marrow edema.]

Marrow: [There is no abnormal marrow edema or marrow replacing lesions.]

Soft tissues: [There is no lymphadenopathy or abnormal masses. Neurovascular structures are within normal limits.]

IMPRESSION:

[Normal MRI examination of the knee.]

KNEE ARTHROGRAM

EXAMINATION:

[MRI KNEE ARTHROGRAM]

INDICATION: [ ]

TECHNIQUE:

Multiplanar images of the knee were performed after the intra-articular injection of dilute gadolinium contrast using a MR knee arthrogram protocol. Sequences include: Axial PD FS, Sagittal T1 FS, Sagittal T2 FS, Coronal T1 FS, Coronal T1.

COMPARISON:

Compared to prior studies from [ ].

FINDINGS:

[There is good distention of the knee joint space with dilute gadolinium contrast.]

Medial meniscus: [There is normal morphology without focal tear.] [There is no abnormal contrast signal extending into the meniscal substance.]
Lateral meniscus: [There is normal morphology without focal tear.] [There is no abnormal contrast signal extending into the meniscal substance.]

Anterior cruciate ligament: [There is normal alignment without focal tear.]
Posterior cruciate ligament: [There is normal alignment without focal tear.]

Medial collateral ligament: [Normal]
Lateral collateral ligamentous complex: [The iliotibial band, fibular collateral ligament, biceps femoris tendon, and popliteus are normal.]

Extensor mechanism: [The quadriceps tendon and patellar tendon are normal. There is normal fatty signal in Hoffa's fat pad. There is no prepatellar bursitis.]

Baker's cyst: [None]
Joint effusion: [There is good joint distension with contrast.]

Patellofemoral articular cartilage: [The cartilage is preserved without focal defects or subchondral marrow edema.]
Medial articular cartilage: [The cartilage is preserved without focal defects or subchondral marrow edema.]
Lateral compartment cartilage: [The cartilage is preserved without focal defects or subchondral marrow edema.]

Marrow: [There is no abnormal marrow edema or marrow replacing lesions.]

Soft tissues: [There is no lymphadenopathy or abnormal masses. Neurovascular structures are within normal limits.]

IMPRESSION:

[Normal MR arthrogram examination of the knee.]

ANKLE

EXAMINATION:

MRI ANKLE

INDICATION: [ ]

TECHNIQUE:
Multiplanar images of the ankle were performed without the administration of intravenous contrast using a routine MR ankle protocol. Sequences include: Axial PD, Axial T2 FS, Sagittal T1, Sagittal STIR, Coronal PD FS.

COMPARISON:

Compared to prior study from [ ].

FINDINGS:
Achilles tendon: [Normal, there is no tendinosis or focal tear. There is no edema in Kager's pad fat. No fluid is seen in the retrocalcaneal or retro-Achilles bursae].

Posterior tibial tendon: [Normal. There is no tendinosis, focal tear or tenosynovitis].
Flexor digitorum tendon: [Normal. There is no tendinosis, focal tear or tenosynovitis].
Flexor hallucis tendon: [Normal. There is no tendinosis, focal tear or tenosynovitis].

Peroneal tendons: [Normal. There is no tendinosis, focal tear or tenosynovitis].

Anterior tibialis tendon: [Normal. There is no tendinosis, focal tear or tenosynovitis].
Extensor digitorum tendon: [Normal. There is no tendinosis, focal tear or tenosynovitis].
Extensor hallucis longus: [Normal. There is no tendinosis, focal tear or tenosynovitis].

Anterior tibiofibular ligament: [Normal].
Posterior tibiofibular ligament: [Normal].

Anterior talofibular ligament: [Normal].
Posterior talofibular ligament: [Normal].
Calcaneofibular ligament: [Normal.]

Tibiotalar ligament: [Normal.]
Tibiospring Ligament: [Normal.]
Spring ligament: [Normal].

Sinus tarsi: [Normal. There is preservation of the normal fatty signal without edema or focal mass].
Plantar fascia: [Normal. There is no thickening of the fascial cords or surrounding edema.]

Tibiotalar joint space: [There is no joint effusion or osteochondral lesions].

Marrow signal: [Normal].

IMPRESSION:

[Normal MRI of the ankle.]

ANKLE ARTHROGRAM

EXAMINATION:

MRI ANKLE ARTHROGRAM

INDICATION: [ ]

TECHNIQUE:

Multiplanar images of the ankle were performed after the intra-articular injection of dilute gadolinium contrast using a MR arthrogram ankle protocol. Sequences include: Axial PD, Axial T2 FS, Sagittal T1, Sagittal STIR, Coronal PD FS. Or Ankle arthrogram: Axial T1 FS, Sagittal T1 FS, Coronal T1 FS, Axial PD, Axial T2 FS, Sagittal T1, Sagittal STIR

COMPARISON:

Compared to prior study from [ ].

FINDINGS:

[There is good distention of the tibiotalar joint space with dilute gadolinium contrast.]

Achilles tendon: [Normal, there is no tendinosis or focal tear. There is no edema in Kager's pad fat. No fluid is seen in the retrocalcaneal or retro-Achilles bursae].

Posterior tibial tendon: [Normal. There is no tendinosis, focal tear or tenosynovitis].
Flexor digitorum tendon: [Normal. There is no tendinosis, focal tear or tenosynovitis].
Flexor hallucis tendon: [Normal. There is no tendinosis, focal tear or tenosynovitis].

Peroneal tendons: [Normal. There is no tendinosis, focal tear or tenosynovitis].

Anterior tibialis tendon: [Normal. There is no tendinosis, focal tear or tenosynovitis].
Extensor digitorum tendon: [Normal. There is no tendinosis, focal tear or tenosynovitis].
Extensor hallucis longus: [Normal. There is no tendinosis, focal tear or tenosynovitis].

Anterior tibiofibular ligament: [Normal].
Posterior tibiofibular ligament: [Normal].

Anterior talofibular ligament: [Normal].
Posterior talofibular ligament: [Normal].
Calcaneofibular ligament: [Normal.]

Tibiotalar ligament: [Normal.]
Tibiospring Ligament: [Normal.]
Spring ligament: [Normal].

Sinus tarsi: [Normal. There preservation of the normal fatty signal without edema or focal mass].
Plantar fascia: [Normal. There is no thickening of the fascial cords or surrounding edema.]

Tibiotalar joint space: [There is no joint effusion or osteochondral lesions].

Marrow signal: [Normal].

IMPRESSION:

[Normal MR arthrogram of the ankle.]

FOREFOOT

EXAMINATION:

MRI of the forefoot without contrast

INDICATION: [ ]

TECHNIQUE:

Multiplanar images of the forefoot were performed without the administration of intravenous or intra-articular contrast using a routine forefoot protocol. Sequences include: Coronal T1, Coronal STIR, Axial T2, Axial STIR, Sagittal T1, Sagittal STIR

COMPARISON:

Compared to prior study from [ ].

FINDINGS:

[There is no abnormal marrow signal to indicate a stress fracture or marrow replacing lesion.]

[Joint spaces are preserved without significant degenerative changes or joint effusions. [No erosions are seen.]

[No masses or fluid are seen between the metatarsal head to suggest a Morton's neuroma or intermetatarsal bursitis.]

[LisFranc Ligament complex is normal.] [Soft tissues of the forefoot are normal.]

IMPRESSION:

Normal MRI examination of the forefoot.

CALVES/LOWER LEG

EXAMINATION:

[MRI CALVES]

INDICATION: [ ]

TECHNIQUE:

Multiplanar images of bilateral calves were performed without the administration of intravenous or intra-articular contrast using a routine bilateral calves protocol. Sequences include: Axial T1, Axial T2 FS, Coronal T1, Coronal STIR, Sagittal STIR (symptomatic side only).

COMPARISON:

Compared to prior study from [ ].

FINDINGS:

[There is normal marrow signal throughout both lower legs.] [No stress fractures or marrow replacing lesions are seen.] [The muscles of the lower legs are symmetric without edema or focal masses.] [There is no muscle atrophy or fatty replacement.]

[The visualized portions of the knee and ankle are within normal limits.] [Subcutaneous soft tissues are normal.]

IMPRESSION:

Normal MRI examination of the lower legs.

INFECTION/MASS PROTOCOL

EXAMINATION:

MRI OF [ ] WITH INTRAVENOUS CONTRAST

INDICATION: [ ]

TECHNIQUE:

Multiplanar images of the [ ] were performed before and after the administration of intravenous contrast to evaluate for suspected infection and/or focal mass. Sequences include: Axial T1, Axial STIR, Sagittal or Coronal T1, Sagittal or Coronal STIR, Axial T1 FS Pre, Axial T1 FS Post, Sagittal or Coronal T1 FS Post, Subtractions (of Axial T1 FS Pre/Post).

COMPARISON:

Compared to prior study from [ ].

FINDINGS:

At the site of skin marker indicating site of concern, there is no discrete mass seen. There is no abnormal enhancement. The bone marrow signal is normal without marrow edema or marrow replacing lesions. The subcutaneous soft tissues are normal without edema or discrete mass.

The adjacent joint spaces are normal without joint effusion or bony erosions. Neurovascular structures are normal.

IMPRESSION:

Normal MRI examination of [ ]. No discrete mass or abnormal enhancement is seen.

Index

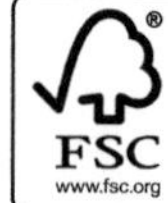

MIX
Papier aus verantwortungsvollen Quellen
Paper from responsible sources
FSC® C105338

If you have any concerns about our products,
you can contact us on
ProductSafety@springernature.com

In case Publisher is established outside the EU,
the EU authorized representative is:
Springer Nature Customer Service Center GmbH
Europaplatz 3, 69115 Heidelberg, Germany

Printed by Libri Plureos GmbH
in Hamburg, Germany